Resent Results
in Cancer Research   **172**

Managing Editors
P. M. Schlag, Berlin · H.-J. Senn, St. Gallen

Associate Editors
P. Kleihues, Zürich · F. Stiefel, Lausanne
B. Groner, Frankfurt · A. Wallgren, Göteborg

Founding Editor
P. Rentchnik, Geneva

B. Groner (Ed.)

Targeted Interference with Signal Transduction Events

With 35 Figures in 45 Separate Illustrations, 23 in Color and 13 Tables

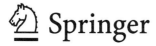

Professor Dr. Bernd Groner
Director, Georg-Speyer-Haus
Institute for Biomedical Research
Paul-Ehrlich-Str. 42–44
60596 Frankfurt am Main
Germany
groner@em.uni-frankfurt.de

ISSN 0080-0015
ISBN 978-3-642-06834-8   e-ISBN 978-3-540-31209-3

This work is subject to copyright. All rights are reserved, whether the whole or part of the material is concerned, specifically the rights of translation, reprinting, reuse of illustrations, recitations, broadcasting, reproduction on microfilm or in any other way, and storage in data banks. Duplication of this publication or parts thereof is permitted only under the provisions of the German Copyright Law of September 9, 1965, in its current version, and permission for use must always be obtained from Springer-Verlag. Violations are liable for prosecution under the German Copyright Law.

Springer is part of Springer Science+Business Media

http//www.springer.com
© Springer-Verlag Berlin Heidelberg 2010
Printed in Germany

The use of general descriptive names, trademarks, etc. in this publication does not imply, even in the absence of a specific statement, that such names are exempt from the relevant protective laws and regulations and therefore free for general use.

Product liability: The publishers cannot guarantee the accuracy of any information about dosage and application contained in this book. In every case the user must check such information by consulting the relevant literature.

Editor: Dr. Ute Heilmann, Heidelberg
Desk Editor: Dörthe Mennecke-Bühler, Heidelberg
Cover-design: Frido Steinen Broo, eStudio Calamar, Spain

Printed on acid-free paper – 21/3151xq – 5 4 3 2 1 0

Contents

1 Introduction: The Rationale for the Development of Targeted Drugs in Cancer Therapy
Bernd Groner 1

2 Identifying Critical Signaling Molecules for the Treatment of Cancer
Constadina Arvanitis, Pavan Bendapudi, Pavan Bachireddy, and Dean W. Felsher 5

3 Tyrosine Kinase Inhibitors and Cancer Therapy
Srinivasan Madhusudan and Trivadi S. Ganesan 25

4 Targeting ERBB Receptors in Cancer
Nancy E. Hynes 45

5 Inhibition of the IGF-I Receptor for Treatment of Cancer. Kinase Inhibitors and Monoclonal Antibodies as Alternative Approaches
Yan Wang, Qun-sheng Ji, Mark Mulvihill, and Jonathan A. Pachter 59

6 Inhibition of the TGF-β Signaling Pathway in Tumor Cells
Klaus Podar, Noopur Raje, and Kenneth C. Anderson 77

7 The Mammalian Target of Rapamycin Kinase and Tumor Growth Inhibition
Anne Boulay and Heidi A. Lane........................... 99

8 The Ras Signalling Pathway as a Target in Cancer Therapy
Kathryn Graham and Michael F. Olson 125

9 The Mitogen-Activated Protein Kinase Pathway for Molecular-Targeted Cancer Treatment
Judith S. Sebolt-Leopold, Roman Herrera, and
Jeffrey F. Ohren 155

10 Clinical Relevance of Targeted Interference with Src-Mediated Signal Transduction Events
Quan P. Ly and Timothy J. Yeatman 169

List of Contributors

Kenneth C. Anderson, MD
Department of Medical Oncology
Dana-Farber Cancer Institute
Jerome Lipper Multiple Myeloma Center
44 Binney Street
Boston, MA 02115
USA

Constadina Arvanitis
Graduate Student, Molecular Pharmacology
Division of Oncology
Departments of Medicine and Pathology
Stanford University School of Medicine
269 Campus Drive, CCSR 1120
Stanford, CA 94305–5151
USA

Pavan Bachireddy
Division of Oncology
Departments of Medicine and Pathology
Stanford University School of Medicine
269 Campus Drive, CCSR 1120
Stanford, CA 94305–5151
USA

Pavan Bendapudi
Division of Oncology
Departments of Medicine and Pathology
Stanford University School of Medicine
269 Campus Drive, CCSR 1120
Stanford, CA 94305–5151
USA

Anne Boulay, PhD
Post-doctoral Fellow
Friedrich Miescher Institute for
Biomedical Research
Maulbeerstr. 66
4059 Basel
Switzerland

Dean W. Felsher, MD, PhD
Assistant Professor, Division of Oncology
Departments of Medicine and Pathology
Stanford University School of Medicine
269 Campus Drive, CCSR 1120
Stanford, CA 94305–5151
USA

Trivadi S. Ganesan, MA (Oxon), MD, MNAMS, PhD (London), FRCP
Professor, Chairman
Cancer Institute and Institute of
Molecular Medicine
Amrita Institute of Medical Sciences
Elamakkara P.O. Kochi
Kerala 682026
India

Kathryn Graham, BSc, MB ChB, MRCP
Clinical Research Fellow
Honorary Specialist Registrar in Clinical
Oncology
The Beatson Institute for Cancer Research
Garscube Estate
Switchback Road
Glasgow, G61 1BD
UK

Bernd Groner, Professor, Dr.
Director
Georg-Speyer-Haus
Institute for Biomedical Research
Paul-Ehrlich-Str. 42–44
60596 Frankfurt am Main
Germany

Roman Herrera, PhD
Pfizer Global Research and Development
Michigan Laboratories
2800 Plymouth Road
Ann Arbor, MI 48105
USA

Nancy E. Hynes
Professor
Friedrich Miescher Institute for
Biomedical Research
Maulbeerstr. 66
4059 Basel
Switzerland

Qun-sheng Ji, PhD, MD
Senior Research Investigator, Cancer Biology
OSI Pharmaceuticals, Inc.
1 Bioscience Park Drive
Farmingdale, NY 11735
USA

Heidi A. Lane, PhD
Unit Head, Director
Novartis Pharma AG
4002 Basel
Switzerland

Quan P. Ly, MD
Assistant Professor of Surgery
H. Lee Moffitt Cancer Center and
Research Institute
12902 Magnolia Drive
Tampa, FL 33612
USA

Srinivasan Madhusudan
Specialist Registrar
Cancer Research UK
Medical Oncology Unit
The Churchill Hospital
Oxford OX3 7LJ
UK

Mark Mulvihill, PhD
Associate Director, Cancer Chemistry
OSI Pharmaceuticals, Inc.
1 Bioscience Park Drive
Farmingdale, NY 11735
USA

Jeffrey F. Ohren, PhD
Pfizer Global Research and Development
Michigan Laboratories
2800 Plymouth Road
Ann Arbor, MI 48105
USA

Michael F. Olson, BSc, PhD
Group Leader
The Beatson Institute for Cancer Research
Garscube Estate
Switchback Road
Glasgow G61 1BD
UK

Jonathan A. Pachter, PhD
Senior Director, Cancer Biology
OSI Pharmaceuticals, Inc.
1 Bioscience Park Drive
Farmingdale, NY 11735
USA

Klaus Podar, MD, MSc, PhD
Department of Medical Oncology
Dana-Farber Cancer Institute
Jerome Lipper Multiple Myeloma Center
44 Binney Street
Boston, MA 02115
USA

Noopur Raje
Director
Multiple Myeloma Program
Department of Adult Oncology
Massachusetts General Hospital
Assistant Professor of Medicine
Harvard Medical School
Boston, MA 02115
USA

Judith S. Sebolt-Leopold, PhD
Pfizer Global Research and Development
Michigan Laboratories
2800 Plymouth Road
Ann Arbor, MI 48105
USA

Yan Wang, PhD
Senior Principal Scientist, Oncology
Schering-Plough Research Institute
2015 Galloping Hill Road
Kenilworth, NJ 07033
USA

Timothy J. Yeatman, MD
Professor of Surgery
H. Lee Moffitt Cancer Center and
Research Institute
12902 Magnolia Drive
Tampa, FL 33612
USA

Introduction: The Rationale for the Development of Targeted Drugs in Cancer Therapy

Bernd Groner

Recent Results in Cancer Research, Vol. 172
© Springer-Verlag Berlin Heidelberg 2007

Cancer remains a leading cause of death in the developed world. Survival rates for patients with common cancers detected at an advanced stage are still low. Only about 10% of patients with metastatic colon cancer and about 5% of patients with pancreatic cancer survive for more than 5 years. Cancer therapies are still largely chosen on the basis of diagnostic categories, and all patients of a particular tumor type and stage of disease receive the same treatment. Biological heterogeneity among patients has long been recognized, but the significance of these differences with respect to the course of disease and drug responsiveness is just starting to be understood. In addition, the limited repertoire of available drugs has made it difficult to exploit these differences for different treatment strategies.

Cancer is being considered as a genetic disease. Multiple mutations are thought to be present in tumor cells that alter the gene functions responsible for the manifestation of the transformed phenotype. Although the analysis of mutated genes has already become useful for diagnostic and therapeutic applications, the number of relevant mutations and the identity of the affected genes still have not been determined (Futreal et al. 2004). Cancer cells are constantly subject to mutations in their DNA. These changes occasionally produce cells that can escape their normal growth constraints and form a tumor. The tumor cells are being selected for their ability to divide, trigger the growth of vessels to provide for their blood supply, and invade the bloodstream and other tissues to form metastases. Defects in their cell cycle and apoptosis regulation are due to mutations in proto-oncogenes and tumor suppressor genes. Genomic instability due to defects in DNA repair enzymes increases the rate of mutations and contributes to cancer evolution. More than 350 human genes have been found to be mutated in cancer cells: 90% of these exhibit mutations in somatic cells, 20% can be found mutated in germline cells and thus contribute to the predisposition to cancer, and 10% are mutated both in somatic and in germline cells (Futreal et al. 2004). Loss of gene functions can not only be caused by changes in the primary DNA sequence, but also by epigenetic control mechanisms of gene expression. Secondary modifications of DNA, histones, or transcription factors can underlie such events (Esteller 2006).

To obtain a comprehensive view of the genetic alterations causing and accompanying the emergence of tumor cells in a particular tissue, it is necessary to derive global sequence information. Sjöblom and colleagues (Sjoblom et al. 2006) analyzed the protein coding sequences in 13,023 genes from 11 breast cancer samples and 11 colon cancer samples and found that individual tumors accumulate about 90 mutated genes on average and that at least 11 of them are thought to be cancer promoting. Altogether the number of 189 «candidate» cancer genes that affect gene transcription, cell adhesion, and invasion might not seem too encouraging when we are looking for the general principles of cancer etiology and a small number of promising drug targets. The cancer genes differed between colon and breast cancers, and each tumor had a different pattern of mutations. This complexity in mutational patterns and the differences among tumors of a distinct histological type have important implications for the variability of current treatment regimens and for the design of new drugs.

The heterogeneity in the genetic changes and the context dependence by which these mutations are causally involved in cancer development and progression makes it difficult to design effective drugs. In addition, the possibility that only a subset of cancer cells with stem cell properties is really relevant for effective eradication of the disease further complicates their design. Tumor cells constantly communicate with normal, neighboring host cells in reciprocal interactions. Factors secreted into the microenvironment of cancer cells by host cells can promote the proliferation of tumor cells, and factors secreted by tumor cells can impede the host immune response (Sawyers 2004).

Which phenotypes are affected in cancer cells, and which mutations can be linked to a particular phenotype? The signaling pathways that control cell cycle progression and cell growth, apoptosis, replicative potential and senescence, motility and invasiveness, metabolic activity, and genome integrity are often deregulated in cancer cells, and the activities of many oncogenes and tumor suppressor genes have been associated with these functions (Vogelstein and Kinzler 2004). The identification of activated oncogenic pathways in particular tumor cells yields a signature that might act as a guide for targeted therapies (Bild et al. 2006).

The concept that the cooperation of oncogenes and tumor suppressor genes, augmented by signals from the tumor microenvironment and stress signals such as DNA damage, can be regarded as the molecular basis of cancer provides the framework for the design of new drugs. These drugs are selected on the basis of their ability to interfere with specific molecules, believed to have a limiting role in the emergence, growth, or progression of tumors. The identification of the appropriate targets for such drugs very much depends on detailed understanding of the molecular alterations causing cancer. The description of cancer in molecular terms will also have profound effects on prevention measures, the early detection of tumors, the improvement of diagnosis complementing histopathological criteria, and the monitoring of treatment.

Despite the discouraging complexity of the genetic basis of cellular transformation, therapeutic advances have been made exploiting insights into genes that have causal and limiting roles in the cancer process. The integration of such genes into signaling pathways that regulate cell growth and cell fate and the development of agents that interfere with such components in a targeted fashion have led to significant gains for cancer patients. Hormones, antibodies, and low-molecular-weight compounds acting as enzyme inhibitors have been used to target oncogene products. Intuitively, it appears reasonable to interfere with the function of cellular components that are distinguishable in amount or functional properties between normal and tumor cells. The selective estrogen receptor modulators, partial agonists of the natural ligand (Ariazi et al. 2006); trastuzumab (Herceptin), an antibody that interferes with the action of the ErbB2 growth factor receptor (Pegram et al. 2000); imatinib (Glivec), a low-molecular-weight tyrosine kinase inhibitor that blocks the activity of the abl kinase (O'Hare et al. 2006); and gefitinib (Iressa), a tyrosine kinase inhibitor of the EGF receptor (Mendelsohn and Baselga 2006), serve as pioneering examples for the benefits that are emanating from targeted drugs. These drugs are not necessarily curative, and only selected subpopulations of patients respond to them. However, they show that a combination of molecular diagnostics, which reveals the gene defects underlying the transformation process, and the deployment of drugs aimed at individual deregulated signaling components emerges as a viable and promising therapeutic strategy.

Can the lessons from these examples be extrapolated? Other target structures are already being exploited in a comparable fashion (Dietel and Sers 2006), but it remains to be determined how many limiting components there are that are druggable (Keller et al. 2006). The development of new, powerful agents able to interfere with cell surface growth factor receptors, intracellular signaling kinases, and signal transduction components that are described in this book embodies the hope of many tumor patients and will lead the way to further improvements in treatment.

References

Ariazi EA, Ariazi JL, Cordera F, Jordan VC (2006) Estrogen receptors as therapeutic targets in breast cancer. Curr Top Med Chem 6:181–202

Bild AH, Yao G, Chang JT, Wang Q, Potti A, Chasse D, Joshi MB, Harpole D, Lancaster JM, Berchuck A, et al. (2006) Oncogenic pathway signatures in human cancers as a guide to targeted therapies. Nature 439:353–357

Dietel M, Sers C (2006) Personalized medicine and development of targeted therapies: The upcoming challenge for diagnostic molecular pathology. A review. Virchows Arch 448:744–755

Esteller M (2006) Epigenetics provides a new generation of oncogenes and tumour-suppressor genes. Br J Cancer 94:179–183

Futreal PA, Coin L, Marshall M, Down T, Hubbard T, Wooster R, Rahman N, Stratton MR (2004) A census of human cancer genes. Nat Rev Cancer 4:177--183

Keller TH, Pichota A, Yin Z (2006) A practical view of 'druggability'. Curr Opin Chem Biol 10:357–361

Mendelsohn J, Baselga J (2006) Epidermal growth factor receptor targeting in cancer. Semin Oncol 33:369–385

O'Hare T, Corbin AS, Druker BJ (2006) Targeted CML therapy: controlling drug resistance, seeking cure. Curr Opin Genet Dev 16:92–99

Pegram MD, Konecny G, Slamon DJ (2000) The molecular and cellular biology of HER2/neu gene amplification/overexpression and the clinical development of herceptin (trastuzumab) therapy for breast cancer. Cancer Treat Res 103:57–75

Sawyers C (2004) Targeted cancer therapy. Nature 432:294–297

Sjoblom T, Jones S, Wood LD, Parsons DW, Lin J, Barber TD, Mandelker D, Leary RJ, Ptak J, Silliman N, et al. (2006) The consensus coding sequences of human breast and colorectal cancers. Science 314:268–274

Vogelstein B, Kinzler KW (2004) Cancer genes and the pathways they control. Nat Med 10:789–799

Identifying Critical Signaling Molecules for the Treatment of Cancer

Constadina Arvanitis, Pavan K. Bendapudi, Pavan Bachireddy, and Dean W. Felsher

Recent Results in Cancer Research, Vol. 172
© Springer-Verlag Berlin Heidelberg 2007

2.1 Overview

Tumorigenesis is a multistep process whereby an individual cell acquires a series of mutant gene products. These genetic changes culminate in proliferation, growth, blocked differentiation, induction of angiogenesis, tissue invasion, and loss of genomic stability. Given the genetic complexity of tumorigenesis, it is perhaps surprising that there are circumstances in which cancer can be reversed through the repair or inactivation of individual mutant genes. However, recent experiments in transgenic mouse models and clinical results with new pharmacological agents demonstrate that cancer can be treated through the targeted repair and/or inactivation of mutant proteins. Hence, cancers appear to be dependent upon particular oncogenes to maintain their neoplastic properties, thus exhibiting the phenomenon of "oncogene addiction."

We will focus on the notion that critical oncogenes mediate signaling processes that underlie the etiology of cancer. These mutant oncogenes are likely to represent the best targets for the treatment of cancer. We will summarize the major signaling pathways that may be most effectively targeted for the treatment of cancer. Then, we will describe how conditional transgenic model systems have been exploited as innovative avenues for discovery and validation of drug targets and therapeutic agents. Next, we will explore the successes to date of targeted therapeutics and possible approaches to the

successful targeting of transcription factors. Finally, we will discuss current thoughts on why the targeted inactivation of specific cell signaling molecules results in tumor regression.

2.2 Critical Signaling Pathways

At least four different classes of signaling molecules are commonly involved in the pathogenesis of cancer including receptors such as ErbB, small GTPases such as Ras, kinases such as BCR-ABL, and transcription factors such as MYC. The proteins in these interacting signaling pathways have been some of the most intensely studied as potential targets and in many cases successfully targeted for the treatment of cancer (Fig. 2.1).

2.2.1 Receptor Signaling

Cell surface receptors are the starting point for all signaling cascades, so it is not surprising that receptors for growth factors were some of the first proto-oncogenes discovered (Olayioye et al. 2000). A multitude of cell surface receptors have been implicated in tumorigenesis including the epithelial growth factor receptor (EGFR), the platelet-derived growth factor receptor (PDGFR), and the insulin-like growth factor receptor (IGFR) (Tibes et al. 2005).

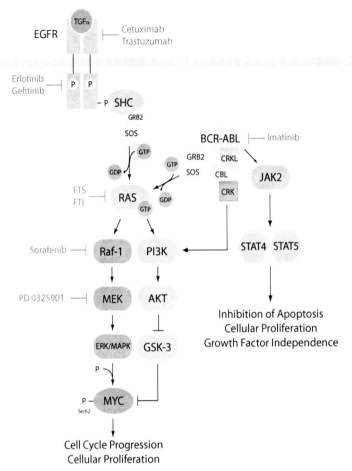

Fig. 2.1 Critical signaling pathways as drug targets for cancer therapy. A Surface receptors dimerize and activate downstream effectors such as RAS (a GTPase). Many surface receptors are targeted by antibodies, and EGFR has been targeted through cetuximab and trastuzumab. B RAS activation is caused by SOS-mediated exchange of GDP for GTP on RAS. G protein signaling molecules, such as RAS, have been targeted by farnesyltransferase inhibitors (FTI) and S-farnesylthiosalicylic acid (FTS). C The BCR-ABL fusion protein activates RAS, PI3K, and other oncogenic signaling molecules. Tyrosine kinases are often targeted with small molecules. BCR-ABL has been targeted by imanitib mesylate. D Transcription factors are often the terminal effectors of a pathway. To date, transcription factors have yet to be successfully targeted. All drugs are in red at their sites of action

A prototypical example of receptors is the ErbB family of transmembrane tyrosine kinase receptors, which includes four family members: EGFR (ErbB1), HER2/NEU (ErbB2 hereafter referred to as HER2), ErbB3, and ErbB4. Ligands have been identified for each of the ErbB family members except for HER2, which likely heterodimerizes with EGFR or HER3. Downstream effectors of these molecules include the MAPK pathways, PI3K/AKT pathways, Janus signaling, RAS signaling, and STAT signaling. Activation of these receptor pathways induces cellular proliferation, survival, and motility (Bianco et al. 2006). Each of these receptors exhibits tissue-specific expression. Correspondingly, mutated receptors have been implicated in particular types of human cancer (Yarden and Sliwkowski 2001). For example, EGFR is commonly overexpressed in lung carcinoma (Hirsch et al. 2003), while Her2 overexpression is more commonly associated with breast cancer (Ross et al. 2004).

There are several reasons why cell surface receptors are attractive candidates for drug targets. First, receptors are specific to particular tissue types, thus allowing for target specificity. Second, pharmacologically blocking a ligand-binding site is an obvious and frequently successful strategy to inactivate a receptor. Finally, drugs that target receptor molecules do not need to be able to transit through cellular membranes.

2.2.2 GTPases

Receptor signaling is frequently mediated through small GTPases (Bourne et al. 1991). A characteristic feature of GTPases is that they must first be modified to localize to the plasma membrane, where they are active (Downward 1996). The RAS family represents a prototypical example of small GTPases consisting of three members: H-RAS, K-RAS, and N-RAS (Bourne et al. 1991). RAS family members are some of the most commonly mutated genes associated with human cancers. At least 25% of human tumors exhibit activating point mutations of a RAS gene (Bos 1989). RAS proteins are known to regulate many cellular processes including cellular growth, proliferation, apoptosis, and angiogenesis (Lowy and Willumsen 1993; Downward 1996).

2.2.3 Kinases

Kinases are among the most abundant signaling molecules, with approximately 500 members, many of which when mutated function as oncogenes (Manning et al. 2002). The ability to readily pharmacologically target the ATP-binding domains of kinases has made these gene products attractive drug targets (Schlessinger 2000; Ventura and Nebreda 2006). The most well-known example of a kinase associated with neoplasia is the BCR-ABL fusion protein, which results from a chromosomal translocation between the ABL proto-oncogene and the BCR locus. BCR-ABL overexpression has been implicated in the pathogenesis of chronic myelogenous leukemia (CML) and ALL. The

targeted inactivation of BCR-ABL through the drug imatinib mesylate (Gleevec, STI-571) is the most cited example of a successful targeted therapeutic (Sawyers 2002; Daley 2003; Druker 2004; Deininger et al. 2005).

2.2.4 Transcription Factors

Nuclear transcription factors are among the proteins most frequently implicated in cancer. The family of MYC proto-oncogenes (c-, n-, l-MYC) are overexpressed in up to half of all human cancers (Nesbit et al. 1999). MYC has been shown to regulate the transcription of thousands of target genes (http://www.myc-cancer-gene.org; Dang et al. 1999; Oster et al. 2002), suggesting that these gene products function as grand coordinators of gene expression programs.

c-MYC was the first family member to be discovered (Bishop 1982). c-MYC is expressed in most cell types and is found to be overexpressed in most types of human cancers. In particular, c-MYC is found to be activated through chromosomal translocation in Burkitt lymphoma. n-MYC is expressed in neuronal cells and is often amplified in neuroblastoma. l-MYC was first identified in lung tissue and is associated with small cell lung carcinoma (Nesbit et al. 1999). To date, transcription factors have yet to be successfully targeted with small molecules.

2.3 Conditional Transgenic Mouse Models

Although the last couple of decades have led to a remarkable amount of insight into the molecular etiology of cancer, to date most conventional therapies for cancer are purely empiric. Only recently have targeted strategies become incorporated into the treatment of cancer. The development of transgenic mouse models has provided the unprecedented opportunity to model the contribution of specific gene products to the pathogenesis of neoplasia Italics. Moreover, the recent development of conditional transgenic models has made it possible to directly interrogate when and how the inactivation of oncogenes can result in tumor regression. Many reviews have extensively described the application of conventional transgenic mouse models for the development of therapeutics for cancer (Van Dyke and Jacks 2002; Weiss and Shannon 2003; Gutmann et al. 2006). Here we will focus on the use of conditional transgenic models to define when and how oncogenes can be used as targets for the treatment of cancer.

2.3.1 Experimental Approaches

Three different strategies have been most commonly utilized to conditionally regulate gene expression in transgenic mouse models: the Tet system, the tamoxifen system, and the TVA system (Jonkers and Berns 2002; Van Dyke and Jacks 2002; Giuriato et al. 2004).

2.3.1.1 The Tet System

The tetracycline regulatory system (Tet system) was developed as a strategy to regulate the transcription of genes in eukaryotic cells by utilizing prokaryotic transcriptional regulatory proteins (Gossen and Bujard 1992; Gossen et al. 1994). There are two variations of this system: One activates transgene expression in the presence of a tetracycline such as doxycycline (Tet-On), while the other system shuts off transgene expression upon doxycycline addition (Tet-Off). In both variations, two different transgenes are generated. The first transgene uses a tissue-specific promoter to drive the expression of a tetracycline transactivator (tTA or rtTA). The second transgene contains a tetracycline response element (Tet-O) adjacent to a target gene of interest. The tTA or rtTA protein binds to the Tet-O promoter regulating gene transcription. The presence of doxycycline prevents binding of the tTA protein to the Tet-O element, turning off gene expression (Tet-Off), or promotes the binding of the rtTA protein to the Tet-O element, turning gene expression on (Tet-On). The Tet system facilitates monitoring of transgene expression at the transcription level in specific tissues within the mouse.

2.3.1.2 The Tamoxifen System

The tamoxifen system also has been employed to conditionally regulate gene activation post-transcriptionally. MYC fused with the estradiol receptor exhibited conditional oncogene activation (Eilers et al. 1989). A mutant version of the estradiol receptor, which binds tamoxifen, is utilized to prevent endogenous estradiol from activating gene function (Littlewood et al. 1995). Upon addition of tamoxifen, MYC is active, and withdrawal leads to an inactive product.

2.3.1.3 The RCAS-TVA-Tet System

The Tet system can be combined with the RCAS-TVA system (Lewis et al. 2003; Pao et al. 2003). In this approach a tissue-specific promoter is used to drive the expression of the avian retroviral receptor (TVA) in transgenic mice. The cells of these mice also contain a Tet-O regulated transgene, but lack the rtTA protein. Avian retroviral vectors (RCAS) are used to deliver the rtTA transactivator to cells that express the TVA. The successfully infected cells now contain a transgene whose expression can be regulated by doxycycline.

2.3.2 Defining When Cancer Is Reversible

Conditional transgenic models have been used to evaluate the consequences of oncogene inactivation italics. From these studies, several general themes emerge regarding the role of oncogenes in the initiation and maintenance of tumorigenesis, as we have described (Felsher 2003, 2004a, 2004b; Giuriato et al. 2004; Bachireddy et al. 2005; Shachaf and Felsher 2005a, 2005b). Oncogene inactivation can reverse tumorigenesis by inducing sustained tumor regression through differentiation, proliferative arrest, and/or apoptosis (see Table 2.1). The specific consequences of the inactivation of an oncogene depend on the type of tumor. In some cases, even briefly in-

2 Identifying Critical Signaling Molecules for the Treatment of Cancer

Table 2.1 Consequences of oncogene inactivation in transgenic mouse models

Oncogene	Model	System	Tumor type	Response to inactivation	Mechanism of tumor regression	References
BCL2	MMTV-tTA Tet-O-BCL-2 Eμ-MYC	Tet-off	Lymphoblastic leukemia	Regression	Apoptosis	Letai et al. 2004
BCR-ABL	MMTV-tTA Tet-O-BCR-ABL	Tet-Off	B-cell leukemia	Regression[a]	Apoptosis	Huettner et al. 2000
	SCL-tTA Tet-O-BCR-ABL	Tet-Off	CML	Regression	ND	Koschmieder et al. 2005
FGF-10	CCSP-rtTA or SPC-rtTA Tet-O-CMV-FGF10	Tet-on	Pulmonary adenomas	Regression	ND	Clark et al. 2001
HER2/NEU	MMTV-rtTA Tet-O-NeuNT	Tet-On	Mammary carcinomas	Regression[a]	Decreased proliferation and apoptosis	Moody et al. 2002
MET	LAP-tTA Tet-O-MET	Tet-On	Hepatocellular carcinoma	Regression	Decreased proliferation and apoptosis	Wang et al. 2001
c-MYC	EμSRα-tTA Tet-O-MYC	Tet-Off	T- and B-cell lymphoma, acute myeloid leukemia	Regression[a]	Cell cycle arrest, differentiation and apoptosis	Felsher and Bishop 1999a, 1999b; Marinkovic et al. 2004
	EμSRα-tTA Tet-O-MYC	Tet-Off	Osteosarcoma	Regression	Differentiation	Jain et al. 2002
	MMTV-rtTA Tet-O-MYC	Tet-On	Breast adenoma	Partial Regression	ND	D'Cruz et al. 2001; Boxer et al. 2004
	LAP-tTA Tet-O-MYC	Tet-Off	Hepatocellular carcinoma	Regression	Apoptosis and differentiation	Beer et al. 2004; Shachaf et al. 2004
	Plns- MycER^Tam	Tamoxifen	Pancreatic islet cell	Regression	Growth arrest, differentiation, cellular adhesion, vascular collapse	Pelengaris et al. 2002
	Involucrin-MycER^Tam	Tamoxifen	Papillomas	Regression	Growth arrest and differentiation	Pelengaris et al. 1999; Flores et al. 2004
RAS	Tyr-rtTA H-Ras^(V12G) Ink4a^-/-	Tet-On	Melanoma	Regression[a]	Apoptosis, EGFR expression required	Chin et al. 1999; Wong and Chin 2000
	SP-r-rtTTA RtTA-KiRas^(G12C)	Tet-On	Lung adenoma	Regression	ND	Floyd et al. 2005
	CCSP-rtTA Tet-O-KiRas^(G12C)	Tet-On	Lung adenoma	Regression	ND	Floyd et al. 2005
	CCSP-rtTA Tet-op-K-Ras4B^(G12D)	Tet-On	Lung adenoma	Regression	Apoptosis	Fisher et al. 2001
	Nestin-TVA RCAS-tTA RCAS-Akt RCAS-Tet-O-KRas	RCAS	Glioblastoma	Regression	Apoptosis	Holmen and Williams 2005
WNT	MMTV-rtTA Tet-O-WNT1 P53^-/-	Tet	Mammary adenoma	Regression[a]	ND	Gunther et al. 2003

[a] While most of the tumors regressed on oncogene inactivation, some of the mice relapsed while the oncogene was inactivated

ND, not determined

activating an oncogene may be sufficient to induce sustained tumor regression (Jain et al. 2002; Flores et al. 2004), but in other cases, this has not been observed (Boxer et al. 2004). Oncogene inactivation may uncover the stem cell properties of tumor cells and induce a state of tumor dormancy (Boxer et al. 2004; Jonkers and Berns 2004; Pelengaris et al. 2004; Shachaf et al. 2004; Yu et al. 2005). Finally, the genetic context can affect whether inactivation of an oncogene will induce sustained regression, or whether the tumors can relapse, acquiring additional genetic events (D'Cruz et al. 2001; Karlsson et al. 2003b; Boxer et al. 2004; Moody et al. 2005).

2.3.2.1 Conditional Models of Receptor-Induced Tumorigenesis

The Tet system has been used to conditionally overexpress receptors including an oncogenic form of HER2 containing an activating point mutation in its transmembrane domain (Moody et al. 2002, 2005). Expression was directed to the breast by utilizing the mouse mammary tumor virus (MMTV) promoter to drive the expression of the rtTA protein. Within 4 days of HER2 activation by doxycycline administration, the mice developed hyperplastic abnormalities. Six weeks after oncogene activation, all of the mice developed multiple invasive mammary carcinomas. The tumors were solid invasive carcinomas that often metastasized to the lung. After 48 h of HER2 inactivation through doxycycline withdrawal, the tumor cells exhibited proliferation arrest and increased apoptosis. The primary carcinomas rapidly and completely regressed in over 90% of the mice, with a mean regression time of 17 days. Within 30 days, the pulmonary metastases had also completely and rapidly regressed. However, a majority of the mice that had a complete regression upon HER2 repression eventually relapsed. Furthermore, when the primary tumors and metastases were transplanted into syngeneic hosts, they completely regressed only 55%–70% of the time. The relapsed tumors all uniformly lacked both endogeneous and transgene protein expression, indicating that the tumors had all become HER2 independent (Moody et al. 2002). Subsequently, Snail, a transcriptional repressor, was found to be activated in relapsed tumors (Moody et al. 2005). Therefore, although oncogene inactivation can cause tumor regression, some transgenic tumors are capable of becoming independent of their initiating oncogenic event.

2.3.2.2 GTPases and Tumor Regression

The Tet-On system has been used to generate a conditional model of mutant H-RAS-induced melanomas (Chin et al. 1999; Wong and Chin 2000). The tyrosinase gene promoter (Tyr) was used to conditionally overexpress an H-RAS bearing an activating point mutation (V12G) in an Ink4a-deficient background. Approximately 25% of the mice developed melanomas within 60 days of H-RAS activation. The melanomas were invasive, highly vascular, and amelanotic. The tumors exhibited expression of tyrosinase-related-protein-1 (TRP-1), an early melanocyte-specific maker. Within 48 h of H-RAS inactivation through doxycycline withdrawal, the tumors decreased their proliferation and exhibited robust apoptosis. Within 14 days of H-RAS inactivation, the tumors had completely regressed, with only microscopically detectable scattered tumor foci. Notably, melanomas transplanted into SCID hosts also regressed on inactivation of mutant H-RAS. Approximately 30% of the melanomas resumed growth, even in the absence of H-RAS, but relapsed tumors failed to express TRP-1, suggesting that these tumors were phenotypically different from the primary tumors (Chin et al. 1999). Additionally, studies have shown that EGFR signaling is required for maintenance of a tumorigenic phenotype in H-RAS-induced melanomas. A dominant-negative EGFR reduced the tumorigenicity of melanomas, and sustained expression of EGFR can delay tumor regression (Bardeesy et al. 2005).

The Tet system has also been used to generate conditional models of mutant K-RAS-induced lung adenocarcinoma (Fisher et al. 2001; Floyd et al. 2005). The Clara cell secretory protein (CCSP) promoter was used to regulate gene expression in alveolar epithelial cells. Within 7–14 days after induction of K-RAS overexpression, type II pneumocytes exhibited focal hyperplasia, and after 2 months multiple solid adenomas or adenocarcinomas were present in the lung. The solid adenomas contained a population of macrophages, but lacked invasive growth and stromal elements. The adenocarcinomas had fewer macrophages and cytoplasmic inclusions, but had local invasion of the pleura. Within 3 days of K-RAS inactivation through doxycycline withdrawal, tumors exhibited decreased cellular density and an increased rate of apoptosis. Within 7 days of K-RAS inactivation, only a few patches of hyperplasia were found, and within a month no residual tumor tissue was found in five of five mice. The same mice were generated in either a p53- or an Ink4A/Arf-deficient background. Tumors grew rapidly in these mice after K-RAS induction but regressed with the same kinetics. TUNEL assays revealed that regardless of the genetic context, tumor regression was associated with apoptosis (Fisher et al. 2001). Similarly, CCSP-regulated K-RAS (G12C)-induced lung adenomas regressed upon oncogene inactivation (Floyd et al. 2005). Hence, even aggressive lung tumors in a tumor suppressor-deficient background regress on the inactivation of a single oncogene.

2.3.2.3 Tumor Regression in a Kinase Model

A conditional transgenic model for BCR-ABL leukemias was generated by using either the MMTV or SCL (stem cell leukemia) promoter to drive the expression of tTA (Huettner et al. 2000; Koschmieder et al. 2005). Upon induction of BCR-ABL the mice developed B-cell leukemia associated with lymphadenopathy, splenomegaly, and bone marrow infiltration. A third of mice with BCR-ABL under the control of the SCL promoter developed B-cell lymphoblastic disease resembling blast crisis, closely mimicking what is observed in patients with chronic myelogenous leukemia (CML). Inactivation of BCR-ABL induced rapid tumor regression in all mice. BCR-ABL inactivation was associated with the apoptosis of 80% of the tumor cells within 20 h and complete tumor regression within 5 days. Sustained regression of tumors was observed in tumors arising from three of the four founder lines, as long as the mice had BCR-ABL continuously inactivated. Upon reactivation of BCR-ABL the tumors rapidly reoccurred. Interestingly, all the mice derived from the fourth founder relapsed within 4 weeks after complete regression. Relapsed tumors lacked continued expression of BCR-ABL protein and mRNA, suggesting that they had become independent of BCR-ABL expression.

2.3.2.4 Nuclear Transcription Factors

The Tet and tamoxifen systems have been used to demonstrate that MYC inactivation can induce tumor regression in a multitude of different types of cancer (see Table 2.1). The Tet-Off system was used to regulate human c-MYC in lymphoid cells under the regulation of the EμSRα promoter (Felsher and Bishop 1999a, 1999b; Marinkovic et al. 2004). When MYC is constitutively activated, 100% of the mice developed hematopoietic tumors within 5 months. On gross examination, the mice exhibited enlargement of the thymus, liver, spleen, and gastrointestinal lymph nodes. Histological examination revealed that tumor cells had invaded all hematopoietic organs as well as liver, kidney, blood, and the lamina propia of the intestines. In one study, tumors were generally immature CD4+/CD8+ T-cell lymphomas and were rarely acute myeloid leukemias (Felsher and Bishop 1999a). In another study, tumors were either B- or T-cell lymphomas (Marinkovic et al. 2004). In both studies, the resulting hematopoietic tumors exhibited a high degree of genomic instability reflected by chromosomal gains, losses, or translocations (Felsher and Bishop 1999a; Marinkovic et al. 2004). Despite this genomic complexity, the inactivation of MYC resulted in rapid and sustained tumor regression. Upon MYC inactivation, tumor cells arrested, differentiated, and then underwent apoptosis. Over 50% of tumors exhibited sustained regression for over 30 weeks. Thus MYC inactivation can induce sustained regression of hematopoietic tumors.

Table 2.2 Oncogene inactivation in the therapeutic setting

Target	Target type	Drug	Cancer	Clinical efficacy	References
EGFR	Receptor tyrosine kinase	Cetuximab	Colorectal cancer	Synergism with irinotecan in irinotecan-refractory colorectal cancer	Cunningham et al. 2004
		Erlotinib (Tarceva)	NSCLC	Approved for refractory NSCLC; disappointing results of addition to chemotherapy in initial treatment of NSCLC	Shepherd et al. 2005
		Gefitinib (Iressa)	NSCLC	Approved for refractory NSCLC; disappointing results of addition to chemotherapy in initial treatment of NSCLC	Kris et al. 2003; Giaccone et al. 2004; Herbst et al. 2004
ERBB2 (Her2/Neu)	Receptor tyrosine kinase	Trastuzumab (Herceptin)	Breast cancer	Increases response rates and improves survival when added to chemotherapy for metastatic HER2 overexpressing breast cancer	Slamon et al. 2001
VEGF	Receptor tyrosine kinase ligand	Bevacizumab (Avastin)	Metastatic colorectal cancer	Significant prolongation of survival in combination therapy	Hurwitz et al. 2004
RAS	GTPase	Zanestra	Colorectal and pancreatic cancer	No effect	End et al. 2001
		ISIS 2503	Pancreatic adenocarcinoma	Unclear benefit in combination therapy	Alberts et al. 2004
BCR-ABL	Tyrosine kinase	Imatinib mesylate (Gleevec/STI-571)	CML; GIST	Complete hematologic and cytogenetic remissions in most CML patients; partial response in more than half of GIST patients	Demetri et al. 2002; O'Brien et al. 2003
RAF-1	Tyrosine kinase	Sorafenib	Metastatic renal cell carcinoma; advanced melanoma	Improves time to progression in metastatic renal cell carcinoma and produces partial responses in combination therapy against advanced melanoma	Flaherty 2004; Escudier et al. 2005

Conditional transgenic mice expressing c-MYC under the control of the Eμ-promoter occasionally developed highly metastatic osteosarcomas (Jain et al. 2002). Histological examination of the primary tumor revealed the presence of disorganized bone matrix. MYC inactivation induced rapid tumor regression associated with the differentiation of tumor into mature bone. Continuous video time-lapsed microscopy (CVTL) revealed that upon MYC inactivation tumor cells ceased to proliferate and differentiated. Identically, MYC inactivation in tumors italics was associated with the differentiation of malignant cells into mature osteoid. Upon MYC reactivation fewer than 1% of the cells were able to regain a proliferative phenotype. Surprisingly, MYC reactivation was also associated with the apoptosis of the now differentiated tumor cells. Moreover, even the transient inactivation of MYC was found to increase the survival of mice with these tumors. Hence, at least in some circumstances, even brief oncogene inactivation can induce sustained loss of a neoplastic state.

The tamoxifen system also has been used to evaluate the consequences of MYC inactivation in different types of tumors with MycERTAM (see Table 2.1). MycERTAM has been expressed in the skin through the involucrin promoter

(Pelengaris et al. 1999; Flores et al. 2004). MYC activation resulted in increased proliferation and blocked differentiation of the suprabasal epidermis. Sustained MYC activation resulted in hyperplasia, dysplasia, angiogenesis, and papillomatosis. MYC inactivation resulted in regression of blood vessels, restoration of cellular differentiation, and the regression of papillomas. A brief inactivation of MYC in keratinocytes caused the cells to differentiate and become unresponsive to MYC reactivation. MYC reactivation could not restore a proliferative phenotype to the differentiated keratinocytes, and eventually the cells were sloughed off the skin (Flores et al. 2004). Hence, brief inactivation of MYC can induce the sustained loss of neoplastic features in some skin tumors.

MycERTAM was also expressed under the control of the insulin (plns) promoter to induce pancreatic islet cell carcinomas (Pelengaris et al. 2002). Within 24 h of MYC activation, virtually all β-islet cells were rapidly proliferating. By 72 h of MYC activation 4%–7% of β-cells were undergoing apoptosis, and within 6–10 days almost no β-cells were detectable. MycERTAM was expressed in the presence of BCL-xL to address the consequences of MYC activation when apoptosis is repressed. Within 7 days of MYC activation β-cells became hyperplastic, ceased insulin production, and decreased expression of the intercellular adhesion molecule E-cadherin. Within 6 weeks pancreatic islet cell carcinomas had formed highly vascularized tumors. Upon MYC inactivation, these tumors regressed completely. The tumors decreased proliferation, differentiated, increased expression of E-cadherin, and exhibited vascular collapse. While these tumors initially regressed upon MYC inactivation, transient MYC inactivation did not result in sustained tumor regression.

The Tet system has been used to explore the role of MYC in the initiation and maintenance of liver cancer by utilizing the liver activator protein (LAP) promoter to express tTA (Beer et al. 2004; Shachaf et al. 2004). The latency of tumorigenesis was inversely correlated with the age at which MYC was activated (Beer et al. 2004). When MYC was activated during embryonic development, mice would succumb to neoplasia within 10 days of birth. In contrast, if MYC was activated in adult mice, the mean latency of tumor onset was 35 weeks. The tumors generated in adult mice histologically resembled hepatocellular carcinomas (HCC) and/or hepatoblastomas. MYC was found to be able to induce proliferation in embryonic or neonatal liver cells but to induce cellular hypertrophy without cellular proliferation in adult liver cells. In part, this was explained by the observation that MYC induced a p53-dependent arrest in cellular division in adult hepatocytes. Thus it appears that the ability of MYC to induce tumorigenesis depends on epigenetic parameters dictated by developmental state.

The same Tet system model was used to examine the consequences of MYC inactivation in liver tumors (Shachaf et al. 2004). The liver tumors were locally invasive, occasionally metastasized to the lung, and were readily transplantable into SCID mice. Within 4 days of MYC inactivation, tumor cells stopped proliferating, differentiated into normal liver cells, and subsequently underwent apoptosis (Shachaf et al. 2004). Even after 5 months of continuous MYC inactivation, a residual population of tumor-derived cells remained detectable. However, MYC reactivation immediately resulted in resumption of a tumorigenic phenotype. Thus these results were in marked contrast to earlier reports that brief inactivation of MYC can result in a permanent loss of a neoplastic phenotype. One possible explanation for these results is that MYC inactivation uncovers the latent stem cell properties of tumor cells that now can differentiate into normal liver, but some of these cancer stem cells retain the capacity to regain their neoplastic features. In support of this hypothesis, upon MYC inactivation some of the residual cells expressed the liver stem cell marker cytokeratin 19 (CK-19) (Shachaf et al. 2004)

MYC also has been conditionally expressed in mammary epithelium by using a Tet-On system with the MMTV promoter (D'Cruz et al. 2001; Boxer et al. 2004). MYC activation resulted in mammary adenocarcinomas with a mean latency of 22 weeks in approximately 86% of mice. Histologically, the tumors exhibited focal hyperplasia, increased proliferation, and dysplasia. Upon MYC inactivation, fewer than half of the adenocarcinomas completely regressed, and a majority of the tumors that completely regressed spontaneously relapsed. Some relapsed tumors either had sustained expression of transgenic MYC in the absence of doxycycline or had reactivated MYC target genes in the absence of transgenic MYC. The majority of tumors relapsed by becoming independent of MYC. Half of the tumors exhibited an activating mutation in either K-RAS2(17/23) or H-RAS2(6/23). Thus MYC inactivation can induce sustained regression of breast cancers unless they have acquired mutations in K- or H-RAS. These important results underscore the importance of genetic context in the consequences of oncogene inactivation in a tumor.

2.4 Themes of Successful Targeted Therapeutics

In many cases, nontoxic therapies have been identified that are directed against specific elements of signaling pathways for the treatment of cancer including acute promyelocytic leukemia, breast cancer, colorectal cancer, and lung adenocarcinoma (see Table 2.2). Two general concepts have emerged: (1) Small molecules can be used to target mutant signaling proteins, and (2) receptors can be targeted with monoclonal antibodies. However, many gene products have yet to be successfully targeted, most notably, transcription factors.

2.4.1 Erlotinib, Gefitinib, and EGFR

Several drugs have been identified that target EGFR. Gefitinib (ZD1839, Iressa) and erlotinib (OSI-774, Tarceva) were approved by the FDA in 2004 as single agents for the treatment of non-small cell lung carcinoma (NSCLC) that had proven refractory to standard chemotherapy. Both agents are members of the anilinoquinazoline class of small molecules and act by competitively inhibiting ATP

binding to the intracellular tyrosine kinase domain of EGFR, thereby preventing the autophosphorylation that is necessary for receptor tyrosine kinases to initiate their signaling cascades (Fig. 2.1). Gefitinib was approved on the basis of two studies conducted at institutions in the United States, Japan, and Europe (the IDEAL-1 and -2 trials) that showed an 11%–19% partial response rate for the drug as a single agent in patients with refractory disease (Fukuoka et al. 2003; Kris et al. 2003; Cohen et al. 2004).

In another study, erlotinib yielded partial responses in 9% of patients when administered as a single agent to those who had failed one or two regimens of standard chemotherapy (Shepherd et al. 2005). Advanced or metastatic NSCLC entails very poor survival, so gefitinib and erlotinib were at first considered to provide real benefits over existing therapy despite the low response rates associated with their use. However, subsequent studies (the INTACT trials) showed that addition of these two drugs to regimens consisting of standard chemotherapy agents yielded no additional benefit (Giaccone et al. 2004; Herbst et al. 2004). Moreover, almost all patients who showed an initial response eventually relapsed with disease that was resistant to EGFR inhibitors (Pao and Miller 2005).

The prospect of successfully inhibiting EGFR with small molecules was thus cast in doubt, and a concerted effort was made to explain the contradictory findings of the IDEAL and INTACT studies. It has been proposed that a tumor's response to gefitinib is dependent on activating mutations in exons 19 and 21 of EGFR (Lynch et al. 2004). Analysis of the crystal structure of EGFR revealed that these mutations occurred in a crucial ATP binding pocket where the anilinoquinazolines act as competitive inhibitors (Stamos et al. 2002). This finding indicates that although gefitinib therapy may not be broadly applicable to all lung tumors, genetic subpopulations may be identified that exhibit an increased susceptibility to EGFR inhibitors. It was also reported that cells transfected with mutant EGFR uniquely activate antiapoptotic pathways involving Akt and STAT signaling (Sordella et al. 2004). Therefore, cells carrying the mutant receptor are resistant to the apoptotic effects of standard chemotherapeutic agents, and EGFR inhibitors may synergize with traditional chemotherapy.

One such synergistic effect between a targeted therapy and a conventional chemotherapy has been reported for cetuximab, a monoclonal antibody to EGFR, and irinotecan, a topoisomerase I inhibitor. Patients with irinotecan-refractory colorectal cancer had higher response rates and modestly prolonged survival when treated with cetuximab in combination with irinotecan than patients treated with cetuximab alone (Cunningham et al. 2004). Therefore, cetuximab may reverse resistance to irinotecan. Similarly, both preclinical and clinical studies have shown synergy between platinum-based chemotherapy and trastuzumab, a monoclonal antibody against the ErbB family member HER2 (Pegram et al. 2004a, 2004b)

EGFR acts upstream of RAS signaling pathways (see Fig. 2.1). Ras and EGFR mutations seem to be mutually exclusive, implying that they are interchangeable in tumorigenesis (Pao and Miller 2005). RAS mutations may allow tumors to circumvent EGFR inhibition (Pao et al. 2005), and thus targeting the RAS pathway may also be required for inhibitors of EGFR to prevent tumor growth.

2.4.2 Targeting RAS

RAS signaling pathways have been targeted by several strategies. RAS must be localized to the plasma membrane to become activated, so pharmacological strategies that prevent localization have been developed. Farnesyltransferase inhibitors (FTIs) were developed to interfere with the posttranslational farnesylation process and thereby abrogate native RAS activity (Cox and Der 2002). While these compounds showed promise against tumors driven by activated H-RAS (Kohl et al. 1995), their activity was not reproduced in cancer cells with K-RAS and N-RAS, the two isotypes that are much more common in human malignancies. N- and K-RAS are resistant to FTIs because they can alternatively be geranylgeranylated when

farnesylation is not possible and can subsequently carry out their tumorigenic functions (Lerner et al. 1997). Unfortunately, inhibitors of geranylgeranyltransferase (GGTIs) were found to be exceedingly toxic in mice when used in combination with FTIs (Lobell et al. 2001) and therefore are not a treatment option.

More recently, S-farnesylthiosalicylic acid (FTS) has been identified as a drug that dislodges activated RAS from the plasma membrane. FTS has been shown to inhibit growth of human tumors xenografted into nude mice (Haklai et al. 1998; Weisz et al. 1999). Clinical studies of FTS in human trials are pending.

RAS has also been targeted at the transcriptional level through the use of antisense RNA. One antisense oligonucleotide, ISIS 2503, has been administered to patients with very little toxicity. In a phase II trial ISIS 2503 exhibited some clinical activity in patients with pancreatic cancer (Alberts et al. 2004).

2.4.3 Imatinib Mesylate and BCR-ABL

The discovery of imatinib mesylate for the treatment of CML has revolutionized targeted therapeutics (Sawyers 2002; Daley 2003; Druker 2004; Deininger et al. 2005). The appreciation that BCR-ABL has constitutive tyrosine kinase activity essential for its transforming ability (Daley et al. 1990; Lugo et al. 1990) suggested a possible strategy for targeted inactivation. Imatinib mesylate is derived from a 2-phenyl-aminopyrimidine backbone that exhibits inhibition of multiple kinases including ABL tyrosine kinases, PDGFR, and the c-kit tyrosine kinase (Buchdunger et al. 2000; Heinrich et al. 2000; Deininger et al. 2005). Imatinib mesylate restricts enzyme activity by competitively inhibiting ATP access to the binding pocket of the kinase, thereby preventing substrate phosphorylation. Preclinical studies confirmed that imatinib mesylate inhibits BCR-ABL activity (Druker et al. 1996).

Early phase I trials of imatinib mesylate revealed that the drug was well tolerated, and almost all patients exhibited a positive clinical response (Druker et al. 2001). Subsequently, a phase II trial in patients with late chronic-phase

CML that failed to respond to interferon-based therapy reported that 41% experienced a complete cytogenetic response, 60% showed a major cytogenetic response, and 89.2% benefited from progression-free survival at 18 months (Kantarjian et al. 2002). Based on the results of these trials, the FDA approved imatinib mesylate for the treatment of CML in advanced-phase disease and after failure of interferon therapy. The results of a phase III study (the IRIS trial) proved imatinib mesylate was significantly superior to interferon alpha plus cytarabine in achieving complete hematologic response, major cytogenetic response, complete cytogenetic response, and progression-free survival (Kantarjian et al. 2003a). Imatinib mesylate was then approved as a first-line treatment for CML in the United States and Europe.

Unfortunately, tumors can become resistant to imatinib mesylate through multiple mechanisms. First, mutations occur in the kinase domain of the BCR-ABL oncoprotein that confer varying degrees of drug insensitivity (Deininger et al. 2005). Sometimes tumors with mutant BCR-ABL will respond to increased doses of imatinib mesylate (Kantarjian et al. 2003b). Resistant tumors also appear to respond to new drugs that are not affected by these mutations (Daub et al. 2004; Prenen et al. 2006). Second, tumors can also become resistant to imatinib mesylate through BCR-ABL gene amplification and mRNA overexpression (Gorre et al. 2001; Hochhaus et al. 2002). Importantly, resistance to imatinib mesylate is almost always associated with reactivation of BCR-ABL signaling, suggesting that this oncogene is required to sustain tumorigenesis in CML (Gorre et al. 2002).

2.4.4 Future Directions: Targeting Transcription Factors

Although there is encouraging experimental and clinical evidence that the targeted inactivation of specific gene products may be useful in cancer treatment, many gene products cannot be targeted with existing pharmacological approaches. In particular, there are no drugs that clinically target MYC and other transcription factors. We will discuss some of the possible approaches to target MYC that have been employed in experimental models such as the following: (1) Antisense oligonucleotides (ASOs), RNAi, and cationic porphyrin TMPyP4 have been used to target MYC at the transcriptional level. (2) Peptides and small molecules have been used to disrupt MYC binding to MAX. (3) Triple helix-forming oligonucleotides (TFOs) have been used to target MYC at the posttranslational level (Felsher and Bradon 2003; Prochownik 2004; Ponzielli et al. 2005). Additionally, MYC may be targeted at the posttranslational level by targeting its phosphorylation sites.

ASOs and RNAi both work by hybridizing to MYC's RNA and targeting it for degradation. ASO and RNAi treatments have led to decreased MYC protein levels both italics and italics (Wickstrom et al. 1991, 1992; Wang et al. 2005). The decrease in MYC results in cellular differentiation, reduced proliferation, and inhibition of G1/S progression in leukemia and lymphoma cells (Heikkila et al. 1987; Holt et al. 1988; Prochownik et al. 1988; Wickstrom et al. 1988, 1989; Carroll et al. 2002). In transgenic mouse models, ASOs have prevented or delayed the onset of Burkitt lymphoma (Huang et al. 1995; Smith and Wickstrom 1998b, 1998a). An ASO-type molecule with a morpholino backbone (AVI-4126) has been administered to patients in a phase I clinical trial and was found to concentrate in the tumor tissues of breast and prostate cancer patients, with little toxicity, thus making it a viable treatment option (Iversen et al. 2003; Devi et al. 2005). Cationic porphyrin TMPyP4 has also been used to target MYC at the transcriptional level. TMPyP4 blocks DNA structures formed during transcription in G-rich regions of DNA (G-quadruplexes) where MYC binds (Lemarteleur et al. 2004; Seenisamy et al. 2005). Additionally, TMPyP4 was able to inhibit italics transcription of MYC and decreased growth of Burkitt lymphoma cells (Simonsson and Henriksson 2002).

Peptides and small molecules have been used to disrupt MYC binding to its dimerization partner MAX. Small peptides that mimic the helix-loop-helix (HLH) domain of MYC were found to sequester MYC and prevent

MYC-MAX dimerization (Soucek et al. 1998; Pescarolo et al. 2001; Soucek et al. 2002). Interference with this protein-protein interaction led to decreased proliferation of breast cancer and colon cancer cell lines (Giorello et al. 1998; Nieddu et al. 2005). Peptide inhibitors are also capable of achieving high concentrations in mouse organs and may therefore be used to treat cancers (Nieddu et al. 2005). Unfortunately, peptides tend to be unstable and must be administered through intravenous injection, leaving a need for the development of small chemical molecules that can effectively prevent MYC-MAX dimerization. Peptidomimetics are an attempt to increase the stability and activity of peptides. Several peptidomimetics have been made that increase stability and activity of proteins that inhibit MYC-MAX dimerization but have not been used in human trials (Pescarolo et al. 2001; Nieddu et al. 2005). Additionally, there has been an effort to target MYC-MAX interaction with small chemical molecules (Berg et al. 2002; Mo and Henriksson 2006; Xu et al. 2006). One of these approaches uses molecular "credit cards," which are planar chemicals designed to physically prevent protein-protein interaction by sliding between the two protein surfaces. In one study, potent inhibitors of MYC-MAX interaction were identified that partially prevented oncogenic transformation of chicken embryonic fibroblasts (Xu et al. 2006).

MYC has also been targeted at the DNA-protein interaction level. Triple helix-forming oligonucleotides (TFOs) can disrupt transcription factor binding to DNA by attaching to purine-rich regions of DNA often found in promoter regions (Kim et al. 1998; McGuffie and Catapano 2002). TFOs against the promoter for MYC have been able to induce apoptosis and cell cycle arrest in several cancer cell lines (Thomas et al. 1995; Catapano et al. 2000; McGuffie et al. 2000). TFOs may also be conjugated to DNA-damaging agents such as daunomycin. This combination agent leads to MYC downregulation in prostate and breast cancer cell lines (Carbone et al. 2004).

MYC may be marked for degradation at the posttranslational level by targeting its phosphorylation sites. MYC has two phosphorylation sites: Thr58 and Ser62. Phosphorylation of Ser62 increases MYC stability and occurs in a Ras-dependent manner. The phosphorylation of Ser62 is followed by phosphorylation of Thr58 and leads to the degradation of MYC (Sears et al. 2000; Sears 2004). Thus it may possible to screen for small molecules that inhibit MYC stabilization, or facilitate MYC degradation.

2.5 Cancer Therapy and Oncogene Addiction

Observations in experimental transgenic mouse models and in the clinic have a central theme: Although cancers are genetically complex and genomically unstable, they appear to be dependent on the continued activation of specific oncogenes to maintain their neoplastic properties, exhibiting the phenomenon of "oncogene addiction". Thus specific gene products that mediate critical signaling processes appear to be the most likely best targets for the treatment of cancer. Conditional transgenic mouse models have been particularly useful for validating which signaling molecules are the most useful targets, for gaining insight into the mechanism of tumor regression, and for anticipating mechanisms by which tumors can escape dependence on signaling processes. In several cases, drugs have been identified that target receptors, GTPases, and/or kinases to successfully treat humans with cancer. However, these drugs, although effective in prolonging the survival of some patients, do not cure cancer. The hope is that in the future, with the correct combination of drugs we will be able to cure cancer. However, there are several potential difficulties.

One major difficulty is that many gene products, in particular transcription factors, have yet to be successfully targeted. Although we may not be able yet to target the most critical gene products, many new approaches suggest that even these gene products can be inhibited through small molecules. It may be possible to develop effective pharmacological strategies to target critical signaling molecules for the treatment of cancer.

Another problem is that we as yet do not understand why the repair or inactivation of specific gene products induces tumor regression. Several possible mechanisms could account for "oncogene addiction". Bernard Weinstein, who was one of the first to articulate the notion of oncogene addiction. He proposed that because oncogenes in cancer cells upregulate cellular programs that drive proliferation and block apoptosis, compensatory programs such as proliferative arrest and proapoptotic programs are also upregulated. Thus when a mutant oncogene is inactivated, the balance in the cancer cell shifts to proliferative arrest and/or apoptosis (Weinstein 2002).

A final issue to consider is that cancer is not just caused by genetic events, therefore reversing these events may not be sufficient to reverse the process of tumorigenesis. Thus it has recently been suggested that cancers consist of cancer stem cells, of generally low abundance, and progenitor cells, that are the majority of the tumor. The cancer stem cells have the capacity for self-renewal, whereas the progenitor cells have a limited capacity of self-renewal. Such a model provides just one example of a circumstance in which the properties that are essential to the neoplastic phenotype are not necessarily dictated by genetic events involving signaling molecules.

Observations in transgenic mouse models have led investigators to reflect on several non-exclusive mechanisms for oncogene addiction. One possibility is that oncogenes initiate tumorigenesis by hijacking stem cell features in cells such as proliferation and self-renewal (Beer et al. 2004; Shachaf et al. 2004), driving cell cycle transit despite ongoing genomic instability (Karlsson et al. 2003a). Hence, upon oncogene inactivation, tumor cells recover their differentiative physiologic program, undergo proliferative arrest, become aware of their genomic damage, and/or undergo apoptosis. Additionally, Chin, Baudino, and Knies-Bamforth have illustrated that upon oncogene inactivation cell nonautonomous programs such as angiogenesis are shut down, which may also contribute to tumor regression (Chin et al. 1999; Baudino et al. 2002; Knies-Bamforth et al. 2004). Hence, cell-autonomous and cell-dependent mechanisms may play a role in oncogene addiction. Other mechanisms could also be involved, such as the potential role of immune or inflammatory mechanisms or the possibility that cellular homeostatic regulatory mechanisms are important. Ultimately, insights into the mechanism of oncogene addiction will be essential in the development of true targeted therapeutics for the treatment and cure of cancer.

Acknowledgements. We thank the members of the Felsher laboratory for their many helpful discussions. This work was supported from grants from the NCI and related programs (ICBP, ICMIC, CCNE), Emerald Foundation, Leukemia and Lymphoma Society, Damon Runyon Foundation, Burroughs Wellcome Fund, and Stanford Digestive Disease Center (D.W.F.), as well as the Developmental and Neonatal Biology NIH Training Grant (C.A).

References

Alberts SR, Schroeder M, Erlichman C, Steen PD, Foster NR, Moore DF, Jr., Rowland KM, Jr., Nair S, Tschetter LK, Fitch TR (2004) Gemcitabine and ISIS-2503 for patients with locally advanced or metastatic pancreatic adenocarcinoma: a North Central Cancer Treatment Group phase II trial. J Clin Oncol 22:4944–4950

Bachireddy P, Bendapudi PK, Felsher DW (2005) Getting at MYC through RAS. Clin Cancer Res 11:4278–4281

Bardeesy N, Kim M, Xu J, Kim RS, Shen Q, Bosenberg MW, Wong WH, Chin L (2005) Role of epidermal growth factor receptor signaling in RAS-driven melanoma. Mol Cell Biol 25:4176–4188

Baudino TA, McKay C, Pendeville-Samain H, Nilsson JA, Maclean KH, White EL, Davis AC, Ihle JN, Cleveland JL (2002) c Myc is essential for vasculogenesis and angiogenesis during development and tumor progression. Genes Dev 16:2530–2543

Beer S, Zetterberg A, Ihrie RA, McTaggart RA, Yang Q, Bradon N, Arvanitis C, Attardi LD, Feng S, Ruebner B, Cardiff RD, Felsher DW (2004) Developmental context determines latency of MYC-induced tumorigenesis. PLoS Biol 2:E332

Berg T, Cohen SB, Desharnais J, Sonderegger C, Maslyar DJ, Goldberg J, Boger DL, Vogt PK (2002) Small-molecule antagonists of Myc/Max dimerization inhibit Myc-induced transformation of chicken embryo fibroblasts. Proc Natl Acad Sci USA 99:3830–385

Bianco R, Melisi D, Ciardiello F, Tortora G (2006) Key cancer cell signal transduction pathways as therapeutic targets. Eur J Cancer 42:290–294

Bishop JM (1982) Retroviruses and Cancer Genes. Advances in Cancer Research. S. W. George Kline. New York, Academic Press Inc. 37:1–32

Bos JL (1989) ras oncogenes in human cancer:a review. Cancer Res 49:4682–4689

Bourne HR, Sanders DA, McCormick F (1991) The GTPase superfamily: conserved structure and molecular mechanism. Nature 349:117–127

Boxer RB, Jang JW, Sintasath L, Chodosh LA (2004) Lack of sustained regression of c-MYC-induced mammary adenocarcinomas following brief or prolonged MYC inactivation. Cancer Cell 6:577–586

Buchdunger E, Cioffi CL, Law N, Stover D, Ohno-Jones S, Druker BJ, Lydon NB (2000) Abl protein-tyrosine kinase inhibitor STI571 inhibits in vitro signal transduction mediated by c-kit and platelet-derived growth factor receptors. J Pharmacol Exp Ther 295:139–145

Carbone GM, McGuffie E, Napoli S, Flanagan CE, Dembech C, Negri U, Arcamone F, Capobianco ML, Catapano CV (2004) DNA binding and antigene activity of a daunomycin-conjugated triplex-forming oligonucleotide targeting the P2 promoter of the human c-myc gene. Nucleic Acids Res 32:2396–2410

Carroll JS, Swarbrick A, Musgrove EA, Sutherland RL (2002) Mechanisms of growth arrest by c-myc antisense oligonucleotides in MCF-7 breast cancer cells: implications for the antiproliferative effects of antiestrogens. Cancer Res 62:3126–3131

Catapano CV, McGuffie EM, Pacheco D, Carbone GM (2000) Inhibition of gene expression and cell proliferation by triple helix-forming oligonucleotides directed to the c-myc gene. Biochemistry 39:5126–5138

Chin L, Tam A, Pomerantz J, Wong M, Holash J, Bardeesy N, Shen Q, O'Hagan R, Pantginis J, Zhou H, Horner JW 2nd, Cordon-Cardo C, Yancopoulos GD, DePinho RA (1999) Essential role for oncogenic Ras in tumour maintenance. Nature 400:468–472

Cohen MH, Williams GA, Sridhara R, Chen G, McGuinn WD Jr, Morse D, Abraham S, Rahman A, Liang C, Lostritto R, Baird A, Pazdur R (2004) United States Food and Drug Administration Drug Approval summary: Gefitinib (ZD1839; Iressa) tablets. Clin Cancer Res 10:1212–1218

Cox AD, Der CJ (2002) Farnesyltransferase inhibitors: promises and realities. Curr Opin Pharmacol 2:388–393

Cunningham D, Humblet Y, Siena S, Khayat D, Bleiberg H, Santoro A, Bets D, Mueser M, Harstrick A, Verslype C, Chau I, Van Cutsem E (2004) Cetuximab monotherapy and cetuximab plus irinotecan in irinotecan-refractory metastatic colorectal cancer. N Engl J Med 351:337–345

D'Cruz CM, Gunther EJ, Boxer RB, Hartman JL, Sintasath L, Moody SE, Cox JD, Ha SI, Belka GK, Golant A, Cardiff RD, Chodosh LA (2001) c-MYC induces mammary tumorigenesis by means of a preferred pathway involving spontaneous Kras2 mutations. Nat Med 7:235–239

Daley GQ (2003) Gleevec resistance:lessons for target-directed drug development. Cell Cycle 2:190–191

Daley GQ, Van Etten RA, Baltimore D (1990) Induction of chronic myelogenous leukemia in mice by the P210bcr/abl gene of the Philadelphia chromosome. Science 247:824–830

Dang CV, Resar LM, Emison E, Kim S, Li Q, Prescott JE, Wonsey D, Zeller K (1999) Function of the c-Myc oncogenic transcription factor. Exp Cell Res 253:63–77

Daub H, Specht K, Ullrich A (2004) Strategies to overcome resistance to targeted protein kinase inhibitors. Nat Rev Drug Discov 3:1001–1010

Deininger M, Buchdunger E, Druker BJ (2005) The development of imatinib as a therapeutic agent for chronic myeloid leukemia. Blood 105:2640–2653

Demetri GD, von Mehren M, Blanke CD, Van den Abbeele AD, Eisenberg B, Roberts PJ, Heinrich MC, Tuveson DA, Singer S, Janicek M, Fletcher JA, Silverman SG, Silberman SL, Capdeville R, Kiese B, Peng B, Dimitrijevic S, Druker BJ, Corless C, Fletcher CD, Joensuu H (2002) Efficacy and safety of imatinib mesylate in advanced gastrointestinal stromal tumors. N Engl J Med 347:472–480

Devi GR, Beer TM, Corless CL, Arora V, Weller DL, Iversen PL (2005) In vivo bioavailability and pharmacokinetics of a c-MYC antisense phosphorodiamidate morpholino oligomer, AVI-4126, in solid tumors. Clin Cancer Res 11:3930–3938

Downward J (1996) Control of ras activation. Cancer Surv 27:87–100

Druker BJ (2004) Imatinib as a paradigm of targeted therapies. Adv Cancer Res 91:1–30

Druker BJ, Talpaz M, Resta DJ, Peng B, Buchdunger E, Ford JM, Lydon NB, Kantarjian H, Capdeville R, Ohno-Jones S, Sawyers CL (2001) Efficacy and safety of a specific inhibitor of the BCR-ABL tyrosine kinase in chronic myeloid leukemia. N Engl J Med 344:1031–1037

Druker BJ, Tamura S, Buchdunger E, Ohno S, Segal GM, Fanning S, Zimmermann J, Lydon NB (1996) Effects of a selective inhibitor of the Abl tyrosine kinase on the growth of Bcr-Abl positive cells. Nat Med 2:561–566

Eilers M, Picard D, Yamamoto KR, Bishop JM (1989) Chimaeras of myc oncoprotein and steroid receptors cause hormone-dependent transformation of cells. Nature 340:66–68

End DW, Smets G, Todd AV, Applegate TL, Fuery CJ, Angibaud P, Venet M, Sanz G, Poignet H, Skrzat S, Devine A, Wouters W, Bowden C (2001) Characterization of the antitumor effects of the selective farnesyl protein transferase inhibitor R115777 in vivo and in vitro. Cancer Res 61:131–137

Escudier B, Szczylik C, Eisen T, Stadler WM, Schwartz B, Shan M, Bukowski RM (2005) Randomized phase III trial of the Raf kinase and VEGFR inhibitor sorafenib (BAY 43-9006) in patients with advanced renal cell carcinoma (RCC). J Clin Oncol 23:1093S

Felsher DW (2003) Cancer revoked:oncogenes as therapeutic targets. Nat Rev Cancer 3:375–380

Felsher DW (2004a) Putting oncogenes into a developmental context. Cancer Biol Ther 3:942–944

Felsher DW (2004b) Reversibility of oncogene-induced cancer. Curr Opin Genet Dev 14:37–42

Felsher DW, Bishop JM (1999a) Reversible tumorigenesis by MYC in hematopoietic lineages. Mol Cell 4:199–207

Felsher DW, Bishop JM (1999b) Transient excess of MYC activity can elicit genomic instability and tumorigenesis. Proc Natl Acad Sci USA 96:3940–3944

Felsher DW, Bradon N (2003) Pharmacological inactivation of MYC for the treatment of cancer. Drug News Perspect 16:370–374

Fisher GH, Wellen SL, Klimstra D, Lenczowski JM, Tichelaar JW, Lizak MJ, Whitsett JA, Koretsky A, Varmus HE (2001) Induction and apoptotic regression of lung adenocarcinomas by regulation of a K-Ras transgene in the presence and absence of tumor suppressor genes. Genes Dev 15:3249–3262

Flaherty KT, Brose M, Schuchter L, Tuveson D, Lee R, Schwartz B, Lathia C, Weber B, O'Dwyer P (2004) Phase I/II trial of BAY 43-9006, carboplatin and paclitaxel demonstrates preliminary antitumor activity in the expansion cohort of patients with metastatic melanoma. J Clin Oncol 22:711s

Flores I, Murphy DJ, Swigart LB, Knies U, Evan GI (2004) Defining the temporal requirements for Myc in the progression and maintenance of skin neoplasia. Oncogene 23:5923–5930

Floyd HS, Farnsworth CL, Kock ND, Mizesko MC, Little JL, Dance ST, Everitt J, Tichelaar J, Whitsett JA, Miller MS (2005) Conditional expression of the mutant Ki-rasG12C allele results in formation of benign lung adenomas:development of a novel mouse lung tumor model. Carcinogenesis 26:2196–2206

Fukuoka M, Yano S, Giaccone G, Tamura T, Nakagawa K, Douillard JY, Nishiwaki Y, Vansteenkiste J, Kudoh S, Rischin D, Eek R, Horai T, Noda K, Takata I, Smit E, Averbuch S, Macleod A, Feyereislova A, Dong RP, Baselga J (2003) Multi-institutional randomized phase II trial of gefitinib for previously treated patients with advanced non-small-cell lung cancer (The IDEAL 1 Trial) [corrected]. J Clin Oncol 21:2237–2246

Giaccone G, Herbst RS, Manegold C, Scagliotti G, Rosell R, Miller V, Natale RB, Schiller JH, Von Pawel J, Pluzanska A, Gatzemeier U, Grous J, Ochs JS, Averbuch SD, Wolf MK, Rennie P, Fandi A, Johnson DH (2004) Gefitinib in combination with gemcitabine and cisplatin in advanced non-small-cell lung cancer: a phase III trial–INTACT 1. J Clin Oncol 22:777–784

Giorello L, Clerico L, Pescarolo MP, Vikhanskaya F, Salmona M, Colella G, Bruno S, Mancuso T, Bagnasco L, Russo P, Parodi S (1998) Inhibition of cancer cell growth and c-Myc transcriptional activity by a c-Myc helix 1-type peptide fused to an internalization sequence. Cancer Res 58:3654–3659

Giuriato S, Rabin K, Fan AC, Shachaf CM, Felsher DW (2004) Conditional animal models:a strategy to define when oncogenes will be effective targets to treat cancer. Semin Cancer Biol 14:3–11

Gorre ME, Ellwood-Yen K, Chiosis G, Rosen N, Sawyers CL (2002) BCR-ABL point mutants isolated from patients with imatinib mesylate-resistant chronic myeloid leukemia remain sensitive to inhibitors of the BCR-ABL chaperone heat shock protein 90. Blood 100:3041–3044

Gorre ME, Mohammed M, Ellwood K, Hsu N, Paquette R, Rao PN, Sawyers CL (2001) Clinical resistance to STI-571 cancer therapy caused by BCR-ABL gene mutation or amplification. Science 293:876–880

Gossen M, Bonin AL, Freundlieb S, Bujard H (1994) Inducible gene expression systems for higher eukaryotic cells. Curr Opin Biotechnol 5:516–520

Gossen M, Bujard H (1992) Tight control of gene expression in mammalian cells by tetracycline-responsive promoters. Proc Natl Acad Sci USA 89:5547–5551

Gutmann DH, Hunter-Schaedle K, Shannon KM (2006) Harnessing preclinical mouse models to inform human clinical cancer trials. J Clin Invest 116:847–852

Haklai R, Weisz MG, Elad G, Paz A, Marciano D, Egozi Y, Ben-Baruch G, Kloog Y (1998) Dislodgment and accelerated degradation of Ras. Biochemistry 37:1306–1314

Heikkila R, Schwab G, Wickstrom E, Loke SL, Pluznik DH, Watt R, Neckers LM (1987) A c-myc antisense oligodeoxynucleotide inhibits entry into S phase but not progress from G0 to G1. Nature 328:445–449

Heinrich MC, Griffith DJ, Druker BJ, Wait CL, Ott KA, Zigler AJ (2000) Inhibition of c-kit receptor tyrosine kinase activity by STI 571, a selective tyrosine kinase inhibitor. Blood 96:925–932

Herbst RS, Giaccone G, Schiller JH, Natale RB, Miller V, Manegold C, Scagliotti G, Rosell R, Oliff I, Reeves JA, Wolf MK, Krebs AD, Averbuch SD, Ochs JS, Grous J, Fandi A, Johnson DH (2004) Gefitinib in combination with paclitaxel and carboplatin in advanced non-small-cell lung cancer: a phase III trial–INTACT 2. J Clin Oncol 22:785–794

Hirsch FR, Scagliotti GV, Langer CJ, Varella-Garcia M, Franklin WA (2003) Epidermal growth factor family of receptors in preneoplasia and lung cancer: perspectives for targeted therapies. Lung Cancer 41 Suppl 1:S29–S42

Hochhaus A, Kreil S, Corbin AS, La Rosee P, Muller MC, Lahaye T, Hanfstein B, Schoch C, Cross NC, Berger U, Gschaidmeier H, Druker BJ, Hehlmann R (2002) Molecular and chromosomal mechanisms of resistance to imatinib (STI571) therapy. Leukemia 16:2190–2196

Holt JT, Redner RL, Nienhuis AW (1988) An oligomer complementary to c-myc mRNA inhibits proliferation of HL-60 promyelocytic cells and induces differentiation. Mol Cell Biol 8:963–973

http://www.myc-cancer-gene.org. from http://www.myc-cancer-gene.org

Huang Y, Snyder R, Kligshteyn M, Wickstrom E (1995) Prevention of tumor formation in a mouse model of Burkitt's lymphoma by 6 weeks of treatment with anti-c-myc DNA phosphorothioate. Mol Med 1:647–658

Huettner CS, Zhang P, Van Etten RA, Tenen DG (2000) Reversibility of acute B-cell leukaemia induced by BCR-ABL1. Nat Genet 24:57–60

Hurwitz H, Fehrenbacher L, Novotny W, Cartwright T, Hainsworth J, Heim W, Berlin J, Baron A, Griffing S, Holmgren E, Ferrara N, Fyfe G, Rogers B, Ross R, Kabbinavar F (2004) Bevacizumab plus irinotecan, fluorouracil, and leucovorin for metastatic colorectal cancer. N Engl J Med 350:2335–2342

Iversen PL, Arora V, Acker AJ, Mason DH, Devi GR (2003) Efficacy of antisense morpholino oligomer targeted to c-myc in prostate cancer xenograft murine model and a Phase I safety study in humans. Clin Cancer Res 9:2510–2519

Jain M, Arvanitis C, Chu K, Dewey W, Leonhardt E, Trinh M, Sundberg CD, Bishop JM, Felsher DW (2002) Sustained loss of a neoplastic phenotype by brief inactivation of MYC. Science 297:102–104

Jonkers J, Berns A (2002) Conditional mouse models of sporadic cancer. Nat Rev Cancer 2:251–265

Jonkers J, Berns A (2004) Oncogene addiction:sometimes a temporary slavery. Cancer Cell 6:535–538

Kantarjian H, Sawyers C, Hochhaus A, Guilhot F, Schiffer C, Gambacorti-Passerini C, Niederwieser D, Resta D, Capdeville R, Zoellner U, Talpaz M, Druker B, Goldman J, O'Brien SG, Russell N, Fischer T, Ottmann O, Cony-Makhoul P, Facon T, Stone R, Miller C, Tallman M, Brown R, Schuster M, Loughran T, Gratwohl A, Mandelli F, Saglio G, Lazzarino M, Russo D, Baccarani M, Morra E (2002) Hematologic and cytogenetic responses to imatinib mesylate in chronic myelogenous leukemia. N Engl J Med 346:645–652

Kantarjian HM, O'Brien S, Cortes J, Giles FJ, Rios MB, Shan J, Faderl S, Garcia-Manero G, Ferrajoli A, Verstovsek S, Wierda W, Keating M, Talpaz M (2003a) Imatinib mesylate therapy improves survival in patients with newly diagnosed Philadelphia chromosome-positive chronic myelogenous leukemia in the chronic phase: comparison with historic data. Cancer 98:2636–2642

Kantarjian HM, Talpaz M, O'Brien S, Giles F, Garcia-Manero G, Faderl S, Thomas D, Shan J, Rios MB, Cortes J (2003b) Dose escalation of imatinib mesylate can overcome resistance to standard-dose therapy in patients with chronic myelogenous leukemia. Blood 101:473–475

Karlsson A, Deb-Basu D, Cherry A, Turner S, Ford J, Felsher DW (2003a) Defective double-strand DNA break repair and chromosomal translocations by MYC overexpression. Proc Natl Acad Sci USA 100:9974–9979

Karlsson A, Giuriato S, Tang F, Fung-Weier J, Levan G, Felsher DW (2003b) Genomically complex lympho-

mas undergo sustained tumor regression upon MYC inactivation unless they acquire novel chromosomal translocations. Blood 101:2797–2803

Kim HG, Reddoch JF, Mayfield C, Ebbinghaus S, Vigneswaran N, Thomas S, Jones DE Jr, Miller DM (1998) Inhibition of transcription of the human c-myc protooncogene by intermolecular triplex. Biochemistry 37:2299–2304

Knies-Bamforth UE, Fox SB, Poulsom R, Evan GI, Harris AL (2004) c-Myc interacts with hypoxia to induce angiogenesis in vivo by a vascular endothelial growth factor-dependent mechanism. Cancer Res 64:6563–6570

Kohl NE, Omer CA, Conner MW, Anthony NJ, Davide JP, deSolms SJ, Giuliani EA, Gomez RP, Graham SL, Hamilton K, et al. (1995) Inhibition of farnesyltransferase induces regression of mammary and salivary carcinomas in ras transgenic mice. Nat Med 1:792–797

Koschmieder S, Gottgens B, Zhang P, Iwasaki-Arai J, Akashi K, Kutok JL, Dayaram T, Geary K, Green AR, Tenen DG, Huettner CS (2005) Inducible chronic phase of myeloid leukemia with expansion of hematopoietic stem cells in a transgenic model of BCR-ABL leukemogenesis. Blood 105:324–334

Kris MG, Natale RB, Herbst RS, Lynch TJ, Jr., Prager D, Belani CP, Schiller JH, Kelly K, Spiridonidis H, Sandler A, Albain KS, Cella D, Wolf MK, Averbuch SD, Ochs JJ, Kay AC (2003) Efficacy of gefitinib, an inhibitor of the epidermal growth factor receptor tyrosine kinase, in symptomatic patients with non-small cell lung cancer:a randomized trial. JAMA 290:2149–2158

Lemarteleur T, Gomez D, Paterski R, Mandine E, Mailliet P, Riou JF (2004) Stabilization of the c-myc gene promoter quadruplex by specific ligands' inhibitors of telomerase. Biochem Biophys Res Commun 323:802–808

Lerner EC, Zhang TT, Knowles DB, Qian Y, Hamilton AD, Sebti SM (1997) Inhibition of the prenylation of K-Ras, but not H- or N-Ras, is highly resistant to CAAX peptidomimetics and requires both a farnesyltransferase and a geranylgeranyltransferase I inhibitor in human tumor cell lines. Oncogene 15:1283–1288

Lewis BC, Klimstra DS, Varmus HE (2003) The c-myc and PyMT oncogenes induce different tumor types in a somatic mouse model for pancreatic cancer. Genes Dev 17:3127–3138

Littlewood TD, Hancock DC, Danielian PS, Parker MG, Evan GI (1995) A modified oestrogen receptor ligand-binding domain as an improved switch for the regulation of heterologous proteins. Nucleic Acids Res 23:1686–1690

Lobell RB, Omer CA, Abrams MT, Bhimnathwala HG, Brucker MJ, Buser CA, Davide JP, deSolms SJ, Dinsmore CJ, Ellis-Hutchings MS, Kral AM, Liu D, Lumma WC, Machotka SV, Rands E, Williams TM, Graham SL, Hartman GD, Oliff AI, Heimbrook DC, Kohl NE (2001) Evaluation of farnesyl: protein transferase and geranylgeranyl:protein transferase inhibitor combinations in preclinical models. Cancer Res 61:8758-8768

Lowy DR, Willumsen BM (1993) Function and regulation of ras. Annu Rev Biochem 62:851-891

Lugo TG, Pendergast AM, Muller AJ, Witte ON (1990) Tyrosine kinase activity and transformation potency of bcr-abl oncogene products. Science 247:1079-1082

Lynch TJ, Bell DW, Sordella R, Gurubhagavatula S, Okimoto RA, Brannigan BW, Harris PL, Haserlat SM, Supko JG, Haluska FG, Louis DN, Christiani DC, Settleman J, Haber DA (2004) Activating mutations in the epidermal growth factor receptor underlying responsiveness of non-small-cell lung cancer to gefitinib. N Engl J Med 350:2129-3219

Manning G, Whyte DB, Martinez R, Hunter T, Sudarsanam S (2002) The protein kinase complement of the human genome. Science 298:1912-1934

Marinkovic D, Marinkovic T, Mahr B, Hess J, Wirth T (2004) Reversible lymphomagenesis in conditionally c-MYC expressing mice. Int J Cancer 110:336-342

McGuffie EM, Catapano CV (2002) Design of a novel triple helix-forming oligodeoxyribonucleotide directed to the major promoter of the c-myc gene. Nucleic Acids Res 30:2701-2709

McGuffie EM, Pacheco D, Carbone GM, Catapano CV (2000) Antigene and antiproliferative effects of a c-myc-targeting phosphorothioate triple helix-forming oligonucleotide in human leukemia cells. Cancer Res 60:3790-3799

Mo H, Henriksson M (2006) Identification of small molecules that induce apoptosis in a Myc-dependent manner and inhibit Myc-driven transformation. Proc Natl Acad Sci USA 103:6344-6349

Moody SE, Perez D, Pan TC, Sarkisian CJ, Portocarrero CP, Sterner CJ, Notorfrancesco KL, Cardiff RD, Chodosh LA (2005) The transcriptional repressor Snail promotes mammary tumor recurrence. Cancer Cell 8:197-209

Moody SE, Sarkisian CJ, Hahn KT, Gunther EJ, Pickup S, Dugan KD, Innocent N, Cardiff RD, Schnall MD, Chodosh LA (2002) Conditional activation of Neu in the mammary epithelium of transgenic mice results in reversible pulmonary metastasis. Cancer Cell 2:451-461

Nesbit CE, Tersak JM, Prochownik EV (1999) MYC oncogenes and human neoplastic disease. Oncogene 18:3004-3016

Nieddu E, Melchiori A, Pescarolo MP, Bagnasco L, Biasotti B, Licheri B, Malacarne D, Tortolina L, Castagnino N, Pasa S, Cimoli G, Avignolo C, Ponassi R, Balbi C, Patrone E, D'Arrigo C, Barboro P, Vasile F, Orecchia P, Carnemolla B, Damonte G, Millo E, Palomba D, Fassina G, Mazzei M, Parodi S (2005) Sequence specific peptidomimetic molecules inhibitors of a protein-protein interaction at the helix 1 level of c-Myc. FASEB J 19:632-634

O'Brien SG, Guilhot F, Larson RA, Gathmann I, Baccarani M, Cervantes F, Cornelissen JJ, Fischer T, Hochhaus A, Hughes T, Lechner K, Nielsen JL, Rousselot P, Rei-

ffers J, Saglio G, Shepherd J, Simonsson B, Gratwohl A, Goldman JM, Kantarjian H, Taylor K, Verhoef G, Bolton AE, Capdeville R, Druker BJ (2003) Imatinib compared with interferon and low-dose cytarabine for newly diagnosed chronic-phase chronic myeloid leukemia. N Engl J Med 348:994-1004

Olayioye MA, Neve RM, Lane HA, Hynes NE (2000) The ErbB signaling network: receptor heterodimerization in development and cancer. EMBO J 19:3159-3167

Oster SK, Ho CS, Soucie EL, Penn LZ (2002) The myc oncogene: MarvelouslY Complex. Adv Cancer Res 84:81-154

Pao W, Klimstra DS, Fisher GH, Varmus HE (2003) Use of avian retroviral vectors to introduce transcriptional regulators into mammalian cells for analyses of tumor maintenance. Proc Natl Acad Sci USA 100:8764-8769

Pao W, Miller VA (2005) Epidermal growth factor receptor mutations, small-molecule kinase inhibitors, and non-small-cell lung cancer: current knowledge and future directions. J Clin Oncol 23:2556-2568

Pao W, Wang TY, Riely GJ, Miller VA, Pan Q, Ladanyi M, Zakowski MF, Heelan RT, Kris MG, Varmus HE (2005) KRAS mutations and primary resistance of lung adenocarcinomas to gefitinib or erlotinib. PLoS Med 2:e17

Pegram MD, Konecny GE, O'Callaghan C, Beryt M, Pietras R, Slamon DJ (2004a) Rational combinations of trastuzumab with chemotherapeutic drugs used in the treatment of breast cancer. J Natl Cancer Inst 96:739-749

Pegram MD, Pienkowski T, Northfelt DW, Eiermann W, Patel R, Fumoleau P, Quan E, Crown J, Toppmeyer D, Smylie M, Riva A, Blitz S, Press MF, Reese D, Lindsay MA, Slamon DJ (2004b) Results of two open-label, multicenter phase II studies of docetaxel, platinum salts, and trastuzumab in HER2-positive advanced breast cancer. J Natl Cancer Inst 96:759-769

Pelengaris S, Abouna S, Cheung L, Ifandi V, Zervou S, Khan M (2004) Brief inactivation of c-Myc is not sufficient for sustained regression of c-Myc-induced tumours of pancreatic islets and skin epidermis. BMC Biol 2:26

Pelengaris S, Khan M, Evan GI (2002) Suppression of Myc-induced apoptosis in beta cells exposes multiple oncogenic properties of Myc and triggers carcinogenic progression. Cell 109:321-334

Pelengaris S, Littlewood T, Khan M, Elia G, Evan G (1999) Reversible activation of c-Myc in skin:induction of a complex neoplastic phenotype by a single oncogenic lesion. Mol Cell 3:565-577

Pescarolo MP, Bagnasco L, Malacarne D, Melchiori A, Valente P, Millo E, Bruno S, Basso S, Parodi S (2001) A retro-inverso peptide homologous to helix 1 of c-Myc is a potent and specific inhibitor of proliferation in different cellular systems. FASEB J 15:31-33

Ponzielli R, Katz S, Barsyte-Lovejoy D, Penn LZ (2005) Cancer therapeutics:targeting the dark side of Myc. Eur J Cancer 41:2485-2501

Prenen H, Cools J, Mentens N, Folens C, Sciot R, Schoffski P, Van Oosterom A, Marynen P, Debiec-Rychter M (2006) Efficacy of the kinase inhibitor SU11248 against gastrointestinal stromal tumor mutants refractory to imatinib mesylate. Clin Cancer Res 12:2622–2627

Prochownik EV (2004) c-Myc as a therapeutic target in cancer. Expert Rev Anticancer Ther 4:289–302

Prochownik EV, Kukowska J, Rodgers C (1988) c-myc antisense transcripts accelerate differentiation and inhibit G1 progression in murine erythroleukemia cells. Mol Cell Biol 8:3683–3695

Ross JS, Fletcher JA, Bloom KJ, Linette GP, Stec J, Symmans WF, Pusztai L, Hortobagyi GN (2004) Targeted therapy in breast cancer: the HER-2/neu gene and protein. Mol Cell Proteomics 3:379–398

Sawyers CL (2002) Finding the next Gleevec:FLT3 targeted kinase inhibitor therapy for acute myeloid leukemia. Cancer Cell 1:413–415

Schlessinger J (2000) Cell signaling by receptor tyrosine kinases. Cell 103:211–225

Sears R, Nuckolls F, Haura E, Taya Y, Tamai K, Nevins JR (2000) Multiple Ras-dependent phosphorylation pathways regulate Myc protein stability. Genes Dev 14:2501–2514

Sears RC (2004) The life cycle of C-myc:from synthesis to degradation. Cell Cycle 3:1133–1137

Seenisamy J, Bashyam S, Gokhale V, Vankayalapati H, Sun D, Siddiqui-Jain A, Streiner N, Shin-Ya K, White E, Wilson WD, Hurley LH (2005) Design and synthesis of an expanded porphyrin that has selectivity for the c-MYC G-quadruplex structure. J Am Chem Soc 127:2944–2959

Shachaf CM, Felsher DW (2005a) Rehabilitation of cancer through oncogene inactivation. Trends Mol Med 11:316–321

Shachaf CM, Felsher DW (2005b) Tumor dormancy and MYC inactivation: pushing cancer to the brink of normalcy. Cancer Res 65:4471–4474

Shachaf CM, Kopelman AM, Arvanitis C, Karlsson A, Beer S, Mandl S, Bachmann MH, Borowsky AD, Ruebner B, Cardiff RD, Yang Q, Bishop JM, Contag CH, Felsher DW (2004) MYC inactivation uncovers pluripotent differentiation and tumour dormancy in hepatocellular cancer. Nature

Shepherd FA, Rodrigues Pereira J, Ciuleanu T, Tan EH, Hirsh V, Thongprasert S, Campos D, Maoleekoonpiroj S, Smylie M, Martins R, van Kooten M, Dediu M, Findlay B, Tu D, Johnston D, Bezjak A, Clark G, Santabarbara P, Seymour L (2005) Erlotinib in previously treated non-small-cell lung cancer. N Engl J Med 353:123–132

Simonsson T, Henriksson M (2002) c-myc Suppression in Burkitt's lymphoma cells. Biochem Biophys Res Commun 290:11–15

Slamon DJ, Leyland-Jones B, Shak S, Fuchs H, Paton V, Bajamonde A, Fleming T, Eiermann W, Wolter J, Pegram M, Baselga J, Norton L (2001) Use of chemotherapy plus a monoclonal antibody against HER2 for metastatic breast cancer that overexpresses HER2. N Engl J Med 344:783–792

Smith JB, Wickstrom E (1998a) Antisense c-myc and immunostimulatory oligonucleotide inhibition of tumorigenesis in a murine B-cell lymphoma transplant model. J Natl Cancer Inst 90:1146–1154

Smith JB, Wickstrom E (1998b) Inhibition of tumorigenesis in a murine B-cell lymphoma transplant model by c-Myc complementary oligonucleotides. Adv Exp Med Biol 451:17–22

Sordella R, Bell DW, Haber DA, Settleman J (2004) Gefitinib-sensitizing EGFR mutations in lung cancer activate anti-apoptotic pathways. Science 305:1163–1167

Soucek L, Helmer-Citterich M, Sacco A, Jucker R, Cesareni G, Nasi S (1998) Design and properties of a Myc derivative that efficiently homodimerizes. Oncogene 17:2463–2472

Soucek L, Jucker R, Panacchia L, Ricordy R, Tato F, Nasi S (2002) Omomyc, a potential Myc dominant negative, enhances Myc-induced apoptosis. Cancer Res 62:3507–3510

Stamos J, Sliwkowski MX, Eigenbrot C (2002) Structure of the epidermal growth factor receptor kinase domain alone and in complex with a 4-anilinoquinazoline inhibitor. J Biol Chem 277:46265–46272

Thomas TJ, Faaland CA, Gallo MA, Thomas T (1995) Suppression of c-myc oncogene expression by a polyamine-complexed triplex forming oligonucleotide in MCF-7 breast cancer cells. Nucleic Acids Res 23:3594–3599

Tibes R, Trent J, Kurzrock R (2005) Tyrosine kinase inhibitors and the dawn of molecular cancer therapeutics. Annu Rev Pharmacol Toxicol 45:357–384

Van Dyke T, Jacks T (2002) Cancer modeling in the modern era: progress and challenges. Cell 108:135–144

Ventura JJ, Nebreda AR (2006) Protein kinases and phosphatases as therapeutic targets in cancer. Clin Transl Oncol 8:153–160

Wang YH, Liu S, Zhang G, Zhou CQ, Zhu HX, Zhou XB, Quan LP, Bai JF, Xu NZ (2005) Knockdown of c-Myc expression by RNAi inhibits MCF-7 breast tumor cells growth in vitro and in vivo. Breast Cancer Res 7:R220–R228

Weinstein IB (2002) Cancer. Addiction to oncogenes-the Achilles heal of cancer. Science 297:63–64

Weiss B, Shannon K (2003) Mouse cancer models as a platform for performing preclinical therapeutic trials. Curr Opin Genet Dev 13:84–89

Weisz B, Giehl K, Gana-Weisz M, Egozi Y, Ben-Baruch G, Marciano D, Gierschik P, Kloog Y (1999) A new functional Ras antagonist inhibits human pancreatic tumor growth in nude mice. Oncogene 18:2579–2588

Wickstrom E, Bacon TA, Wickstrom EL (1992) Down-regulation of c-MYC antigen expression in lymphocytes of Emu-c-myc transgenic mice treated with anti-c-myc DNA methylphosphonates. Cancer Res 52:6741–6745

Wickstrom E, Bacon TA, Wickstrom EL, Werking CM, Palmiter RD, Brinster RL, Sandgren EP (1991) Antisense oligodeoxynucleoside methylphosphonate inhibition of mouse c-myc p65 protein expression in E mu-c-myc transgenic mice. Nucleic Acids Symp Ser:151–154

Wickstrom EL, Bacon TA, Gonzalez A, Freeman DL, Lyman GH, Wickstrom E (1988) Human promyelocytic leukemia HL-60 cell proliferation and c-myc protein expression are inhibited by an antisense pentadecadeoxynucleotide targeted against c-myc mRNA. Proc Natl Acad Sci USA 85:1028–1032

Wickstrom EL, Bacon TA, Gonzalez A, Lyman GH, Wickstrom E (1989) Anti-c-myc DNA increases differentiation and decreases colony formation by HL-60 cells. In Vitro Cell Dev Biol 25:297–302

Wong AK, Chin L (2000) An inducible melanoma model implicates a role for RAS in tumor maintenance and angiogenesis. Cancer Metastasis Rev 19:121–129

Xu Y, Shi J, Yamamoto N, Moss JA, Vogt PK, Janda KD (2006) A credit-card library approach for disrupting protein-protein interactions. Bioorg Med Chem 14:2660–2673

Yarden Y, Sliwkowski MX (2001) Untangling the ErbB signalling network. Nat Rev Mol Cell Biol 2:127–137

Yu D, Dews M, Park A, Tobias JW, Thomas-Tikhonenko A (2005) Inactivation of Myc in murine two-hit B lymphomas causes dormancy with elevated levels of interleukin 10 receptor and CD20: implications for adjuvant therapies. Cancer Res 65:5454–5461

Tyrosine Kinase Inhibitors and Cancer Therapy

Srinivasan Madhusudan and Trivadi S. Ganesan

Recent Results in Cancer Research, Vol. 172
© Springer-Verlag Berlin Heidelberg 2007

3.1 Introduction

Cancer is the second leading cause of death in the western world and is an increasing health problem in the developing world. Overall survival of patients with advanced cancer is poor. Until recently, surgery, chemotherapy, radiotherapy and endocrine therapy have been the mainstay in the treatment of cancer patients. This has improved outcomes in certain tumour types but treatment-related toxicity and emergence of drug resistance have been the major cause of morbidity and mortality. This need to improve outcomes has stimulated intense scientific research in recent years. Several novel drug targets have been identified. Amongst these, tyrosine kinases have emerged as the new promising anti-cancer drug target. Inhibitors of BCR-ABL, EGFR and VEGFR tyrosine kinases have now been licenced for use in cancers. In this chapter, we will discuss how this has been achieved in recent years.

3.2 Human Protein Tyrosine Kinases

Human genome sequence analysis has identified at least 90 tyrosine kinase genes [58 receptor tyrosine kinases (RTKs) and 32 non-receptor tyrosine kinases (NRTKs)] (Manning et al. 2002; Krupa and Srinivasan 2002). Based on their extracellular and non-catalytic domain sequences, both the RTKs and NRTKs have been further grouped into 20 and 10 subfamilies, respectively (Tables 3.1 and 3.2) (Robinson et al. 2000; Barbieri et al. 2004). Protein tyrosine kinases are found only in metazoans and the signalling pathways they initiate are complex (Schlessinger 2000; Hunter 2000; Yarden and Sliwkowski 2001). Receptor tyrosine kinases (RTKs) contain an amino-terminal extracellular ligand binding domain (usually glycosylated), a hydrophobic transmembrane helix and a cytoplasmic domain, which contains a conserved protein tyrosine kinase core and additional regulatory sequences (that contain crucial carboxy-terminal tyrosine residues and receptor regulatory motifs). Ligand binding (EGF or others) to the extracellular domain results in receptor dimerisation/oligomerisation, leading to activation of cytoplasmic tyrosine kinase activity and phosphorylation of tyrosine residues. Autophosphorylated tyrosine residues serve as a platform for the recognition and recruitment of a specific set of signal-transducing proteins [such as proteins containing Src homology 2 (SH2) and phosphotyrosine binding (PTB) domains] that modulate diverse cell signalling responses (Yarden and Sliwkowski 2001; Normanno et al. 2006; Zaczek et al. 2005; Fischer et al. 2003; Sakurada et al. 2006). Non-receptor tyrosine kinases (NRTKs) have a common conserved catalytic domain (similar to RTKs) with a modular amino-terminal, which has different adapter protein motifs (Neet and Hunter 1996). Tyrosine kinases play

Table 3.1 Receptor tyrosine kinases and cancer

Tyrosine Kinase		Cancer associations
EGFR family	EGFR (HER-1)	Breast, ovary, lung, glioblastoma multiforme and others
	ERBB2 (HER-2)	Breast, ovary, stomach, lung, colon and others
	ERBB3 (HER-3)	Breast
	ERBB4 (HER-4)	Breast, granulosa cell tumours
InsulinR family	IGF-1R	Cervix, kidney (clear cell), sarcomas and others
	IRR, INSR	–
PDGFR family	PDGFR-α	Glioma, glioblastoma, ovary
	PDGFR-β	Chronic myelomonocytic leukaemia (CMML), glioma
	CSF-1R	CMML, malignant histiocytosis, glioma, endometrium
	KIT/SCFR	GIST, AML, myelodysplasia, mastocytosis, seminoma, lung
	FLK2/FLT3	Acute myeloid leukaemia (AML)
VEGFR family	VEGFR1	Tumour angiogenesis
	VEBFR2	Tumour angiogenesis
	VEGFR3	tumour angiogenesis, Kaposi sarcoma, haemangiosarcoma
FGFR family	FGFR-1	AML, lymphoma, several solid tumours
	FGFR-2	Stomach, breast, prostate
	FGFR-3	Multiple myeloma
	FGFR-4	–
KLG/CCK family (CCK4)		–
NGFR family	TRKA	Papillary thyroid cancer, neuroblastoma
	TRKB	–
	TRKC	Congenital fibrosarcoma, acute myeloid leukaemia
HGFR family	MET	Papillary thyroid, rhabdomyosarcoma, liver, kidney
	RON	Colon, liver
EPHR family	EPHA2	Melanoma
	EPHA1, 3, 4, 5, 6, 7, 8	–
	EPHB2	Stomach, oesophagus, colon
	EPHB4	Breast
	EPHB1, 3, 5&6	–
AXL family	AXL	AML
	MER, TYRO3	–
TIE family	TIE	Stomach, capillary haemagioblastoma
	TEK	Tumour angiogenesis
RYK family (RYK)		Ovarian cancer
DDR family (DDR1&DDR2)		Breast, ovarian cancer
RET family (RET)		Thyroid (papillary and medullary),multiple endocrine neoplasia
ROS family (ROS)		Glioblastoma, astrocytoma
LTK family	ALK	Non-Hodgkin lymphoma
	LTK	–
ROR family (ROR1&ROR2)		–
MUSK family (MUSK)		–
LMR family (AATYK, AATYK 2&3)		–
RTK106		–

Table 3.2 Non-receptor tyrosine kinases and cancer

Tyrosine Kinase		Cancer associations
ABL family	ABL1	Chronic myeloid leukaemia (CML), AML, ALL, CMML
	ARG	AML
FRK family	BRK	Breast
	FRK	–
	SRMS	–
JAK family	JAK1	Leukaemias
	JAK2	AML, ALL, T- cell childhood ALL, atypical CML
	JAK3	Leukaemia, B-cell malignancies
	JAK4	–
SRC-A family	FGR	AML, CLL, EBV associated lymphoma
	FYN	–
	SRC	Colon, breast, pancreas, neuroblastoma
	YES1	Colon, melanoma
SRC-B family	BLK	–
	HCK	–
	LCK	T cell ALL, CLL
	LYN	–
SYK family	SYK	Breast
	ZAP70	–
FAK family	FAK	Adhesion, invasion and metastasis of several tumours
	PYK2	Adhesion, invasion and metastasis of several tumours
ACK family	ACK1	–
	TNK1	–
CSK family	CSK	–
	MATK	–
FES family	FER	–
	FES	–
TEC family	BMX	–
	BTK	–
	ITK	–
	TEC	–
	TXK	–

a critical role in the regulation of fundamental cellular processes including cell development, differentiation, proliferation, survival, growth, apoptosis, cell shape, adhesion, migration, cell cycle control, T-cell and B-cell activation, angiogenesis, responses to extracellular stimuli, neuro-transmitter signalling, platelet activation, transcription and glucose uptake (Hunter 1998). Aberrant tyrosine kinase signalling has been implicated in several human disorders including developmental anomalies, immunodeficiency state, non-insulin-dependent diabetes mellitus (NIDDM), atherosclerosis, psoriasis, renal disease, neurological disorders, leukaemia and solid tumours (Hunter 1998; Weiner and Zagzag 2000; Ben-Bassat 2001; Lee et al. 2002; Indo 2002).

3.3 Role of Tyrosine Kinases in Human Cancer

Aberrant tyrosine kinase signalling plays a critical role in oncogenic transformation and this may be achieved in several ways (Blume-Jensen and Hunter 2001). Gene amplification and/or overexpression of tyrosine kinases may lead to enhanced kinase activity that may quantitatively and qualitatively alter downstream signalling (e.g. EGFR and HER-2 over-expression is commonly seen in several cancers). Chromosomal translocations can result in fusion proteins with constitutively active kinase activity (e.g. p210 Bcr-Abl fusion protein is commonly seen in chronic myeloid leukaemia). Gain-of-function mutations or deletion in PTKs within the kinase domain or extracellular domain result in constitutively active tyrosine kinase (e.g. EGFRvIII mutant that lacks amino acids 6–273 of the extracellular domain is constitutively active and is observed in solid tumours). Over-expression of ligands may result in excessive receptor activation (e.g. TGF-α is over-expressed in glioblastoma and head and neck cancer (Grandis et al. 1998)). Finally, retroviral transduction of a proto-oncogene corresponding to a PTK concomitant with deregulating structural changes is a frequent mechanism by which oncogenic transformation occurs in animals (rodents and chicken) (Blume-Jensen and Hunter 2001). Whether a similar mechanism exists in human cancer remains to be established.

There is convincing evidence to suggest that protein tyrosine kinases are associated with human cancer pathogenesis. This association is summarised in Table 3.1. Clinical studies also suggest that over-expression and/or dys-regulation of tyrosine kinase activity may be of prognostic and/or of predictive significance in patients. Prognostic factors are measurements available at the time of diagnosis or surgery which are associated with recurrence, death or other clinical outcomes and determine how patients will fare irrespective of treatment. Predictive factors are measures which help determine which patients do well with particular types of treatment. Though only a few new prognostic or predictive factors have been validated in the past 10 years in cancer diagnosis, several recent clinical studies have reported the prognostic or predictive value of tyrosine kinases in cancer diagnosis. Discussion of individual studies is beyond the scope of this chapter and a brief overview will be provided here.

EGFR (HER-1) over-expression is associated with a poor prognosis in several human tumours such as ovarian, head and neck, oesophageal, cervical, bladder, breast, colorectal, gastric and endometrial cancer (Nicholson et al. 2001). HER-2 over-expression is associated with poorer outcome in patients with breast (Tandon et al. 1989), ovary (Meden and Kuhn 1997), prostate (Sadasivan et al. 1993), lung (Selvaggi et al. 2002) and bone cancer (Zhou et al. 2003). VEGF is a central growth factor which drives tumour angiogenesis and is an important prognostic marker in solid tumours (Fox et al. 2001). VEGFR-1 expression is associated with poor prognosis in breast carcinoma (Meunier-Carpentier et al. 2005). VEGFR 3 expression in lung cancer (Arinaga et al. 2003) and colorectal carcinoma (Parr and Jiang 2003) may be associated with poor prognosis. The expression of IGF-1R along with IGF-1 and IGF-2 may have prognostic value in a subset of colorectal cancer patients (Peters et al. 2003). BCR-ABL tyrosine kinase

is of prognostic value in chronic myeloid and acute lymphoblastic leukaemia (ALL) (Gleissner et al. 2002). Mutation in C-KIT tyrosine kinase is associated with inferior survival in patients with gastrointestinal stromal tumours (Taniguchi et al. 1999) and adversely affects relapse rate in acute myeloid leukaemia (Care et al. 2003). In small-cell lung cancer C-KIT expression was linked to poor survival (Naeem et al. 2002). In acute myeloid leukaemia, FLT 3 mutation predicts higher relapse rate and a shorter event-free survival (Schnittger et al. 2002). Trk tyrosine kinase is an important marker for neuroblastoma (NB). TrkA is present in NB with favourable biological features and highly correlated with patient survival, whereas TrkB is mainly expressed on unfavourable, aggressive NB with MYCN-amplification (Eggert et al. 2000). HGFR (c-Met) over-expression is associated with disease progression, recurrence, and inferior survival in early-stage invasive cervical cancer (Baykal et al. 2003), correlates with poor prognosis in synovial sarcoma (Oda et al. 2000) and predicts a significantly shorter 5-year survival in hepatocellular carcinoma (Ueki et al. 1997). Axl tyrosine kinase expression was associated with poor outcome in acute myeloid leukaemia (Rochlitz et al. 1999). Tie-1 kinase expression inversely correlates with survival in gastric cancer (Lin et al. 1999) and in early chronic-phase chronic myeloid leukaemia (Verstovsek et al. 2002). Soluble Tie-2 receptor levels independently predict loco-regional recurrence in head and neck squamous cell carcinoma (Homer et al. 2002). ALK protein expression is an independent predictor of survival and serves as a useful biologic marker of a specific disease entity within the spectrum of anaplastic large-cell lymphoma (ALCL) (Gascoyne et al. 1999). Src tyrosine kinase is an independent indicator of poor clinical prognosis in all stages of human colon carcinoma (Aligayer et al. 2002). FAK over-expression is correlated with tumour invasiveness and lymph node metastasis in oesophageal squamous cell carcinoma (Miyazaki et al. 2003) and reduced expression of the Syk gene is correlated with poor prognosis in breast cancer (Toyama et al. 2003).

3.4 Tyrosine Kinase Inhibitors for Cancer Therapy

Given the essential role played by tyrosine kinase signalling pathway in cancer, several approaches to target this pathway have been developed in recent years (Table 3.3) (Krause and Van Etten 2005; Baselga and Cortes 2005; Rhee and Hoff 2005; Speake et al. 2005; Ranson 2004; Hynes and Lane 2005; Pal and Pegram 2005; Tibes et al. 2005; Madhusudan and Ganesan 2004). The catalytic domain (Mg-ATP complex binding site) of tyrosine kinases is the most important target for drug design. High-throughput screening, combinatorial chemistry, in silico cloning, structure-based drug design and computational chemistry approaches have been used to identify potent tyrosine kinase inhibitors. Most small molecules in clinical development bind in the vicinity of the ATP-binding site of their target kinases. Such ATP mimics are competitive inhibitors of the substrate-binding sites within the catalytic domain (Stamos et al. 2002; Laird and Cherrington 2003; Fry 2003) and compete with endogenous ATP for binding. Recombinant antibody technology has allowed the design, selection and production of humanised/human antibodies, human-mouse chimeric or bispecific antibodies against tyrosine kinase receptors (Mendelsohn 2002; Farah et al. 1998; Hudson 1999).

Small-molecule tyrosine inhibitors such as imatinib, geftinib, erlotinib, sorafenib and sunitnib are now licenced for use in human cancer. In addition, several other small-molecule inhibitors are in advanced stage of clinical development. Monoclonal antibodies such as Trastuzumab, Bevacizumab and Cetuximab have also been licenced for cancer therapy. We will focus on these drugs in this chapter and review how this has been achieved in recent years.

3.5 Small-Molecule Tyrosine Kinase Inhibitors

3.5.1 Imatinib

Imatinib (STI571, Gleevec; Novartis Pharmaceuticals, East Hanover, NJ, USA) is a potent orally available small-molecule inhibitor of c-Abl, PDGFR-β and c-Kit tyrosine kinases (Druker et al. 1996; Buchdunger et al. 1996; Manley et al. 2002). It has been extensively investigated in chronic myelogenous leukaemia (CML), where reciprocal translocation between the long arms of chromosomes 9 and 22 results in an abnormally short chromosome 22 called the Philadelphia chromosome (Ph). The Ph chromosome links the BCR gene of chromosome 22 with the ABL gene of chromosome 9 and the Bcr-Abl gene product (Bcr-Abl fusion protein) is a constitutively activated tyrosine kinase which is critical role in the pathogenesis of CML (Sawyers 1999). Imatinib inhibits autophosphorylation of Bcr-Abl and suppresses proliferation and tumour formation of Bcr-Abl-expressing myeloid cells (Druker et al. 1996). With oral administration of imatinib, dose-dependent inhibition (Druker et al. 1996) and

Table 3.3 Tyrosine kinase inhibitors licenced for clinical use

Inhibitor	Mode of action	Clinical use
Imatinib	BCR-ABL, c-KIT, PDGFR	CML, GIST
Erlotinib	Inhibitor of EGFR	Metastatic NSCLC, pancreatic cancer
Gefitinib	Inhibitor of EGFR	NSCLC
Sorafanib	Inhibitor of Raf, VEGFR2, VEGFR 3, PDGFR, FLT3, c-KIT	Metatstatic renal cell cancer
Sunitinib	Inhibitor of VEGFR1, VEGFR 2, FLT 3, c-KIT, PDGFR	Metastatic renal cell cancer
Trastuzumab	Monoclonal antibody against HER2	Breast cancer
Cetuximab	Monoclonal antibody against EGFR	Metastatic colorectal cancer
Bevacizumab	Monoclonal antibody against VEGF	Metastatic colorectal cancer

eradication (le Coutre et al. 1999) of Bcr-Abl containing tumours were seen in mice. Phase I dose escalation studies of imatinib were performed in patients with chronic-phase CML who had failed prior interferon therapy. Myelosuppression was the common side effect and there were no other major adverse events. At doses of ≥300 mg, 53/54 patients achieved complete sustained haematologic response (typically within 3 weeks of therapy). A major cytogenetic remission was seen in 31% and complete cytogenetic response was seen in 13% of patients (Druker et al. 2001a). In subsequent phase I studies in CML patients with myeloid or lymphoid blast crisis and relapsed/refractory Ph chromosome-positive ALL, imatinib produced significant but less durable responses (Druker et al. 2001b). An international cooperative group conducted phase II studies in over 1,000 patients with chronic-phase (400 mg of STI571 daily), accelerated-phase (600 mg daily) or blast crisis (600 mg daily) CML. Impressive complete haematological/cytogenetic responses were seen (91%/36%, 53%/17% and 26%/7%, respectively) (Druker 2002). In May 2001, on the basis of phase II data, the US Food and Drug Administration approved imatinib for the treatment of Ph-positive CML in blast crisis, accelerated phase or chronic phase after failure of interferon-α therapy (Johnson et al. 2003). It has now been approved for first-line treatment of CML.

Imatinib-resistant BCR-ABL mutations in leukaemic subclones are an important cause for relapse in previously imatinib-treated patients. Dasatinib, a small-molecule BCR-ABL inhibitor, effectively targets imatinib-resistant BCR-ABL mutations, in CML or Ph-positive ALL (Kantarjian et al. 2006). In a recent phase I study in patients with CML or with Ph-positive ALL who were either resistant or intolerant to imanitib, dasatinib therapy induced impressive haematologic, cytogenetic and clinical response. Complete haematologic response was achieved in 37 of 40 patients with chronic-phase CML, and major haematologic responses were reported in 31 of 44 patients with accelerated-phase CML, CML with blast crisis, or Ph-positive ALL. Myelosuppression was commonly seen in patients but not dose limiting in this study (Talpaz et al. 2006).

Mutations in c-KIT proto-oncogene result in a constitutively activated tyrosine kinase. This activating mutation is frequently seen in gastrointestinal stromal tumours (GISTs) (Demetri 2002; Rubin et al. 2001). Imatinib is also a potent inhibitor of c-KIT. Imatinib inhibited proliferation and induced apoptosis of GIST cells in pre-clinical studies(Tuveson et al. 2001). In an open-label, randomised, multi-centre trial of imatinib in GIST, significant anti-cancer activity was demonstrated (53.7% partial response and 27.9% stable disease). Gastrointestinal or intra-abdominal haemorrhage was seen in about 5% of patients, possibly related to rapid tumour shrinkage. In February 2001, the US Food and Drug Administration approved imatinib (400 mg or 600 mg daily) for the treatment of malignant metastatic and/or unresectable GISTs based on the updated analysis of the above study (Dagher et al. 2002).

Imatinib is also a potent inhibitor of PDGFR tyrosine kinase. PDGFR is involved in the pathogenesis of chronic myelomonocytic leukaemia and dermatofibrosarcoma protruberens. Clinical studies suggest that imatinib may have significant therapeutic effect in these disorders (Gunby et al. 2003; Cortes et al. 2003; Sawyers 2002). A newly described tyrosine kinase created by fusion of PGDFRA and FIP1L1 gene appears to be causative in some patients with hypereosinophilic syndrome and dramatic responses have been seen in patients treated with imatinib (Gleich et al. 2002; Cools et al. 2003). Similar gene rearrangement has recently been described in mast cell disease and eosinophilia where patients have achieved responses to imatinib (Pardanani et al. 2003).

3.5.2 Gefitinib

Gefitinib (ZD1839, Iressa; AstraZeneca Pharmaceuticals LP, Wilmington, DE, USA) is a orally available potent inhibitor of EGFR tyrosine kinase (Grunwald and Hidalgo 2003b). Several pre-clinical studies confirmed the anti-cancer activity of this EGFR inhibitor (Sirotnak 2003). Gefitinib inhibits tumour angiogenesis (Hirata

3 Tyrosine Kinase Inhibitors and Cancer Therapy

et al. 2002), inhibits metastasis (Wells 2000) and promotes apoptosis (Ciardiello et al. 2000). Gefitinib inhibits tumour growth in xenografts studies either alone or in combination with chemotherapy (Ciardiello et al. 2000; Penne et al. 2005; Sirotnak et al. 2000). Gefitinib was well tolerated in phase I human studies. Acneiform skin rash and gastrointestinal toxicity were the most common side effects (Ranson et al. 2002; Negoro et al. 2001; Baselga et al. 2000b; Goss et al. 2001). Pharmacodynamic studies on serial skin biopsies showed that at a dose of >100 mg/day significant inhibition of EGFR activation was achieved (Albanell et al. 2002). In patients with non-small-cell lung cancer who participated in these early phase I studies, a significant number of objective responses were seen (Johnson 2003). A combination of chemotherapy and gefitinib was safe and well tolerated (Grunwald and Hidalgo 2003b). Two major phase II trials in non-small-cell lung cancer have been completed. IDEAL 1 (Iressa dose evaluation in advanced lung cancer) was conducted in Europe and Japan in patients whose lung cancer was resistant to platinum-based chemotherapy and who had previously received one or two lines of chemotherapy (Fukuoka et al. 2002). IDEAL 2 was conducted in the United States in patients with lung cancer resistant to platinum and docetaxel chemotherapy who had received two or more lines of treatment (Kris et al. 2002). An overall response (OR) of 19% and 11% was seen in IDEAL 1 and 2 studies, respectively. In addition, a significant proportion of patients achieved disease stabilisation (SD) (34% in IDEAL 1 and 29% in IDEAL 2). In May 2003, gefitinib was approved for the treatment of patients with advanced non-small-cell lung cancer (NSCLC) previously treated with chemotherapy based on the above phase II studies (Cohen et al. 2004, 2003).

In chemotherapy-naive patients with stage IIIB/IV NSCLC, two large randomised phase III trials (INTACT 1 and 2) comparing chemotherapy alone versus chemotherapy and gefitinib were reported (Giaccone et al. 2004; Herbst et al. 2004). Both INTACT 1 (Giaccone et al. 2004) and INTACT 2 (Herbst et al. 2004) trials failed to show any improvements in survival or response rates in patients receiving gefitinib

in addition to chemotherapy. Several reasons for the negative results have been proposed. Insufficient target modulation due to suboptimal dosing, antagonism between chemotherapy and gefitinib, targeting the same population of cancer cells (chemotherapy thereby masking the effects of gefitinib), inadequate scheduling of treatment or dilution of benefit obtained by a small proportion of patients by a large proportion of unresponsive patients are some of the plausible explanations (Dancey and Sausville 2003). The Iressa Survival Evaluation in advanced lung cancer (ISEL) trial was conducted in previously treated refractory NSCLC to assess best supportive care with gefitinib or placebo. A significantly higher response rate was seen in the gefitinib group but this did not translate into better overall survival (Thatcher et al. 2005). Following the reporting of negative results from the ISEL and INTACT trials, several other phase III trials were prematurely closed (Thatcher et al. 2005). Subsequently gefitinib has been licenced for restricted use for patients who were already receiving and benefiting from gefitinib (Thatcher et al. 2005).

Asian patients, patients with adenocarcinomas, women and 'never smokers' have been found to be particularly responsive to gefitinib. Development of skin rash and good performance may predict response to gefitinib (Dudek et al. 2006; Mohamed et al. 2005). EGFR gene sequencing analysis in this subset of patients has shown gain-of-function somatic mutations around the ATP-binding pocket of the kinase domain of EGFR (Lynch et al. 2004; Pao et al. 2004). This has been confirmed by several studies and predicts response to geftinib. A recent study in which patients were selected to receive geftinib only if they had mutations had a response rate of 75% (Inoue et al. 2006). In addition, DNA microarray analysis can be a useful technique to identify gene expression signature which may predict response to geftinib (Kakiuchi et al. 2004).

3.5.3 Erlotinib

Erlotinib (OSI-774, Tarceva ; Genetech, Inc, South San Francisco, CA, USA) is a potent and highly selective orally available inhibitor of EGFR tyrosine kinase (Moyer et al. 1997). Tumour xenografts studies of head and neck cancer (Pollack et al. 1999), non-small-cell lung cancer (Akita and Sliwkowski 2003) and pancreatic cancer (Ng et al. 2002) showed a direct correlation between EGFR inhibition and tumour growth suppression. Pre-clinical studies also suggest that cells expressing EGFRvIII mutant may be more susceptible to erlotinib (Akita and Sliwkowski 2003). Enhancement of anti-tumour activity was also seen when erlotinib was combined with cytotoxic agents (Pollack et al. 1999), tamoxifen or HER-2 inhibitors in pre-clinical studies (Akita and Sliwkowski 2003; Smith 2005).

In human phase I studies, acneiform skin rash and diarrhoea were the dose-limiting toxicities. A dose of 150 mg/day was the maximum tolerated dose and recommended for phase II studies. Tumour responses were seen in patients with renal, NSCLC, colon, head and neck cancer (Herbst 2003; Hidalgo et al. 2001). Pharmacodynamic studies in serial skin biopsies confirmed inhibition of EGFR activation (Grunwald and Hidalgo 2003a). In phase I studies in combination with chemotherapy (temazolamide, docetaxel, paclitaxel + carboplatin or gemcitabine + cisplatin), the dose-limiting toxicities were neutropoenia, acneiform rash and diarrhoea. Tumour responses were seen in patients with NSCLC, ovarian cancer and head and neck cancer in phase II trials (Herbst 2003).

The National Cancer Institute of Canada (NCIC) conducted a randomised, placebo-controlled, double-blind trial (clinical trial BR.21) to evaluate the role of erlotinib in non-small-cell lung cancer after the failure of first-line or second-line chemotherapy. The response rate was 8.9% in the erlotinib group and less than 1% in the placebo group with a the median duration of response of 7.9 months in the erlotinib group compared to 3.7 months in the placebo group. There was a significant increase in overall survival in patients receiving erlotinib (6.7 months compared to 4.7 months in the placebo group) (Shepherd et al. 2005). Histologic features of adenocarcinoma, female sex, no history of smoking, and Asian ancestry predicted response to erlotinib in this trial.

The NCIC trial is the first randomised study of a tyrosine kinase inhibitor to demonstrate clinical benefit in terms of both symptom relief and prolongation of survival in non-small-cell lung cancer (Doroshow 2005). Erlotinib was approved for use in non-small-cell lung cancer after failure of at least one prior chemotherapy regimen (Johnson et al. 2005; Cohen et al. 2005). Response to erlotinib was significantly associated with EGFR positivity on immunohistochemical analysis and increased numbers of copies of the EGFR gene in the BR.21 trial. In addition, the presence of an EGFR mutation may increase responsiveness to the agent, but it is not indicative of a survival benefit (Tsao et al. 2005). Two large phase III randomised, placebo-controlled trials were conducted in lung cancer, comparing chemotherapy alone or in combination with erlotinib. In the TRIBUTE trial, erlotinib in combination with carboplatin and paclitaxel did not confer a survival advantage over carboplatin and paclitaxel alone (Herbst et al. 2005). In the TALENT trial, erlotinib was combined with cisplatin and gemcirabine but did not confer any survival advantage (Blackhall et al. 2006).

3.5.4 Sorafenib

Sorafenib (BAY 43-9006, Nexavar: Bayer and Onyx Pharmaceuticals, USA) is a novel oral multi-kinase inhibitor of serine/threonine and receptor tyrosine kinases including Raf, VEGFR-2, VEGFR-3, PDGFR-β, FLT-3 and c-kit (Rini 2006; Strumberg 2005). It inhibits angiogenesis and Raf-mediated cell proliferation. In phase I studies in patients with a variety of advanced, refractory solid tumours, including renal cell carcinoma, colorectal cancer and hepatocellular carcinoma, sorafenib was well tolerated and was found to have clinical activity. Diarrhoea, fatigue and skin toxicity were the dose-limiting toxicities (Strumberg et al. 2005; Awada et al. 2005; Moore et al. 2005). In a phase II randomised study in advanced renal cell carcinoma, sorafenib produced significant anti-tumour responses and a significant prolongation of median progression-free survival (Ratain et al. 2006). In recently presented phase III studies, sorafenib

3 Tyrosine Kinase Inhibitors and Cancer Therapy

significantly prolonged progression-free survival over placebo in renal cell cancer patients (Escudier et al. 2005). Sorafenib was approved for clinical use in advanced renal cell carcinoma in December 2005. Sorafenib in combination with chemotherapy has also been investigated and has been found to be safe and well tolerated (Richly et al. 2006; Kupsch et al. 2005).

3.5.5 Sunitinib

Sunitinib (SU11248; SUTENT; Pfizer Inc, New York, NY) is a novel oral multi-targeted tyrosine kinase inhibitor. Sunitinib is a potent inhibitor of VEGFR-1, VEGFR-2, fetal liver tyrosine kinase receptor 3 (FLT3), KIT [stem-cell factor (SCF) receptor] and PDGFR. Pre-clinical data suggest that Sunitinib has anti-angiogenic and anti-proliferative effects. In phase I studies, Sunitinib was well tolerated and showed anti-tumour activity in patients with metastatic renal cell carcinoma (Faivre et al. 2006). In a phase II study in metastatic renal cell cancer, a significant proportion of patients achieved partial responses or stable disease with a median time to progression of about 8.7 months (Motzer et al. 2006). Sunitinib has also shown anti-cancer activity in Gleevec-resistant GIST or patients unable to tolerate Gleevec. Sunitinib significantly prolongs time to disease progression in the patient group (Prenen et al. 2006). Sunitinib received FDA approval for clinical use in renal cancer and GIST recently.

3.6 Other Small-Molecule Inhibitors in Development

3.6.1 Lapatinib

Lapatinib (GW572016; GlaxoSmithklineBeecham, USA) is a potent inhibitor of EGFR and HER2. It is orally bio-available. Phase I studies show that lapatinib is safe and well tolerated. Anti-tumour responses were seen in a proportion of patients, particularly in breast

cancer that overexpresses EGFR and HER2 (Burris et al. 2005; Nelson and Dolder 2006). Diarrhoea, skin rash, nausea and fatigue are the commonly reported side effects. The biological effect was confirmed in tumour tissue (Spector et al. 2005). A phase I trial in combination with trastuzumab in metastatic breast cancer reported partial responses in 22% and stable disease in 37% of patients (Storniolo et al. 2005). Based on these studies several phase II and phase III studies have been initiated in metastatic breast cancer. Preliminary analyses suggest that lapatinib has significant anti-cancer activity (Nelson and Dolder 2006)

3.6.2 Vatalanib

Vatalanib (PTK787/ZK222584; Schering Health Care, USA) is an orally bio-available inhibitor of VEGFR-1, VEGR-1 and PDGF-R (Wood et al. 2000). Phase I studies have confirmed its safety and bio-availability (Thomas et al. 2005). Preliminary results from a large phase III study in colorectal cancer in combination with FOLFOX4 suggest that in a subset of patients with high lactate dehydrogenase, significant improvement in progression-free survival was seen (Tyagi 2005). Phase III studies in combination with FOLFORI are ongoing.

3.6.3 Zactima

Zactima (ZD6474; AstraZeneca, USA) is an orally available small-molecule inhibitor of VEGFR-2, VEGFR-3 and epidermal growth factor receptor with potent anti-tumour activity in pre-clinical studies (Ryan and Wedge 2005; Heymach 2005). In phase I studies, diarrhoea, skin rash, nausea, hypertension and fatigue were the commonly reported side effects. Tumour responses were seen in lung cancer. A series of clinical trials have now been initiated in NSCLC. These studies include investigation of ZD6474 vs Geftinib, combination of ZD6474 and docetaxel, ZD6474 in combination with carboplatin and taxol (Ryan and Wedge 2005).

3.7 Monoclonal Antibodies Targeting Tyrosine Kinase Receptors and Their Ligands

3.7.1 Trastuzumab

Trastuzumab (Herceptin; Genetech Inc, South San Francisco, CA, USA) is a humanised monoclonal antibody which binds with high affinity to the extracellular domain of HER-2. HER-2 is expressed in a wide variety of human cancers including breast, ovarian, lung and prostate cancer. Overexpression of HER-2 has predictive and prognostic value in patients (Agus et al. 2000b; Berchuck et al. 1990; Tsai et al. 1993; Pegram et al. 1998a; Slamon et al. 1987; Slamon et al. 1989; Press et al. 1997). Pre-clinical studies of trastuzumab confirmed its antiproliferative activity either alone or in combination with chemotherapeutic agents (Carter et al. 1992; Baselga et al. 1998; Pegram et al. 2000). In phase I trials either alone or in combination with chemotherapy trastuzumab was found to be safe and showed a prolonged half-life of 8.3 days (Harries and Smith 2002). Phase II studies in heavily pre-treated breast cancer patients showed that trastuzumab as monotherapy or in combination with chemotherapy was active (Baselga et al. 1996; Pegram et al. 1998b; Cobleigh et al. 1999). Patients who overexpressed HER-2 were more likely to respond to therapy. Trastuzumab monotherapy as a first-line treatment produced significant disease responses (Vogel et al. 2002). A pivotal phase III study confirmed the benefit of trastuzumab in combination with chemotherapy in metastatic breast cancer patients (Slamon et al. 2001). In 1998, the US Food and Drug Administration approved trastuzumab for metastatic breast cancer. Two large phase III randomised studies in operable breast cancer were published in 2005. Adjuvant trastuzumab significantly improved disease-free survival among women with HER2-positive breast cancer in these studies (Romond et al. 2005; Piccart-Gebhart et al. 2005; Hortobagyi 2005). Trastuzumab has now been approved for adjuvant therapy in breast cancer.

Trastuzumab has also been investigated in other tumour types. In a recently published large phase II study in ovarian cancer or primary peritoneal carcinoma, modest overall response rate of 7.3% (including one complete and two partial responses) was seen (Bookman et al. 2003). Ongoing phase II trials show that trastuzumab in combination with standard chemotherapy in advanced NSCLC is safe and efficacious in a subset of HER-2-positive (detected by fluorescent in situ hybridisation) tumours. Whether trastuzumab will show a clear benefit for patients with NSCLC, either alone or in combination with established chemotherapy, remains to be proven in phase III testing (Azzoli et al. 2002). Docetaxel/estramustine/trastuzumab appears to be a safe combination when used in the treatment of metastatic androgen independent prostate carcinoma (Small et al. 2001). Trastuzumab is now being investigated in combination with several other chemotherapeutic agents (vinorelbine, epirubicin, capecitabine and hormone therapy). Early reports are promising. Adjuvant trastuzumab trials have also been initiated and results should be available in a few years' time (Harries and Smith 2002). Targeted pro-drug treatment of HER-2-positive breast tumor cells with trastuzumab and paclitaxel linked by A-Z-CINN Linker followed by light exposure adjacent to the tumor in mice caused light-accelerated release of paclitaxel and enhanced anti-tumour activity (Gilbert et al. 2003). Cooperative inhibitory effect of gefitinib (Iressa) in combination with trastuzumab (Herceptin) on human breast cancer cell growth has been reported and may have future therapeutic implications (Normanno et al. 2002).

3.7.2 Cetuximab

Cetuximab (IMC-C225, Erbitux; ImClone System and Bristol-Myers Squibb, USA) is a human-murine chimeric IgG monoclonal antibody which competitively binds to the extracellular domain of EGFR (Ciardiello and Tortora 2001). It inhibits EGFR auto-phosphorylation, promotes receptor internalisation and degradation, inhibits cell cycle progression, induces apoptosis and inhibits tumour angiogenesis (Grunwald and Hidalgo 2003b). Preclinical studies confirm the anti-tumour activity of cetuximab in several xenograft models. Moreover, it also potentiates the cytotoxicity of chemotherapeutic agents and radiation (Bruns et al. 2000; Perrotte et al. 1999; Sato et al. 1983; Fan et al. 1993; Baselga et al. 1993; Harari and Huang 2001; Huang and Harari 2000).

At least three phase I studies of cetuximab either alone or in combination with chemotherapy/radiation have been reported. In all these studies the treatment was well tolerated, with skin toxicity as the most common adverse event. Transfusion reaction-like symptoms have also been reported (Grunwald and Hidalgo 2003b; Baselga et al. 2000a; Shin et al. 2001). Serial tumour biopsy studies showed robust EGFR TK inhibition in a phase I study in head and neck cancer patients (Mendelsohn et al. 1999). In eight phase II studies in various tumour types (kidney, colorectal, NSCLC, head and neck and pancreatic cancer), cetuximab was well tolerated and produced clinical responses (Grunwald and Hidalgo 2003b; Frieze and McCune 2006). In a phase II trial of cetuximab in patients with refractory colorectal cancer which expresses the epidermal growth factor receptor, cetuximab showed modest activity and was well tolerated as a single agent in patients with chemotherapy-refractory colorectal cancer (Saltz et al. 2004). In another trial comparing cetuximab monotherapy and cetuximab plus irinotecan in irinotecan-refractory metastatic colorectal cancer, a response rate of 22.9% was seen in the combination arm compared to 10.8% in the monotherapy arm. In addition, the median time to progression was significantly greater in the combination-therapy group (4.1 vs. 1.5 months) and the median survival time was 8.6 months in the combination-therapy group and 6.9 months in the monotherapy group (Cunningham et al. 2004). In February 2004, it was granted accelerated approval by the US FDA for the treatment of metastatic colorectal cancer on the basis of tumour response rates in phase II trials (Goldberg 2005). Two large phase III studies of cetuximab are ongoing. One trial is comparing cetuximab with best supportive care and best supportive care alone. Another trial is comparing cetuximab with irinotecan and irinotecan alone as second-line treatment in metastatic colorectal cancer (Frieze and McCune 2006). A recently reported phase III study in head and neck cancer patients showed significantly higher objective responses in patients treated with cetuximab and cisplatin compared to cisplatin alone. However, no difference in progression free or overall survival was seen in this study (Burtness et al. 2002). There are ongoing phase III studies in lung cancer and pancreatic cancer in combination with chemotherapy (Frieze and McCune 2006).

3.7.3 Bevacizumab

Bevacizumab (Avastin; Genentech Inc, South San Francisco, CA, USA) is a humanised anti-VEGF monoclonal antibody (also known as rhuMab VEGF or Avastin, Genentech, Inc). It binds to and neutralises VEGF-A isoforms with high affinity but does not neutralise VEGF-B or VEGF-C. Bevacizumab has a long half-life of about 17–21 days (Ferrara et al. 2004, 2005). Bevacizumab inhibits tumour growth in preclinical tumour xenograft models (Ferrara et al. 2004). Bevacizumab monotherapy was found to be safe in phase I human studies and it did not potentiate the toxicity of chemotherapy in combination regimens (Margolin et al. 2001; Gordon et al. 2001). Phase II studies were conducted in several tumour types (Cobleigh et al. 2003; Yang, et al. 2003; Yang 2004; Kabbinavar et al. 2003; Johnson et al. 2004). Bevacizumab showed evidence of anti-tumour activity in phase II studies in combination with chemotherapy in colorectal cancer (Kabbinavar et al. 2003) and non-small-cell lung cancer (Johnson et al. 2004). Bevacizumab showed single-agent activity in renal cell cancer (Yang, et al. 2003). A pivotal phase III trial of bevacizumab in combination with IFL (irinotecan, 5-FU and leucovorin) in colorectal cancer showed that median survival was increased from 15.6 months in the placebo arm to 20.3 months in the bevacizumab arm (Hurwitz et al. 2004, 2005). Preliminary analysis suggests that bevacizumab also prolongs survival in combination with FOLFOX4 chemotherapy (5-FU, leucovorin and oxaliplatin) (Ferrara and Kerbel

2005). Phase III studies of bevacizumab are ongoing in NSCLC, metastatic breast and renal cancer (Ferrara and Kerbel 2005). Although bevacizumab was well tolerated, reported side effects included thrombosis, bleeding, proteinuria, hypertension and gastrointestinal perforation. A pooled analysis of about 1,745 patients treated in randomised studies of bevacizumab has shown that thrombo-embolic events are more common in patients receiving bevacizumab in combination with chemotherapy and patients who were ≥65 years of age and had a previous history of atherosclerosis were particularly at risk of thrombo-embolic events (Zakarija and Soff 2005). It has been proposed that bevacizumab-related adverse events may reflect impaired response of normal endothelial cells to injury due to inhibition of normal VEGF response. In February 2004, bevacizumab was approved for the treatment of metastatic colorectal cancer in combination with 5-FU-based chemotherapy regimes.

Another effective way to inhibit the VEGF signaling pathway is to prevent VEGF from binding to its receptors by administering a decoy-soluble receptor. This so-called VEGF trap (Regeneron/Sanofi-Aventis) involves a fusion protein between the constant region of IgG and the extracellular domain of VEGF receptor (Holash et al. 2002). It is proposed that the binding affinity of the decoy receptor to VEGF is significantly higher than VEGF monoclonal antibody (Lau et al. 2005). Clinical trials are under way to investigate this approach in cancer. Pegaptanib sodium (Macugen; Eyetech/Pfizer) is an aptamer which recognizes the heparin binding domain of VEGF and inhibits VEGF165 and is licenced for use in macular degeneration (Ng et al. 2006).

3.8 Other Monoclonal Antibodies in Clinical Development

MDX-H210 (Medarex Inc, New Jersey, USA) is a bispecific antibody and is constructed from murine monoclonal antibody (mAb 520C9) which recognises HER-2 and the humanised murine monoclonal antibody (mAb H22) which recognises the high-affinity type I Fc receptor CD64 present on monocytes/macrophages. It induces antibody-dependent cellular cytotoxicity against HER-2-positive targets. (Lewis et al. 2001; Posey et al. 1999; James et al. 2001). 2C4 (Pertuzumab, Omnitarg; Genetech Inc, South San Francisco, CA, USA) is a monoclonal antibody which binds to a different epitope of HER2 ectodomain than trastuzumab and sterically hinders HER2 recruitment in heterodimers with other HER receptors. This results in the inhibition of signalling by HER2-based heterodimers in cells with both low and high HER2 expression (Albanell et al. 2003; Agus et al. 2000a, 2003). ABX-EGF (Abgenix, Fremont, CA, USA) is a fully humanised monoclonal antibody which binds to EGFR with high affinity, blocks ligand binding and inhibits auto-phosphorylation of the TK domain of EGFR. It inhibits the growth of human tumour xenografts (breast, epidermal, renal, pancreatic, prostate and ovarian cancers). The anti-tumour effect seems to be related to EGFR expression (no therapeutic effect seen in tumours which express less than 11,000 receptors per cell) (Lynch and Yang 2002). In a recently reported phase I study, ABX-EGF was well tolerated (skin rash was the predominant adverse event). A phase II study in kidney cancer produced disease stabilisation in 50% of patients (Grunwald and Hidalgo 2003b). EMD 72000 (Merck KgaA, Darmstadt, Germany) is a humanised monoclonal antibody which selectively binds to EGFR. Preclinical studies confirm its anti-proliferative activity (Hoffmann et al. 1997; Hambek et al. 2001). MDX-447 is a bispecific antibody (humanised Fab anti-CD64 and humanised Fab anti-EGFR). By recognising CD64 and EGFR it induces antibody-dependent cellular cytotoxicity against EGFR-positive cancer cells. Early-phase trials either alone or in combination with GM-CSF showed that it was well tolerated and produced disease stabilisations (Curnow 1997).

3.9 Toxicity and Resistance to Targeted Agents

Inhibition of EGFR pathway in the skin may be the reason for the characteristic acneiform skin rash induced by tyrosine kinase inhibitors . In addition, gastrointestinal side effects including diarrhoea, nausea and vomiting may be the result of EGFR signal transduction inhibition in the intestinal epithelial cells or may reflect the entero-hepatic circulation of the drug or its metabolite or the effect of the drug on other kinase targets in the epithelium (Dancey and Sausville 2003). Gefitinib induces pulmonary fibrosis in about 2%–4% of patients in Japan. Risk factors include male gender, history of pre-existing pulmonary fibrosis and smoking (Saijo and Nishio 2003). Although bevacizumab was well tolerated, reported side effects included thrombosis, bleeding, proteinuria, hypertension and gastrointestinal perforation. A pooled analysis of about 1,745 patients treated in randomised studies of bevacizumab has shown that thrombo-embolic events are more common in patients receiving bevacizumab in combination with chemotherapy and patients who were ≥65 years of age and had a previous history of atherosclerosis were particularly at risk of thrombo-embolic events (Zakarija and Soff 2005). It has been proposed that bevacizumab-related adverse events may reflect impaired response of normal endothelial cells to injury due to inhibition of normal VEGF response. Thrombo-embolic events have also been reported in a trial of VEGFR inhibitors in combination with cisplatin and gemcitabine (Kuenen et al. 2002; Robert et al. 2005).

Three different types of resistance have been described. The malignant phenotype may be independent of the activity of the target kinase (target-independent resistance). Over-expression or mutation of the tyrosine kinase may counteract the inhibition of tyrosine kinases (target-dependent resistance) by small-molecule inhibitors. Alterations of drug transporters or drug-metabolizing pathways may negatively affect the bio-availability of inhibitors (drug-dependent resistance) (van der Kuip et al. 2005; Ozvegy-Laczka et al. 2005; Cools et al. 2005). Studies of imatinib in chronic myeloid leukaemia provide valuable insights (Paterson et al. 2003). BCR-ABL gene amplification may be an important mechanism for resistance to imatinib in CML. Mutations in the ATP-binding pocket such that it alters the affinity of imatinib to the binding site may also account for resistance in some patients. High levels of alpha-1-glycoprotein (AGP), an extensively glycosylated plasma protein and a drug binder, have also been reported in CML. AGP- imatinib binding may render STI571 biologically unavailable and contribute to resistance. There is also a correlation between increased multi-drug resistance protein (MDR-1) expression and relapse in CML patients on STI571. Single nucleotide polymorphisms in the MDR-1 gene resulting in altered sensitivity to drugs may partly explain imatinib resistance in some patients (Paterson et al. 2003; Deininger 2005).

3.10 Conclusions

Imatinib, gefitinib, erlotinib, sorafenib and sunitnib are the small-molecule tyrosine kinase inhibitors currently licenced for use in cancer. In addition, trastuzumab, cetuximab and bevacizumab are the monoclonal antibodies targeting tyrosine kinase receptors or their ligands which are licenced for use in cancer. This unprecedented advance required huge international effort and a concerted collaboration by academia and the industry.

However, several problems remain to be addressed over the next few years to fully evaluate the potential of tyrosine kinase inhibitors. There are critical issues with regards to trial design for targeted agents (Madhusudan and Ganesan 2004). Resistance to therapy remains a significant clinical problem. The evolving era of pharmacogenomics provides a realistic possibility to individualise patient therapies. Determination of molecular signatures which predict response to targeted therapy may be achieved with genomics, proteomics and metabolomics. Finally, advances in drug discovery technology are likely to identify new targets and new drugs over the next decade.

References

Agus DB et al. (2000a) A potential role for activated HER-2 in prostate cancer. Semin Oncol 27:76–83; discussion 92–100

Agus DB et al. (2000b) HER-2/neu as a therapeutic target in non-small cell lung cancer, prostate cancer, and ovarian cancer. Semin Oncol 27:53–63; discussion 92–100

Agus DB, Gordon M, Taylor RB, Natale B, Karlan B, Mendelson D, et al. (2003) Clinical activity in a phase I trial of HER-2 targeted rhuMAb 2C4 (pertuzumab) in patients with advanced solid tumours. In: Proc ASCO (abstract 771)

Akita RW, Sliwkowski MX (2003) Preclinical studies with Erlotinib (Tarceva). Semin Oncol 30:15–24

Albanell J et al. (2002) Pharmacodynamic studies of the epidermal growth factor receptor inhibitor ZD1839 in skin from cancer patients:histopathologic and molecular consequences of receptor inhibition. J Clin Oncol 20:110–124

Albanell J et al. (2003) Mechanism of action of anti-HER2 monoclonal antibodies:scientific update on trastuzumab and 2C4. Adv Exp Med Biol 532:253–268

Aligayer H et al. (2002) Activation of Src kinase in primary colorectal carcinoma:an indicator of poor clinical prognosis. Cancer 94:344–351

Arinaga M et al. (2003) Clinical significance of vascular endothelial growth factor C and vascular endothelial growth factor receptor 3 in patients with nonsmall cell lung carcinoma. Cancer 97:457–464

Awada A et al. (2005) Phase I safety and pharmacokinetics of BAY 43-9006 administered for 21 days on/7 days off in patients with advanced, refractory solid tumours. Br J Cancer 92:1855–1861

Azzoli CG et al. (2002) Trastuzumab in the treatment of non-small cell lung cancer. Semin Oncol 29:59–65

Barbieri MA et al. (2004) Receptor tyrosine kinase signaling and trafficking–paradigms revisited. Curr Top Microbiol Immunol 286:1–20

Baselga J et al. (1993) Antitumor effects of doxorubicin in combination with anti-epidermal growth factor receptor monoclonal antibodies. J Natl Cancer Inst 85:1327–1333

Baselga J et al. (1996) Phase II study of weekly intravenous recombinant humanized anti-p185HER2 monoclonal antibody in patients with HER2/neu-overexpressing metastatic breast cancer. J Clin Oncol 14:737–744

Baselga J et al. (1998) Recombinant humanized anti-HER2 antibody (Herceptin) enhances the antitumor activity of paclitaxel and doxorubicin against HER2/neu overexpressing human breast cancer xenografts. Cancer Res 58:2825–2831

Baselga J et al. (2000a) Phase I studies of anti-epidermal growth factor receptor chimeric antibody C225 alone and in combination with cisplatin. J Clin Oncol 18:904–914

Baselga J et al. (2000b) Continuous administration of ZD1839 (Iressa), a novel oral epidermal growth factor receptor tyrosine kinase inhibitor (EGFR-TKI), in patients with five selected tumor types:evidence of activity and good tolerability [Abstract No. 686]. In Proc ASCO (Vol. 19)

Baselga J, Cortes J (2005) Epidermal growth factor receptor pathway inhibitors. Cancer Chemother Biol Response Modif 22:205–223

Baykal C et al. (2003) Overexpression of the c-Met/HGF receptor and its prognostic significance in uterine cervix carcinomas. Gynecol Oncol 88:123–129

Ben-Bassat H (2001) Biological activity of tyrosine kinase inhibitors:novel agents for psoriasis therapy. Curr Opin Investig Drugs 2:1539–1545

Berchuck A et al. (1990) Overexpression of HER-2/neu is associated with poor survival in advanced epithelial ovarian cancer. Cancer Res 50:4087–4091

Blackhall F et al. (2006) Where next for gefitinib in patients with lung cancer? Lancet Oncol 7:499–507

Blume-Jensen P, Hunter T (2001) Oncogenic kinase signalling. Nature 411:355–365

Bookman MA et al. (2003) Evaluation of monoclonal humanized anti-HER2 antibody, trastuzumab, in patients with recurrent or refractory ovarian or primary peritoneal carcinoma with overexpression of HER2:a phase II trial of the Gynecologic Oncology Group. J Clin Oncol 21:283–290

Bruns CJ et al. (2000) Epidermal growth factor receptor blockade with C225 plus gemcitabine results in regression of human pancreatic carcinoma growing orthotopically in nude mice by antiangiogenic mechanisms. Clin Cancer Res 6:1936–1948

Buchdunger E et al. (1996) Inhibition of the Abl protein-tyrosine kinase in vitro and in vivo by a 2-phenylaminopyrimidine derivative. Cancer Res 56:100–104

Burris H 3rd et al. (2005) Phase I safety, pharmacokinetics, and clinical activity study of lapatinib (GW572016), a reversible dual inhibitor of epidermal growth factor receptor tyrosine kinases, in heavily pretreated patients with metastatic carcinomas. J Clin Oncol 23:5305–5313

Burtness B, Li Y, Flood W, Mattar BI, Forastiere AA (2002) Phase III trial comparing cisplatin (C) + placebo (P) + anti-epidermal growth factor antibody (EGF-R) C225 in patients (pts) with metastatic/recurrent head and neck cancer (HNC) [Abstract No. 901]. In Proc ASCO (Vol. 21)

Care RS et al. (2003) Incidence and prognosis of c-KIT and FLT3 mutations in core binding factor (CBF) acute myeloid leukaemias. Br J Haematol 121:775–777

Carter P et al. (1992) Humanization of an anti-p185HER2 antibody for human cancer therapy. Proc Natl Acad Sci USA 89:4285–4289

Ciardiello F et al. (2000) Antitumor effect and potentiation of cytotoxic drugs activity in human cancer cells by ZD-1839 (Iressa), an epidermal growth factor receptor-selective tyrosine kinase inhibitor. Clin Cancer Res 6:2053–2063

Ciardiello F, Tortora G (2001) A novel approach in the treatment of cancer:targeting the epidermal growth factor receptor. Clin Cancer Res 7:2958–2970

Cobleigh MA et al. (1999) Multinational study of the efficacy and safety of humanized anti-HER2 monoclonal antibody in women who have HER2-overexpressing metastatic breast cancer that has progressed after chemotherapy for metastatic disease. J Clin Oncol 17:2639–2648

Cobleigh MA et al. (2003) A phase I/II dose-escalation trial of bevacizumab in previously treated metastatic breast cancer. Semin Oncol 30:117–124

Cohen MH et al. (2003) FDA drug approval summary: gefitinib (ZD1839) (Iressa) tablets. Oncologist 8:303–306

Cohen MH et al. (2004) United States Food and Drug Administration drug approval summary:gefitinib (ZD1839; Iressa) tablets. Clin Cancer Res 10:1212–1218

Cohen MH et al. (2005) FDA drug approval summary: erlotinib (Tarceva) tablets. Oncologist 10:461–466

Cools J et al. (2003) A tyrosine kinase created by fusion of the PDGFRA and FIP1L1 genes as a therapeutic target of imatinib in idiopathic hypereosinophilic syndrome. N Engl J Med 348:1201–1214

Cools J et al. (2005) Resistance to tyrosine kinase inhibitors:calling on extra forces. Drug Resist Update 8:119–129

Cortes J et al. (2003) Results of imatinib mesylate therapy in patients with refractory or recurrent acute myeloid leukemia, high-risk myelodysplastic syndrome, and myeloproliferative disorders. Cancer 97:2760–2766

Cunningham D et al. (2004) Cetuximab monotherapy and cetuximab plus irinotecan in irinotecan-refractory metastatic colorectal cancer. N Engl J Med 351:337–345

Curnow RT (1997) Clinical experience with CD64-directed immunotherapy. An overview. Cancer Immunol Immunother 45:210–215

Dagher R et al. (2002) Approval summary:imatinib mesylate in the treatment of metastatic and/or unresectable malignant gastrointestinal stromal tumors. Clin Cancer Res 8:3034–3038

Dancey J, Sausville EA (2003) Issues and progress with protein kinase inhibitors for cancer treatment. Nat Rev Drug Discov 2:296–313

Deininger M (2005) Resistance to imatinib:mechanisms and management. J Natl Compr Canc Netw 3:757–768

Demetri GD (2002) Identification and treatment of chemoresistant inoperable or metastatic GIST:experience with the selective tyrosine kinase inhibitor imatinib mesylate (STI571). Eur J Cancer 38 Suppl 5:S52–S59

Doroshow JH (2005) Targeting EGFR in non-small-cell lung cancer. N Engl J Med 353:200–202

Druker BJ et al. (1996) Effects of a selective inhibitor of the Abl tyrosine kinase on the growth of Bcr-Abl positive cells. Nat Med 2:561–566

Druker BJ et al. (2001a) Efficacy and safety of a specific inhibitor of the BCR-ABL tyrosine kinase in chronic myeloid leukemia. N Engl J Med 344:1031–1037

Druker BJ et al. (2001b) Activity of a specific inhibitor of the BCR-ABL tyrosine kinase in the blast crisis of chronic myeloid leukemia and acute lymphoblastic leukemia with the Philadelphia chromosome. N Engl J Med 344:1038–1042

Druker BJ (2002) Imatinib and chronic myeloid leukemia:validating the promise of molecularly targeted therapy. Eur J Cancer 38 Suppl 5:S70–S76

Dudek AZ et al. (2006) Skin rash and bronchoalveolar histology correlates with clinical benefit in patients treated with gefitinib as a therapy for previously treated advanced or metastatic non-small cell lung cancer. Lung Cancer 51:89–96

Eggert A et al. (2000) Prognostic and biological role of neurotrophin-receptor TrkA and TrkB in neuroblastoma. Klin Padiatr 212:200–205

Escudier B et al. (2005) Randomized phase III trial of the Raf kinase and VEGFR inhibitor sorafenib (BAY 43-9006) in patients with advanced renal cell carcinoma (RCC). Proc Am Soc Clin Oncol 23:1093s

Faivre S et al. (2006) Safety, pharmacokinetic, and antitumor activity of SU11248, a novel oral multitarget tyrosine kinase inhibitor, in patients with cancer. J Clin Oncol 24:25–35

Fan Z et al. (1993) Antitumor effect of anti-epidermal growth factor receptor monoclonal antibodies plus cis-diamminedichloroplatinum on well established A431 cell xenografts. Cancer Res 53:4637–4642

Farah RA et al. (1998) The development of monoclonal antibodies for the therapy of cancer. Crit Rev Eukaryot Gene Expr 8:321–356

Ferrara N et al. (2004) Discovery and development of bevacizumab, an anti-VEGF antibody for treating cancer. Nat Rev Drug Discov 3:391–400

Ferrara N et al. (2005) Bevacizumab (Avastin), a humanized anti-VEGF monoclonal antibody for cancer therapy. Biochem Biophys Res Commun 333:328–335

Ferrara N. and Kerbel RS (2005) Angiogenesis as a therapeutic target. Nature 438:967–974

Fischer OM et al. (2003) EGFR signal transactivation in cancer cells. Biochem Soc Trans 31:1203–1208

Fox SB et al. (2001) Angiogenesis:pathological, prognostic, and growth-factor pathways and their link to trial design and anticancer drugs. Lancet Oncol 2:278–289

Frieze DA, McCune JS (2006) Current status of cetuximab for the treatment of patients with solid tumors. Ann Pharmacother 40:241–250

Fry DW (2003) Mechanism of action of erbB tyrosine kinase inhibitors. Exp Cell Res 284:131–139

Fukuoka M, Yano S, Giaccone G, Tanura T, Nakagawa K, Douillard J et al. (2002) Final results from a phase II trial of ZD1839 (Iressa) for patients with advanced non-small cell lung cancer (IDEAL 1) [Abstract No. 1188]. In Proc ASCO (Vol. 21)

Gascoyne RD et al. (1999) Prognostic significance of anaplastic lymphoma kinase (ALK) protein expression in adults with anaplastic large cell lymphoma. Blood 93:3913–3921

Giaccone G et al. (2004) Gefitinib in combination with gemcitabine and cisplatin in advanced non-small-cell lung cancer:a phase III trial–INTACT 1. J Clin Oncol 22:777–784

Gilbert CW et al. (2003) Targeted prodrug treatment of HER-2-positive breast tumor cells using trastuzumab and paclitaxel linked by A-Z-CINN Linker. J Exp Ther Oncol 3:27–35

Gleich GJ et al. (2002) Treatment of hypereosinophilic syndrome with imatinib mesilate. Lancet 359:1577–1578

Gleissner B et al. (2002) Leading prognostic relevance of the BCR-ABL translocation in adult acute B-lineage lymphoblastic leukemia:a prospective study of the German Multicenter Trial Group and confirmed polymerase chain reaction analysis. Blood 99:1536–1543

Goldberg RM (2005) Cetuximab. Nat Rev Drug Discov Suppl:S10–S11

Gordon MS et al. (2001) Phase I safety and pharmacokinetic study of recombinant human anti-vascular endothelial growth factor in patients with advanced cancer. J Clin Oncol 19:843–850

Goss GD, Hirte H, Lorimer I, Miller W, Stewart DJ, Batish G et al. (2001) Final results of the dose escalation phase of a phase I pharmacokinetic (PK), pharmacodynamic (PD) and biological activity study of ZD1839:NCIC CTG Ind.122 [Abstract No. 335]. In Proc ASCO (Vol. 20)

Grandis JR et al. (1998) Downmodulation of TGF-alpha protein expression with antisense oligonucleotides inhibits proliferation of head and neck squamous carcinoma but not normal mucosal epithelial cells. J Cell Biochem 69:55–62

Grunwald V, Hidalgo M (2003a) Development of the epidermal growth factor receptor inhibitor OSI-774. Semin Oncol 30:23–31

Grunwald V, Hidalgo M (2003b) Developing inhibitors of the epidermal growth factor receptor for cancer treatment. J Natl Cancer Inst 95:851–867

Gunby RH et al. (2003) Sensitivity to imatinib but low frequency of the TEL/PDGFRb fusion protein in chronic myelomonocytic leukemia. Haematologica 88:408–415

Hambek M et al. (2001) Tumor necrosis factor alpha sensitizes low epidermal growth factor receptor (EGFR)-expressing carcinomas for anti-EGFR therapy. Cancer Res 61:1045–1049

Harari PM, Huang SM (2001) Radiation response modification following molecular inhibition of epidermal growth factor receptor signaling. Semin Radiat Oncol 11:281–289

Harries M, Smith I (2002) The development and clinical use of trastuzumab (Herceptin). Endocr Relat Cancer 9:75–85

Herbst RS (2003) Erlotinib (Tarceva):an update on the clinical trial program. Semin Oncol 30:34–46

Herbst RS et al. (2004) Gefitinib in combination with paclitaxel and carboplatin in advanced non-small-cell lung cancer:a phase III trial–INTACT 2. J Clin Oncol 22:785–794

Herbst RS et al. (2005) TRIBUTE:a phase III trial of erlotinib hydrochloride (OSI-774) combined with carboplatin and paclitaxel chemotherapy in advanced non-small-cell lung cancer. J Clin Oncol 23:5892–5899

Heymach JV (2005) ZD6474–clinical experience to date. Br J Cancer 92 Suppl 1:S14–S20

Hidalgo M et al. (2001) Phase I and pharmacologic study of OSI-774, an epidermal growth factor receptor tyrosine kinase inhibitor, in patients with advanced solid malignancies. J Clin Oncol 19:3267–3279

Hirata A et al. (2002) ZD1839 (Iressa) induces antiangiogenic effects through inhibition of epidermal growth factor receptor tyrosine kinase. Cancer Res 62:, 2554–2560

Hoffmann T et al. (1997) Antitumor activity of anti-epidermal growth factor receptor monoclonal antibodies and cisplatin in ten human head and neck squamous cell carcinoma lines. Anticancer Res 17:4419–4425

Holash J et al. (2002) VEGF-Trap:a VEGF blocker with potent antitumor effects. Proc Natl Acad Sci USA 99:11393–11398

Homer JJ et al. (2002) Soluble Tie-2 receptor levels independently predict locoregional recurrence in head and neck squamous cell carcinoma. Head Neck 24:773–778

Hortobagyi GN (2005) Trastuzumab in the treatment of breast cancer. N Engl J Med 353:1734–1736

Huang SM, Harari PM (2000) Modulation of radiation response after epidermal growth factor receptor blockade in squamous cell carcinomas:inhibition of damage repair, cell cycle kinetics, and tumor angiogenesis. Clin Cancer Res 6:2166–2174

Hudson PJ (1999) Recombinant antibody constructs in cancer therapy. Curr Opin Immunol 11:548–557

Hunter T (1998) The Croonian Lecture 1997. The phosphorylation of proteins on tyrosine:its role in cell growth and disease. Philos Trans R Soc Lond B Biol Sci 353:583–605

Hunter T (2000) Signaling–2000 and beyond. Cell 100:113–127

Hurwitz H et al. (2004) Bevacizumab plus irinotecan, fluorouracil, and leucovorin for metastatic colorectal cancer. N Engl J Med 350:2335–2342

Hurwitz HI et al. (2005) Bevacizumab in combination with fluorouracil and leucovorin:an active regimen for first-line metastatic colorectal cancer. J Clin Oncol 23:3502–3508

Hynes NE, Lane HA (2005) ERBB receptors and cancer: the complexity of targeted inhibitors. Nat Rev Cancer 5:341–354

Indo Y (2002) Genetics of congenital insensitivity to pain with anhidrosis (CIPA) or hereditary sensory and autonomic neuropathy type IV. Clinical, biological and molecular aspects of mutations in TRKA(NTRK1) gene encoding the receptor tyrosine kinase for nerve growth factor. Clin Auton Res 12 Suppl 1:I20–I32

Inoue A et al. (2006) Prospective phase II study of gefitinib for chemotherapy-naive patients with advanced non-small-cell lung cancer with epidermal growth factor receptor gene mutations. J Clin Oncol 24:3340–3346

James ND et al. (2001) A phase II study of the bispecific antibody MDX-H210 (anti-HER2 x CD64) with GM-CSF in HER2+ advanced prostate cancer. Br J Cancer 85:152–156

Johnson DH (2003) Gefitinib (Iressa) trials in non-small cell lung cancer. Lung Cancer 41 Suppl 1:S23–S28

Johnson DH et al. (2004) Randomized phase II trial comparing bevacizumab plus carboplatin and paclitaxel with carboplatin and paclitaxel alone in previously untreated locally advanced or metastatic non-small-cell lung cancer. J Clin Oncol 22:2184–2191

Johnson JR et al. (2003) Approval summary:Imatinib mesylate capsules for treatment of adult patients with newly diagnosed Philadelphia chromosome-positive chronic myelogenous leukemia in chronic phase. Clin Cancer Res 9:1972–1979

Johnson JR et al. (2005) Approval summary for erlotinib for treatment of patients with locally advanced or metastatic non-small cell lung cancer after failure of at least one prior chemotherapy regimen. Clin Cancer Res 11:6414–6421

Kabbinavar F et al. (2003) Phase II, randomized trial comparing bevacizumab plus fluorouracil (FU)/leucovorin (LV) with FU/LV alone in patients with metastatic colorectal cancer. J Clin Oncol 21:60–65

Kakiuchi S et al. (2004) Prediction of sensitivity of advanced non-small cell lung cancers to gefitinib (Iressa, ZD1839). Hum Mol Genet 13:3029–3043

Kantarjian H et al. (2006) Dasatinib. Nat Rev Drug Discov 5:717–718

Krause DS, Van Etten RA (2005) Tyrosine kinases as targets for cancer therapy. N Engl J Med 353:172–187

Kris MG et al. (2002) A phase II trial of ZD1839 (Iressa) in advanced non-small cell lung cancer (NSCLC) patients who failed platinum- and docetaxel- based regimens (IDEAL 2) [Abstract No. 1166]. In Proc ASCO (Vol. 21)

Krupa A, Srinivasan N (2002) The repertoire of protein kinases encoded in the draft version of the human genome:atypical variations and uncommon domain combinations. Genome Biol 3:RESEARCH0066

Kuenen BC et al. (2002) Dose-finding and pharmacokinetic study of cisplatin, gemcitabine, and SU5416 in patients with solid tumors. J Clin Oncol 20:1657–1667

Kupsch P et al. (2005) Results of a phase I trial of sorafenib (BAY 43-9006) in combination with oxaliplatin in patients with refractory solid tumors, including colorectal cancer. Clin Colorectal Cancer 5:188–196

Laird AD, Cherrington JM (2003) Small molecule tyrosine kinase inhibitors:clinical development of anti-cancer agents. Expert Opin Investig Drugs 12:51–64

Lau SC et al. (2005) Technology evaluation:VEGF Trap (cancer), Regeneron/sanofi-aventis. Curr Opin Mol Ther 7:493–501

le Coutre P et al. (1999) In vivo eradication of human BCR/ABL-positive leukemia cells with an ABL kinase inhibitor. J Natl Cancer Inst 91:163–168

Lee DC et al. (2002) RET receptor tyrosine kinase isoforms in kidney function and disease. Oncogene 21:5582–5592

Lewis LD et al. (2001) Pharmacokinetic-pharmacodynamic relationships of the bispecific antibody MDX-H210 when administered in combination with interferon gamma:a multiple-dose phase-I study in patients with advanced cancer which overexpresses HER-2/neu. J Immunol Methods 248:149–165

Lin WC et al. (1999) tie-1 protein tyrosine kinase:a novel independent prognostic marker for gastric cancer. Clin Cancer Res 5:1745–1751

Lynch DH, Yang XD (2002) Therapeutic potential of ABX-EGF:a fully human anti-epidermal growth factor receptor monoclonal antibody for cancer treatment. Semin Oncol 29:47–50

Lynch TJ et al. (2004) Activating mutations in the epidermal growth factor receptor underlying responsiveness of non-small-cell lung cancer to gefitinib. N Engl J Med 350:2129–2139

Madhusudan S, Ganesan TS (2004) Tyrosine kinase inhibitors in cancer therapy. Clin Biochem 37:618–635

Manley PW et al. (2002) Imatinib:a selective tyrosine kinase inhibitor. Eur J Cancer 38 Suppl 5:S19–S27

Manning G et al. (2002) The protein kinase complement of the human genome. Science 298:1912–1934

Margolin K et al. (2001) Phase Ib trial of intravenous recombinant humanized monoclonal antibody to vascular endothelial growth factor in combination with chemotherapy in patients with advanced cancer:pharmacologic and long-term safety data. J Clin Oncol 19:851–856

Meden H, Kuhn W. (1997) Overexpression of the oncogene c-erbB-2 (HER2/neu) in ovarian cancer:a new prognostic factor. Eur J Obstet Gynecol Reprod Biol 71:173–179

Mendelsohn J. (2002) Targeting the epidermal growth factor receptor for cancer therapy. J Clin Oncol 20:1S–13S

Mendelsohn J, Shin DM, Donato N, Khuri F, Radinsky R et al. (1999) A phase I study of chimerized anti-epidermal growth factor receptor (EGFr) monoclonal antibody, C225, in combination with cisplatin (CDDP) in patients (PTS) with recurrent head and neck squamous cell carcinoma (SCC) [Abstract No.1502]. In Proc ASCO 1999 (Vol. 18)

Meunier-Carpentier S et al. (2005) Comparison of the prognosis indication of VEGFR-1 and VEGFR-2 and Tie2 receptor expression in breast carcinoma. Int J Oncol 26:977–984

Miyazaki T et al. (2003) FAK overexpression is correlated with tumour invasiveness and lymph node metastasis in oesophageal squamous cell carcinoma. Br J Cancer 89:140–145

Mohamed MK et al. (2005) Skin rash and good performance status predict improved survival with gefitinib in patients with advanced non-small cell lung cancer. Ann Oncol 16:780–785

Moore M et al. (2005) Phase I study to determine the safety and pharmacokinetics of the novel Raf kinase and VEGFR inhibitor BAY 43-9006, administered for 28 days on/7 days off in patients with advanced, refractory solid tumors. Ann Oncol 16:1688–1694

Motzer RJ et al. (2006) Activity of SU11248, a multitargeted inhibitor of vascular endothelial growth factor receptor and platelet-derived growth factor receptor, in patients with metastatic renal cell carcinoma. J Clin Oncol 24:16–24

Moyer J.D et al. (1997) Induction of apoptosis and cell cycle arrest by CP-358,774, an inhibitor of epidermal growth factor receptor tyrosine kinase. Cancer Res 57:4838–4848

Naeem M et al. (2002) Analysis of c-kit protein expression in small-cell lung carcinoma and its implication for prognosis. Hum Pathol 33:1182–1187

Neet K, Hunter, T. (1996) Vertebrate non-receptor protein-tyrosine kinase families. Genes Cells 1:147–169

Negoro S, Nakagawa K, Fukuoka M, Kudoh S, Tamura T, Yoshimura N et al. (2001) Final results of a phase I intermittent dose-escalation trial of ZD1839 ('Iressa') in Japanese patients with various solid tumours [Abstract No. 1292]. In Proc ASCO (Vol. 20)

Nelson MH, Dolder, C.R. (2006) Lapatinib:a novel dual tyrosine kinase inhibitor with activity in solid tumors. Ann Pharmacother 40:261–269

Ng EW et al. (2006) Pegaptanib, a targeted anti-VEGF aptamer for ocular vascular disease. Nat Rev Drug Discov 5:123–132

Ng SS et al. (2002) Effects of the epidermal growth factor receptor inhibitor OSI-774, Tarceva, on downstream signaling pathways and apoptosis in human pancreatic adenocarcinoma. Mol Cancer Ther 1:777–783

Nicholson RI et al. (2001) EGFR and cancer prognosis. Eur J Cancer 37 Suppl 4:S9–S15

Normanno N et al. (2002) Cooperative inhibitory effect of ZD1839 (Iressa) in combination with trastuzumab (Herceptin) on human breast cancer cell growth. Ann Oncol 13:65–72

Normanno N et al. (2006) Epidermal growth factor receptor (EGFR) signaling in cancer. Gene 366:2–16

Oda Y et al. (2000) Expression of hepatocyte growth factor (HGF)/scatter factor and its receptor c-MET correlates with poor prognosis in synovial sarcoma. Hum Pathol 31:185–192

Ozvegy-Laczka C et al. (2005) Tyrosine kinase inhibitor resistance in cancer:role of ABC multidrug transporters. Drug Resist Update 8, 15–26

Pal SK, Pegram M (2005) Epidermal growth factor receptor and signal transduction:potential targets for anticancer therapy. Anticancer Drugs 16:483–494

Pao W et al. (2004) EGF receptor gene mutations are common in lung cancers from "never smokers" and are associated with sensitivity of tumors to gefitinib and erlotinib. Proc Natl Acad Sci USA 101:13306–13311

Pardanani A et al. (2003) CHIC2 deletion, a surrogate for FIP1L1-PDGFRA fusion, occurs in systemic mastocytosis associated with eosinophilia and predicts response to imatinib mesylate therapy. Blood 102:3093–3096

Parr C, Jiang WG (2003) Quantitative analysis of lymphangiogenic markers in human colorectal cancer. Int J Oncol 23:533–539

Paterson SC et al. (2003) Is there a cloud in the silver lining for imatinib? Br J Cancer 88:983–987

Pegram MD et al. (1998a) HER-2/neu as a predictive marker of response to breast cancer therapy. Breast Cancer Res Treat 52:65–77

Pegram MD et al. (1998b) Phase II study of receptor-enhanced chemosensitivity using recombinant humanized anti-p185HER2/neu monoclonal antibody plus cisplatin in patients with HER2/neu-over-expressing metastatic breast cancer refractory to chemotherapy treatment. J Clin Oncol 16:2659–2671

Pegram MD et al. (2000) Trastuzumab and chemotherapeutics:drug interactions and synergies. Semin Oncol 27:21–25; discussion 92–100

Penne K et al. (2005) Gefitinib (Iressa, ZD1839) and tyrosine kinase inhibitors:the wave of the future in cancer therapy. Cancer Nurs 28:481–486

Perrotte P et al. (1999) Anti-epidermal growth factor receptor antibody C225 inhibits angiogenesis in human transitional cell carcinoma growing orthotopically in nude mice. Clin Cancer Res 5:257–265

Peters G et al. (2003) IGF-1R, IGF-1 and IGF-2 expression as potential prognostic and predictive markers in colorectal-cancer. Virchows Arch

Piccart-Gebhart MJ et al. (2005) Trastuzumab after adjuvant chemotherapy in HER2-positive breast cancer. N Engl J Med 353:1659–1672

Pollack VA et al. (1999) Inhibition of epidermal growth factor receptor-associated tyrosine phosphorylation in human carcinomas with CP-358,774:dynamics of receptor inhibition in situ and antitumor effects in athymic mice. J Pharmacol Exp Ther 291:739–748

Posey JA et al. (1999) A pilot trial of GM-CSF and MDX-H210 in patients with erbB-2-positive advanced malignancies. J Immunother 22:371–379

Prenen H et al. (2006) Efficacy of the kinase inhibitor SU11248 against gastrointestinal stromal tumor mutants refractory to imatinib mesylate. Clin Cancer Res 12:2622–2627

Press MF et al. (1997) HER-2/neu gene amplification characterized by fluorescence in situ hybridization: poor prognosis in node-negative breast carcinomas. J Clin Oncol 15:2894–2904

Ranson M et al. (2002) ZD1839, a selective oral epidermal growth factor receptor-tyrosine kinase inhibitor, is well tolerated and active in patients with solid, malignant tumors:results of a phase I trial. J Clin Oncol 20:2240–2250

Ranson M (2004) Epidermal growth factor receptor tyrosine kinase inhibitors. Br J Cancer 90:2250–2255

Ratain MJ et al. (2006) Phase II placebo-controlled randomized discontinuation trial of sorafenib in patients with metastatic renal cell carcinoma. J Clin Oncol 24:2505–2512

Rhee J, Hoff PM (2005) Angiogenesis inhibitors in the treatment of cancer. Expert Opin Pharmacother 6:1701–1711

Richly H et al. (2006) Results of a Phase I trial of sorafenib (BAY 43-9006) in combination with doxorubicin in patients with refractory solid tumors. Ann Oncol 17:866–873

Rini BI (2006) Sorafenib. Expert Opin Pharmacother 7:453–461

Robert C et al. (2005) Cutaneous side-effects of kinase inhibitors and blocking antibodies. Lancet Oncol 6:491–500

Robinson DR et al. (2000) The protein tyrosine kinase family of the human genome. Oncogene 19:5548–5557

Rochlitz C et al. (1999) Axl expression is associated with adverse prognosis and with expression of Bcl-2 and CD34 in de novo acute myeloid leukemia (AML):results from a multicenter trial of the Swiss Group for Clinical Cancer Research (SAKK). Leukemia 13:1352–1358

Romond EH et al. (2005) Trastuzumab plus adjuvant chemotherapy for operable HER2-positive breast cancer. N Engl J Med 353:1673–1684

Rubin BP et al. (2001) KIT activation is a ubiquitous feature of gastrointestinal stromal tumors. Cancer Res 61:8118–8121

Ryan AJ, Wedge SR (2005) ZD6474–a novel inhibitor of VEGFR and EGFR tyrosine kinase activity. Br J Cancer 92 Suppl 1:S6–S13

Sadasivan R et al. (1993) Overexpression of Her-2/neu may be an indicator of poor prognosis in prostate cancer. J Urol 150:126–131

Saijo N, Nishio KN (2003) (Abstract no. O.20) Mechanisms of ZD1839 resistance and ZD1839 induced pulmonary fibrosis. In 2nd International Symposium on Signal Transduction Modulators in Cancer Therapy.

Sakurada A et al. (2006) Epidermal growth factor receptor tyrosine kinase inhibitors in lung cancer:impact of primary or secondary mutations. Clin Lung Cancer 7 Suppl 4:S138–S144

Saltz LB et al. (2004) Phase II trial of cetuximab in patients with refractory colorectal cancer that expresses the epidermal growth factor receptor. J Clin Oncol 22:1201–1208

Sato JD et al. (1983) Biological effects in vitro of monoclonal antibodies to human epidermal growth factor receptors. Mol Biol Med 1:511–529

Sawyers CL (1999) Chronic myeloid leukemia. N Engl J Med 340:1330–1340

Sawyers CL (2002) Imatinib GIST keeps finding new indications:successful treatment of dermatofibrosarcoma protuberans by targeted inhibition of the platelet-derived growth factor receptor. J Clin Oncol 20:3568–3569

Schlessinger J (2000) Cell signaling by receptor tyrosine kinases. Cell 103:211–225

Schnittger S et al. (2002) Analysis of FLT3 length mutations in 1003 patients with acute myeloid leukemia:correlation to cytogenetics, FAB subtype, and prognosis in the AMLCG study and usefulness as a marker for the detection of minimal residual disease. Blood 100:59–66

Selvaggi G et al. (2002) HER-2/neu overexpression in patients with radically resected nonsmall cell lung carcinoma. Impact on long-term survival. Cancer 94:2669–2674

Shepherd FA et al. (2005) Erlotinib in previously treated non-small-cell lung cancer. N Engl J Med 353:123–132

Shin DM et al. (2001) Epidermal growth factor receptor-targeted therapy with C225 and cisplatin in patients with head and neck cancer. Clin Cancer Res 7:1204–1213

Sirotnak FM (2003) Studies with ZD1839 in preclinical models. Semin Oncol 30:12–20

Sirotnak FM et al. (2000) Efficacy of cytotoxic agents against human tumor xenografts is markedly enhanced by coadministration of ZD1839 (Iressa), an inhibitor of EGFR tyrosine kinase. Clin Cancer Res 6:4885–4892

Slamon DJ et al. (1987) Human breast cancer:correlation of relapse and survival with amplification of the HER-2/neu oncogene. Science 235:177–182

Slamon DJ et al. (1989) Studies of the HER-2/neu proto-oncogene in human breast and ovarian cancer. Science 244:707-712

Slamon DJ et al. (2001) Use of chemotherapy plus a monoclonal antibody against HER2 for metastatic breast cancer that overexpresses HER2. N Engl J Med 344:783–792

Small EJ et al. (2001) Docetaxel, estramustine, plus trastuzumab in patients with metastatic androgen-independent prostate cancer. Semin Oncol 28:71–76

Smith J. (2005) Erlotinib:small-molecule targeted therapy in the treatment of non-small-cell lung cancer. Clin Ther 27:1513–1534

Speake G et al. (2005) Recent developments related to the EGFR as a target for cancer chemotherapy. Curr Opin Pharmacol 5:343–349

Spector NL et al. (2005) Study of the biologic effects of lapatinib, a reversible inhibitor of ErbB1 and ErbB2 tyrosine kinases, on tumor growth and survival pathways in patients with advanced malignancies. J Clin Oncol 23:2502–2512

Stamos J et al. (2002) Structure of the epidermal growth factor receptor kinase domain alone and in complex with a 4-anilinoquinazoline inhibitor. J Biol Chem 277:46265–46272

Storniolo A et al. (2005) A Phase I, open-label study of lapatinib (GW572016) plus trastuzumab;a clinically active regimen (abstract). Proc Am Soc Clin Oncol 23:559

Strumberg D. (2005) Preclinical and clinical development of the oral multikinase inhibitor sorafenib in cancer treatment. Drugs Today (Barc) 41:773–784

Strumberg D et al. (2005) Phase I clinical and pharmacokinetic study of the novel Raf kinase and vascular endothelial growth factor receptor inhibitor BAY 43-9006 in patients with advanced refractory solid tumors. J Clin Oncol 23:965–972

Talpaz M et al. (2006) Dasatinib in imatinib-resistant Philadelphia chromosome-positive leukemias. N Engl J Med 354:2531–2541

Tandon AK et al. (1989) HER-2/neu oncogene protein and prognosis in breast cancer. J Clin Oncol 7:1120–1128

Taniguchi M et al. (1999) Effect of c-kit mutation on prognosis of gastrointestinal stromal tumors. Cancer Res 59:4297–4300

Thatcher N et al. (2005) Gefitinib plus best supportive care in previously treated patients with refractory advanced non-small-cell lung cancer:results from a randomised, placebo-controlled, multicentre study (Iressa Survival Evaluation in Lung Cancer). Lancet 366:1527–1537

Thomas A.L et al. (2005) Phase I study of the safety, tolerability, pharmacokinetics, and pharmacodynamics of PTK787/ZK 222584 administered twice daily in patients with advanced cancer. J Clin Oncol 23:4162–4171

Tibes R et al. (2005) Tyrosine kinase inhibitors and the dawn of molecular cancer therapeutics. Annu Rev Pharmacol Toxicol 45:357–384

Toyama T et al. (2003) Reduced expression of the Syk gene is correlated with poor prognosis in human breast cancer. Cancer Lett 189:97–102

Tsai CM et al. (1993) Correlation of intrinsic chemoresistance of non-small-cell lung cancer cell lines with HER-2/neu gene expression but not with ras gene mutations. J Natl Cancer Inst 85:897–901

Tsao MS et al. (2005) Erlotinib in lung cancer – molecular and clinical predictors of outcome. N Engl J Med 353:133–144

Tuveson DA et al. (2001) STI571 inactivation of the gastrointestinal stromal tumor c-KIT oncoprotein:biological and clinical implications. Oncogene 20:5054–5058

Tyagi P. (2005) Vatalanib (PTK787/ZK 222584) in combination with FOLFOX4 versus FOLFOX4 alone as first-line treatment for colorectal cancer:preliminary results from the CONFIRM-1 trial. Clin Colorectal Cancer 5:24–26

Ueki T et al. (1997) Expression of hepatocyte growth factor and its receptor c-met proto-oncogene in hepatocellular carcinoma. Hepatology 25:862–866

van der Kuip H et al. (2005) Mechanisms of clinical resistance to small molecule tyrosine kinase inhibitors targeting oncogenic tyrosine kinases. Am J Pharmacogenomics 5:101–112

Verstovsek S et al. (2002) Prognostic significance of Tie-1 protein expression in patients with early chronic phase chronic myeloid leukemia. Cancer 94:1517–1521

Vogel CL et al. (2002) Efficacy and safety of trastuzumab as a single agent in first-line treatment of HER2-overexpressing metastatic breast cancer. J Clin Oncol 20:719–726

Weiner HL, Zagzag D (2000) Growth factor receptor tyrosine kinases:cell adhesion kinase family suggests a novel signaling mechanism in cancer. Cancer Invest 18:544–554

Wells A (2000) Tumor invasion:role of growth factor-induced cell motility. Adv Cancer Res 78:31–101

Wood JM et al. (2000) PTK787/ZK 222584, a novel and potent inhibitor of vascular endothelial growth factor receptor tyrosine kinases, impairs vascular endothelial growth factor-induced responses and tumor growth after oral administration. Cancer Res 60:2178–2189

Yang JC et al. (2003) A randomized trial of bevacizumab, an anti-vascular endothelial growth factor antibody, for metastatic renal cancer. N Engl J Med 349:427–434

Yang JC (2004) Bevacizumab for patients with metastatic renal cancer:an update. Clin Cancer Res 10:6367S–6370S

Yarden Y, Sliwkowski MX (2001) Untangling the ErbB signalling network. Nat Rev Mol Cell Biol 2:127–137

Zaczek A et al. (2005) The diverse signaling network of EGFR, HER2, HER3 and HER4 tyrosine kinase receptors and the consequences for therapeutic approaches. Histol Histopathol 20:1005–1015

Zakarija A, Soff G (2005) Update on angiogenesis inhibitors. Curr Opin Oncol 17:578–583

Zhou H et al. (2003) Her-2/neu expression in osteosarcoma increases risk of lung metastasis and can be associated with gene amplification. J Pediatr Hematol Oncol 25:27–32

Targeting ERBB Receptors in Cancer

Nancy E. Hynes

Recent Results in Cancer Research, Vol. 172
© Springer-Verlag Berlin Heidelberg 2007

4.1 Introduction

Tyrosine kinases are a large and diverse family of proteins found only in metazoans. The ERBB family, which encompasses subgroup I of the receptor tyrosine kinase (RTK) superfamily, has four members: epidermal growth factor receptor (EGFR)/ErbB1, ErbB2, ErbB3, and ErbB4. ERBB RTKs contain an extracellular domain that binds peptide ligands; they span the membrane once and have an intracellular portion with protein tyrosine kinase activity (Fig. 4.1). Ligand binding induces the formation of receptor dimers, and as a consequence the intrinsic kinase of the receptor is activated and transfers a phosphate group from the bound ATP to specific tyrosine side chains on the receptor proteins and on intracellular signaling proteins that bind the active RTKs. Subsequently, multiple signaling pathways become activated. The ERBB receptor/ligand family has been investigated in depth for many years, and comprehensive signaling maps describing the links between the plasma membrane receptors, the cytoplasmic signaling pathways, and the nucleus are available (Oda 2005).

In many types of human tumors ERBB receptors are aberrantly activated and contribute to cancer development. Thus these receptors have been intensively studied both to understand their roles in cancer biology and to employ them as therapeutic targets. Many ERBB-targeted inhibitors are now in clinical use. In this review I will outline our understanding of how ERBB receptors are activated and contribute to cancer, including a discussion on targeted therapeutics and their effects on the tumor cells. Potential mechanisms that underlie a successful clinical response to inhibition of ERBB RTKs, as well as possible reasons for nonresponse, will be discussed.

4.2 ERBB Receptors and Ligands

Reflecting the complexity of the organisms, the ERBB family has evolved from a single ligand-receptor combination in the nematode Caenorhabditis elegans, with one homolog of EGFR, LET-23, and one ligand, LIN-3 (Moghal and Sternberg 2003), to a complex system in higher vertebrates comprising four receptors and multiple ligands, the EGF-related peptides (Yarden and Sliwkowski 2001). These are divided into three groups based on binding specificity (Fig. 4.1). The first group includes EGF, transforming growth factor (TGF)-α, amphiregulin (AR), and epigen (EPG), which bind specifically to EGFR; the second group includes betacellulin (BTC), heparin-binding EGF (HB-EGF), and epiregulin (EPR), which exhibit dual specificity, binding both EGFR and ErbB4. The third group, composed of the neuregulins (NRGs), forms two subgroups based on their capacity to bind ErbB3 and ErbB4

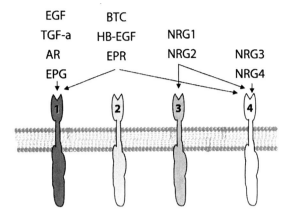

Fig. 4.1 The ERBB receptors and their ligands. The ERBB receptor family has four members: EGFR/ErbB1, ErbB2, ErbB3, and ErbB4, labeled *1–4*, respectively. ERBB ligands can be divided into categories depending on binding specificity toward the ErbB receptors. EGF, transforming growth factor (*TGF*)-α, amphiregulin (*AR*), and epigen (*EPG*) bind EGFR/ErbB1; betacellulin (*BTC*), heparin-binding EGF (*HB-EGF*), and epiregulin (*EPR*) exhibit dual specificity, binding both EGFR/ErbB1 and ErbB4; the neuregulins (*NRGs*) form two subgroups based on their capacity to bind ErbB3 and ErbB4 (*NRG-1* and *NRG-2*) or only ErbB4 (*NRG-3* and *NRG-4*). ErbB2 has no direct ligand

(NRG-1 and NRG-2) or only ErbB4 (NRG-3 and NRG-4) (Kochupurakkal et al. 2005; Riese and Stern 1998). The ERBB receptors are activated in response to binding of EGF-related peptides. On stimulation, the receptors couple to multiple signaling molecules (Jones et al. 2006) and pathways (reviewed in Schlessinger 2004 and http://stke.sciencemag.org/cgi/cm/stkecm;CMP_14987). Intriguingly, despite the fact that none of the EGF-related peptides binds ErbB2, this receptor is an important member of the family and is the preferred dimerization partner for the other ligand-activated ERBBs (Graus-Porta et al. 1997) (Fig. 4.2).

4.3 ERBB Receptor Activation in Cancer

The ERBB receptors, in particular EGFR and ErbB2, are aberrantly activated in a wide variety of human tumors. Three major mechanisms contribute to abnormal ERBB activation. These include enhanced or aberrant expression of EGF-related peptides, overexpression of receptors, usually due to gene amplification, and constitutive activation resulting from mutations.

Many tumor types show expression of EGFR and one or more of its ligands, which are produced by the tumor itself (autocrine) or by stromal cells (paracrine) (reviewed in Salomon et al. 1995; Pollard 2004). Enhanced or aberrant expression of EGF-related peptides promotes constitutive receptor activation. Autocrine EGFR activation is, for example, an early event in the development of head and neck squamous cell carcinoma (HNSCC) (Grandis et al. 2000).

Gene amplification leading to EGFR overexpression has been described in many types of cancer (Ohgaki et al. 2004; Sunpaweravong et al. 2005). For some of these, including bladder and cervical carcinomas and HNSCC, there is a significant association between increased EGFR expression and decreased survival (Nicholson et al. 2001), strongly suggesting that aberrant activation contributes to the malignancy of the cancer. In a high percentage of glioblastomas, EGFR amplification is accompanied by structural rearrangements that cause in-frame deletions in the ectodomain of the receptor, the most common of these being a deletion of exons 2–7 referred to as EGFRvIII

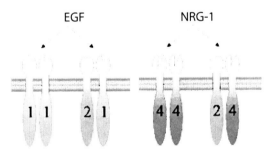

Fig. 4.2 ErbB2 is activated by heterodimerization. Ligand binding to ERBB receptors induces the formation of receptor homo- and heterodimers and the activation of the intrinsic kinase domain. None of the ERBB ligands binds ErbB2, but it is the preferred dimerization partner for all the other ERBB receptors. Shown are some of the numerous potential receptor homo- and heterodimers resulting from ERBB ligand binding

(Ekstrand et al. 1992). In contrast to the wild-type overexpressed EGFR that requires a ligand for activation, EGFRvIII is constitutively active (reviewed in Jorissen et al. 2003).

In 2004 the first somatic mutations in the kinase domain of EGFR were reported in tumors from non-small-cell lung cancer (NSCLC) patients (Lynch et al. 2004; Paez et al. 2004; Pao et al. 2004). The reported missense mutations and in-frame deletions affect residues in the ATP binding pocket and, at least in vitro, appear to enhance the coupling of the mutant receptor to the prosurvival PI3K-Akt and STAT pathways important for tumor cell survival (Sordella et al. 2004; Greulich et al. 2005). To date, kinase domain mutations appear to be most prevalent in lung cancers, since no mutations have been confirmed in other types of tumors (reviewed in Shigematsu and Gazdar 2006). Indeed, a family with multiple cases of NSCLC associated with germline transmission of an exon 20 EGFR mutation has recently been described (Bell et al. 2005), providing genetic evidence for the importance of this receptor in lung cancer. The frequency of kinase domain mutations in EGFR is reported to lie between 24% (477 in >2,000) (Shigematsu and Gazdar 2006) and 31% (350 in 1,108) (Greulich et al. 2005). The impact of EGFR kinase domain mutation on survival in NSCLC is currently under investigation; however, kinase domain mutations have been associated with response to EGFR kinase inhibition (discussed below).

Amplification of ERBB2 was initially described in a subset of breast tumors (Slamon et al. 1987; Berger et al. 1988) and also occurs in cancers arising in the ovaries, gastric system, bladder, and salivary gland. Amplification contributes to ErbB2 overexpression, leading to its constitutive activation, even in the absence of ligands (reviewed in Holbro and Hynes 2004). The clinical significance of ERBB2 amplification and overexpression is most thoroughly documented in breast cancer (reviewed in Ross et al. 2003). The consensus of numerous clinical studies is that high levels of ErbB2 predict poor prognosis in patients with positive lymph nodes (discussed in Mosesson and Yarden 2004). ERBB2 kinase domain mutations have also been found in NSCLC cancer, although at a lower frequency compared to EGFR. Compared to EGFR kinase domain mutations that occur in 24% or more tumors, ERBB2 kinase domain mutations are rarer, at approximately 2% [11 in 671 (Shigematsu et al. 2005) and 5/120 (Stephens et al. 2004)]. The clinical significance of ERBB2 kinase domain mutation has not yet been described.

4.4 Approaches to Block ERBB Receptor Activity

Each of the described alterations promotes constitutive ERBB activation, a process that contributes to cancer development at many levels. Data gleaned mainly from in vitro cancer cell models show that constitutively active ERBB receptors control key intracellular pathways that govern fundamental cellular processes including proliferation, cell migration, metabolism. and survival (Fig. 4.3). Because of this, as well as the clinical studies implicating EGFR and ErbB2 in the pathology of specific tumor types (Nicholson et al. 2001; Ross et al. 2003), an enormous effort has gone into developing ERBB-targeted anticancer agents.

Most efforts for targeting ERBB receptors have focused on either the extracellular domain with antibody-based approaches or blockade of the intracellular kinase domain with small-molecule tyrosine kinase inhibitors (TKIs). Several of these antibodies and targeted TKIs are in clinical use or are in advanced stages of clinical development (reviewed in Hynes and Lane 2005). The ERBB receptors are also being targeted by other approaches, including recombinant immunotoxins (von Minckwitz et al. 2005; reviewed in FitzGerald et al. 2004) and siRNA-based methods to downregulate receptor levels (reviewed in Dorsett and Tuschl 2004).

Considering monoclonal antibodies (mAbs), the first ones that interfered with EGF binding to the EGFR were described more than 20 years ago (Sato et al. 1983; Schreiber et al. 1981). In 2004, cetuximab, a chimeric EGFR-targeted antibody, was approved by the FDA for treatment of advanced colorectal cancer. Shortly after the discovery of ERBB2 (Schechter et al. 1985; Semba et al.

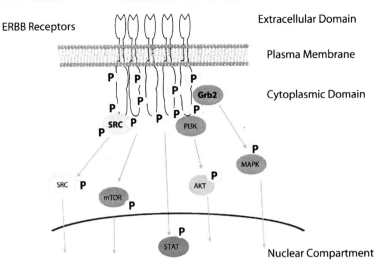

Fig. 4.3 Active ERBB receptors impact on tumor cell characteristics. In tumor cells ERBB receptors are activated by various mechanisms. In this example, ERBB receptor overexpression promotes activation, indicated by high levels of phospho-tyrosine (*circled P*). Active ERBB receptors stimulate numerous signaling pathways by recruiting proteins, such as *Src*, *PI3K*, and *Grb2*, to specific phosphotyrosine residues in their carboxy-terminal domain. The signaling proteins and pathways in this figure are the Src tyrosine kinase, the mammalian target of rapamycin (*mTOR*) serine/threonine kinase, the signal transducer and activator of transcription (*STAT*) transcription factor, the phosphatidylinositol 3-kinase (*PI3K*)- Akt serine/threonine kinase pathway, and the mitogen-activated protein kinase (*MAPK*) pathway. Constitutive activation of signaling proteins and pathways ultimately leads to changes in activity of nuclear transcription factors (for simplicity, only the *STAT* transcription factor is shown), which impinge upon all aspects of cellular physiology, as indicated at the bottom of the figure

1985), ErbB2-specific mAbs with in vitro growth inhibitory activity were described (Hudziak et al. 1989). Trastuzumab, a humanized antibody specific for ErbB2, was approved for treatment of metastatic breast cancer in 1998.

Considering the small-molecule kinase inhibitors, Levitzki and colleagues did some of the pioneering work in designing EGFR-directed TKIs, the tyrphostins (Gazit et al. 1989). Subsequently, optimization of various lead structures including quinazolines, pyrrolopyrimidines, and phenylaminopyrimidines led to the development of several ERBB-targeted TKIs (Traxler 2003; reviewed in Hynes and Lane 2005). Two of these, gefitinib and tarceva, have been approved by the FDA for treatment of NSCLC.

4.5 Clinical Response to ERBB-Targeted Therapeutics

There is now a plethora of signal transduction inhibitors (STIs) directed to EGFR and ErbB2. A mechanistic understanding of how these inhibitors function will be essential to further enhance the initial clinical successes. Furthermore, optimization of factors that predict response or resistance to a specific therapeutic must continue, in order to help in optimal patient selection and interpretation of efficacy data. I will concentrate this discussion on the ERBB-targeted antibodies and TKIs since the greatest amount of clinical data is available on these inhibitors.

4.5.1 Trastuzumab and ErbB2

The pivotal trials on trastuzumab for the treatment of metastatic breast cancer showed an improved response rate and a modest, but significant enhanced survival in patients who received the antibody in combination with chemotherapy (Slamon et al. 2001). Recently, exciting data from phase III clinical trials designed to test the role of trastuzumab as adjuvant therapy after surgical removal of the primary tumor have been published (Piccart-Gebhart et al. 2005; Romond et al. 2005). These analyses showed that the addition of trastuzumab to chemotherapy significantly reduced the risk of breast cancer recurrence by approximately 50% in women with early-stage, ErbB2-overexpressing breast cancer. While there are still many open questions (discussed in Hortobagyi 2005), these are very exciting results since they represent the largest quantitative improvement in outcome for any group of women with breast cancer in the past 25 years.

4.5.2 Mechanisms Underlying Efficacy of Trastuzumab

Understanding the molecular mechanism underlying in vivo response to trastuzumab should ultimately improve its clinical efficacy. There are numerous proposed mechanisms based mainly on results from experiments performed with in vitro cultured tumor cells or with animal models. These include trastuzumab-induced downregulation of ErbB2 protein levels (Hudziak et al. 1989) and/or receptor signaling activity (Lane et al. 2000; Motoyama et al. 2002; Yakes et al. 2002), antibody-induced reduction in tumor-associated vessels necessary for angiogenesis (Izumi et al. 2002), and others (Molina et al. 2001). Furthermore, antibodies targeting the receptors have the inherent ability to recruit immune effector cells such as macrophages and monocytes to the tumor through the binding of the antibody constant Fc domain to specific receptors on these cells. In xenograft models this mechanism is relevant for the antitumor activity of trastuzumab (Clynes et al. 2000).

Evidence to back up some of these proposed mechanisms has been obtained in the trastuzumab neoadjuvant setting, a situation in which the antibody is given to patients whose tumors overexpress ErbB2, before surgery. There are publications describing treatment with trastuzumab in the neoadjuvant setting, given either alone (Gennari et al. 2004; Mohsin et al. 2005) or in combination with chemotherapeutics (Burstein et al. 2003). In addition to monitoring for decrease in the primary tumor size, specific molecular markers were analyzed in these studies. A neoadjuvant trastuzumab trial on 35 patients with ErbB2-overexpressing breast tumors reported a median decrease in tumor size of 20% after a 3-week period (Mohsin et al. 2005). This was accompanied by an increase in the level of cleaved caspase-3, representing a 35% increase in apoptosis. Furthermore, in patients who responded there was a measurable decrease in nuclear P-Akt levels that was not seen in nonresponding patients. A pilot neoadjuvant trastuzumab study carried out on 11 ErbB-2-overexpressing breast cancer patients (Gennari et al. 2004) described a significant decrease in tumor size in 5 patients, without a measurable decrease in CD31-positive vessel staining. A correlation with pathological response and the presence of higher in situ levels of leukocytes was observed. These results suggest that trastuzumab-mediated cell-dependent cytotoxicity might occur in vivo. In striking contrast to the in vitro results (Lane et al. 2000; Motoyama et al. 2002; Yakes et al. 2002), neither of these neoadjuvant studies reported a measurable decrease in tumor cell proliferation (Gennari et al. 2004; Mohsin et al. 2005). However, since Ki67 was used in both studies, it is still possible that tumor cells cycle more slowly, but do not enter G0 in response to trastuzumab. Furthermore, neither study found that trastuzumab treatment led to a decrease in ErbB2 levels in the primary tumors (Gennari et al. 2004; Mohsin et al. 2005). Surface downregulation of ErbB2 has long been promoted as an important antitumor mechanism (Hudziak et al. 1989; Baselga and Albanell 2001) and is often observed in vitro with ErbB2-targeted antibodies (Harwerth et al. 1992; Klapper et al. 1997). A recent publication that described the use of multiple techniques to measure endocytosis and cycling of trastuzumab-bound ErbB2 showed that the surface ErbB2 pool is dynamic, undergoing endocytosis and efficient recycling to the membrane. Trastuzumab appears not to downregulate ErbB2, but efficiently recycles with the receptor (Austin et al. 2004).

Taken together, both studies suggest that in the context of primary ErbB2-overexpressing breast cancer, trastuzumab treatment does cause a reduction in tumor size, most likely due to increased cell death, that could result from downregulation of Akt activity, as well as ADCC. ErbB2 levels do not decrease, at least early after antibody administration. Considering the dramatic results in the trastuzumab adjuvant trials mentioned above, it is tempting to speculate that in early-stage breast cancer the ErbB2-overexpressing tumor cells are dependent on the receptor for survival, in particular in the presence of cytotoxics.

4.5.3 EGFR Mutations and TKIs

Somatic mutations in the kinase domain of EGFR have been detected in NSCLC patients (Lynch et al. 2004; Paez et al. 2004; Pao et al. 2004). The pooled data from these first studies revealed that 81% (25/31) of lung cancer patients who had partial or strong responses to the EGFR-selective TKIs gefitinib or erlotonib expressed EGFRs with gain-of-function mutations in the kinase domain (Pao et al. 2004). The results from three additional studies (Han et al. 2005; Mitsudomi et al. 2005; Takano et al, 2005) (reviewed in Johnson and Janne 2005) describe response rates for patients with EGFR kinase domain mutations ranging from 65% to 83%.

Recent clinical trial results showing that erlotinib provided a 2-month survival advantage to NSCLC patients after failure on chemotherapy were greeted with enthusiasm (Doroshow 2005). This trial, carried out with more than 700 patients and including an untreated control arm, was the first clinical study of an ERBB-targeted TKI that showed substantial benefit to patients (Shepherd et al. 2005). Confirming the above-mentioned studies, the presence of an EGFR mutation correlated with higher response rates to erlotinib (Tsao et al. 2005). However, it should be noted here that only 16% of the patients with kinase domain mutations responded to erlotinib, while 20% of the patients with EGFR amplification as determined by fluorescence in situ hybridization (FISH) responded in this trial. The presence of a kinase domain mutation was not associated with the survival benefit of erlotinib therapy; however, the expression level of EGFR was associated with increased survival (Tsao et al. 2005).

Bronchoalveolar carcinoma (BAC) and adenocarcinomas with BAC features appear to be increasing in incidence, and EGFR might have a particularly important role in the development of this type of lung cancer. It was noted in the first reports of EGFR mutations (Lynch et al. 2004; Paez et al. 2004; Pao et al. 2004) that they were especially prevalent in the BAC subtype. Furthermore, as mentioned above, a family with multiple cases of NSCLC of the BAC subtype, associated with germline transmission of an EGFR mutation, has been described (Bell et al. 2005).

From the point of view of NSCLC patient selection for TKI therapy, the current data suggest that screening for EGFR kinase domain mutations as well as EGFR amplification could be considered. Furthermore, although needing confirmation, another study of ~100 NSCLC patients showed that ErbB2 gene copy number, in combination with high or mutant EGFR, was associated with an enhanced response to gefitinib (Cappuzzo et al. 2005b). Thus ErbB2 activation status might also contribute to the biology of NSCLC and have an impact on response to TKIs. Finally, it is also important to note that objective responses to TKIs have been observed in the absence of EGFR kinase domain mutations or overexpression (Pao et al. 2004; Takano et al. 2005; Tsao et al. 2005). Thus it will be essential to examine other signaling molecules for their contribution to response.

4.5.4 TKI vs. Antibody

The EGFR-specific chimeric recombinant antibody cetuximab has also been intensively studied for its antitumor activity and was approved in 2004 by the FDA for the treatment of advanced colorectal cancer. Cetuximab binds the extracellular domain of EGFR. This binding prevents EGFR from adopting the conformation required for dimerization and partially overlaps with the region that binds ligands (Li et al. 2005), a characteristic that is expected to interfere with the autocrine receptor activation found in many solid tumors. Gefitinib and cetuximab have been compared for their in vitro activity on NSCLC tumor cell lines with mutant and wild-type EGFR. The TKI was more effective in blocking tumor cell proliferation and increasing apoptosis in comparison to the antibody (Mukohara et al. 2005). Clinical data on cetuximab efficacy in NSCLC have been disappointing, although the trials are ongoing (Minna et al. 2005). Furthermore, although only limited comparative clinical data are available, it appears that the TKI is more effective in blocking the disease (Mukohara et al. 2005).

4.6 Factors Influencing Response to ERBB-Directed Inhibitors

4.6.1 Trastuzumab and Breast Cancer

Despite the documented clinical efficacy of trastuzumab discussed above, it was evident quite early in its development that only one-third or fewer of ErbB2-overexpressing metastatic cancer patients responded to trastuzumab monotherapy (see, e.g., Cobleigh et al. 1999). Thus it was assumed that other factors in addition to gene amplification and ErbB2 overexpression must play a role in clinical efficacy. Various hypotheses, ranging from compensatory signaling pathways bypassing oncogenic ErbB2 to signaling aberrations downstream of the receptor, have been proposed.

Data, from in vitro and clinical studies, supporting these hypotheses exist. Considering the first, ERBB ligands might facilitate escape from trastuzumab through activation of alternative ERBB homo- and heterodimers. It has been shown experimentally that trastuzumab-sensitive tumor cells become resistant in the presence of ERBB ligands, since the antibody is unable to prevent formation of ligand-induced ErbB2-containing heterodimers or to prevent the activation of downstream signaling pathways (Agus et al. 2002; Motoyama et al. 2002). Since trastuzumab binds domain IV of ErbB2, a region not involved in receptor dimerization (Cho et al. 2003), this explains why ERBB ligands can induce formation and activation of ErbB2-containing dimers in the presence of the antibody. Clearly, the relevance of these data to the trastuzumab-treated patient will only become apparent when more detailed epidemiology has been carried out, correlating the molecular characteristics of a tumor to patient response. However, considering that many tumors express multiple ERBB receptors and are exposed to ERBB ligands (Rubin Grandis et al. 1998; Salomon et al. 1995), the potential for their involvement in resistance should be kept in mind.

4.6.2 PI3K Pathway Activation and Response to ERBB inhibitors

The in vitro antiproliferative effect of ERBB-targeted therapeutics often correlates with downregulation of signaling pathways including the MAPK and the PI3K/Akt pathways. It is possible that persistent activation of these pathways caused by aberrations downstream of the receptors might also have a role in in vivo resistance to ERBB-targeted inhibitors, both antibodies and TKIs. Indeed, somatic point mutations in the PIK3CA gene, encoding the $p110\alpha$ subunit of the enzyme, have recently been described (Samuels et al. 2004). Considering breast cancer, PIK3CA mutations have been detected in 25% of tumors (Bachman et al. 2004), making this one of the most frequently mutated genes in breast cancer. Furthermore, loss or mutation of PTEN (phosphatase and tensin homolog deleted in chromosome 10), the lipid phosphatase that negatively regulates PI3K activity, may contribute to resistance. The main role of PTEN is to dephosphorylate position D3 of phosphatidylinositol-3,4,5 triphosphate, and thereby antagonize PI3K function, leading to down-regulation of Akt activity. In a small panel of ErbB2-overexpressing primary breast tumors it was shown that the level of PTEN was positively correlated with the clinical efficacy of trastuzumab (Nagata et al. 2004). Loss of PTEN expression (Eng 2003), amplification of chromosomal loci encoding Akt or PI3K (reviewed in Thompson and Thompson 2004), or gain-of-function mutations in PIK3CA (Samuels et al. 2004) are common in solid tumors and might have an important role in modulating the efficacy of ERBB directed therapies. As a consequence combination strategies to alleviate this potential resistance mechanism might be required (discussed in Hynes and Lane, 2005).

ErbB3 has impaired kinase activity due to amino acid substitutions in critical residues in the kinase domain and only becomes phosphorylated and functions as a signaling protein when dimerized with another ERBB receptor (Kim et al. 1998). Furthermore, of all the ERBBs, ErbB3 couples best to the PI3K/Akt pathway since it contains six docking sites for the p85 adaptor subunit of PI3K (Holbro et al. 2003; Olayioye et al. 2000). In a panel of gefitinib-treated NSCLC cell lines, the antiproliferative activity of the TKI correlated with downregulation of Akt signaling, which was dependent on coupling of this pathway to ErbB3; in other words, EGFR employed ErbB3 to couple to this pathway, and activity of ErbB3 was dependent on EGFR activity (Engelman et al. 2005). Importantly, in another EGFR-positive group of NSCLC patients, P-Akt levels correlated with a benefit of gefitinib treatment (Cappuzzo et al. 2005a). These data, as well as others (Sordella et al. 2004), point to the importance of the PI3K/Akt pathway in promoting lung cancer survival in NSCLC culture models. Furthermore, at least in some studies (Engelman et al. 2005) EGFR couples to the pathway via ErbB3.

4.6.3 TKIs and Glioblastoma

Glioblastomas have a number of genetic abnormalities, including amplification of the EGFR gene and expression of the EGFRvarIII deletion as well as loss of PTEN (Ermoian et al. 2002; Smith et al. 2001). Based on clinical results from a phase II trial showing that some glioblastoma patients respond to gefitinib (Rich et al. 2004), a study was initiated to examine whether or not PTEN expression has a role in response. In fact, coexpression of EGFRvIII and PTEN was recently found to correlate highly with clinical response to gefitinib and erlotinib (Mellinghoff et al. 2005). This is an excellent example showing the importance of considering multiple genetic abnormalities when analyzing clinical data. Based on these results it is hoped that prospective validation of EGFRvIII and PTEN as predictors of response to EGFR-targeted inhibitors will be undertaken. Furthermore, the results suggest that the PI3K-Akt pathway may be particularly important for glioblastoma survival and that inhibition of other pathway members, for example, mTOR, might be particularly effective in treatment of glioblastoma (Goudar et al. 2005).

4.7 Acquired Resistance to EGFR-Targeted TKIs

Resistance to TKIs has emerged as a significant clinical problem. Resistance was initially reported in the context of chromic myelogenous leukemia (CML), a cancer associated with the BCR-ABL oncoprotein. Imatinib-treated CML patients who become resistant to the BCR-ABL-targeted TKI often show mutations in the kinase domain. As observed in CML, it has recently been shown that resistance to the EGFR-directed TKIs can be acquired by a mutation in exon 20 of the kinase domain (Kobayashi et al. 2005; Pao et al. 2005). Based on the model of erlotininb bound to the EGFR kinase domain (Kobayashi et al. 2005), the threonine to methionine amino acid change at position 790, the so-called gatekeeper residue, is predicted to keep the receptor active but prevent the drug from binding (Kobayashi et al. 2005). Interestingly, imatinib-resistant

CML patients often show a mutation at position 315, the amino acid structurally corresponding to T790 of EGFR (with isoleucine replacing threonine), and this leads to a similar structural change (Gorre et al. 2001). Fortunately, TKI resistance can be overcome. For example, the irreversible EGFR inhibitor CL-387,785 (Discafani et al. 1999) is able to block kinase activity of the T790M mutant (Greulich et al. 2005).

4.8 Future Perspectives

An understanding of the molecular, structural, and biological characteristics of the ERBB receptor/ligand network has been essential for rational development of ERBB-targeted inhibitors. Despite the clinical success of some ERBB-directed TKIs and antibodies discussed here, a major challenge for the future will be to develop accurate predictors of response to ERBB-targeted therapies. Considering just one therapeutic, trastuzumab, it is known that high ErbB2 expression is a prerequisite for treatment; however, we still do not know why some patients respond and others do not. Thus it is obvious that other factors should be considered in addition to high ErbB2 levels. As discussed above, knowledge of mutations on the PI3K/Akt pathway might help select patients who might better be treated with trastuzumab in combination with a pathway inhibitor. In the future, I am confident that the continuing interchange of information and ideas between basic and clinical research will help us successfully develop these molecular markers.

Acknowledgements. The laboratory of N.E.H. is supported by Novartis Forschungsstiftung Zweigniederlassung Friedrich Miescher Institute for Biomedical Research.

References

Agus DB, Akita RW, Fox WD, Lewis GD, Higgins B, Pisacane PI, Lofgren JA, Tindell C, Evans DP, Maiese K, Scher HI, Sliwkowski MX (2002) Targeting ligand-activated ErbB2 signaling inhibits breast and prostate tumor growth. Cancer Cell 2:127–137

Austin CD, De Maziere AM, Pisacane PI, van Dijk SM, Eigenbrot C, Sliwkowski MX, Klumperman J, Scheller RH (2004) Endocytosis and sorting of ErbB2 and the site of action of cancer therapeutics trastuzumab and geldanamycin. Mol Biol Cell 15:5268–5282

Bachman KE, Argani P, Samuels Y, Silliman N, Ptak J, Szabo S, Konishi H, Karakas B, Blair BG, Lin C, Peters BA, Velculescu VE, Park BH (2004) The PIK3CA gene is mutated with high frequency in human breast cancers. Cancer Biol Ther 3:772–775

Baselga J, Albanell J (2001) Mechanism of action of anti-HER2 monoclonal antibodies. Ann Oncol 12 Suppl 1:S35–S41

Bell DW, Gore I, Okimoto RA, Godin-Heymann N, Sordella R, Mulloy R, Sharma SV, Brannigan BW, Mohapatra G, Settleman J, Haber DA (2005) Inherited susceptibility to lung cancer may be associated with the T790 M drug resistance mutation in EGFR. Nat Genet 37:1315–1316

Berger MS, Locher GW, Saurer S, Gullick WJ, Waterfield MD, Groner B, Hynes NE (1988) Correlation of c-erbB-2 gene amplification and protein expression in human breast carcinoma with nodal status and nuclear grading. Cancer Res 48:1238-1243

Burstein HJ, Harris LN, Gelman R, Lester SC, Nunes RA, Kaelin CM, Parker LM, Ellisen LW, Kuter I, Gadd MA, Christian RL, Kennedy PR, Borges VF, Bunnell CA, Younger J, Smith BL, Winer EP (2003) Preoperative therapy with trastuzumab and paclitaxel followed by sequential adjuvant doxorubicin/cyclophosphamide for HER2 overexpressing stage II or III breast cancer: a pilot study. J Clin Oncol 21:46–53

Cappuzzo F, Hirsch FR, Rossi E, Bartolini S, Ceresoli GL, Bemis L, Haney J, Witta S, Danenberg K, Domenichini I, Ludovini V, Magrini E, Gregorc V, Doglioni C, Sidoni A, Tonato M, Franklin WA, Crino L, Bunn PA Jr, Varella-Garcia M (2005a) Epidermal growth factor receptor gene and protein and gefitinib sensitivity in non-small-cell lung cancer. J Natl Cancer Inst 97:643–655

Cappuzzo F, Varella-Garcia M, Shigematsu H, Domenichini I, Bartolini S, Ceresoli GL, Rossi E, Ludovini V, Gregorc V, Toschi L, Franklin WA, Crino L, Gazdar AF, Bunn PA Jr, Hirsch FR (2005b) Increased HER2 gene copy number is associated with response to gefitinib therapy in epidermal growth factor receptor-positive non-small-cell lung cancer patients. J Clin Oncol 23:5007–5018

Cho HS, Mason K, Ramyar KX, Stanley AM, Gabelli SB, Denney DW Jr, Leahy DJ (2003) Structure of the extracellular region of HER2 alone and in complex with the Herceptin Fab. Nature 421:756–760

Clynes RA, Towers TL, Presta LG, Ravetch JV (2000) Inhibitory Fc receptors modulate in vivo cytotoxicity against tumor targets. Nat Med 6:443–446

Cobleigh MA, Vogel CL, Tripathy D, Robert NJ, Scholl S, Fehrenbacher L, Wolter JM, Paton V, Shak S, Lieberman G, Slamon DJ (1999) Multinational study of the efficacy and safety of humanized anti-HER2 monoclonal antibody in women who have HER2-overexpressing metastatic breast cancer that has progressed after chemotherapy for metastatic disease. J Clin Oncol 17:2639–2648

Discafani CM, Carroll, ML, Floyd MB Jr, Hollander IJ, Husain Z, Johnson BD, Kitchen D, May MK, Malo MS, Minnick AA Jr, Nilakantan R, Shen R, Wang YF, Wissne, A, Greenberger LM (1999) Irreversible inhibition of epidermal growth factor receptor tyrosine kinase with in vivo activity by N-[4-[(3-bromophenyl)amino]-6-quinazolinyl]-2-butynamide (CL-387,785). Biochem Pharmacol 57:917–925

Doroshow JH (2005) Targeting EGFR in non-small-cell lung cancer. N Engl J Med 353:200–202

Dorsett Y, Tuschl T (2004) siRNAs:applications in functional genomics and potential as therapeutics. Nat Rev Drug Discov 3:318–329

Ekstrand AJ, Sugawa N, James CD, Collins VP (1992) Amplified and rearranged epidermal growth factor receptor genes in human glioblastomas reveal deletions of sequences encoding portions of the N- and/or C-terminal tails. Proc Natl Acad Sci USA 89:4309–4313

Eng C (2003) PTEN:one gene, many syndromes. Hum Mutat 22:183–198

Engelman JA, Janne PA, Mermel C, Pearlberg J, Mukohara T, Fleet C, Cichowski K, Johnson BE, Cantley LC (2005) ErbB-3 mediates phosphoinositide 3-kinase activity in gefitinib-sensitive non-small cell lung cancer cell lines. Proc Natl Acad Sci USA 102:3788–3793

Ermoian RP, Furniss CS, Lamborn KR, Basila D, Berger MS, Gottschalk AR, Nicholas MK, Stokoe D, Haas-Kogan DA (2002) Dysregulation of PTEN and protein kinase B is associated with glioma histology and patient survival. Clin Cancer Res 8:1100–1106

FitzGerald DJ, Kreitman R, Wilson W, Squires D, Pastan I (2004) Recombinant immunotoxins for treating cancer. Int J Med Microbiol 293:577–582

Gazit A, Yaish P, Gilon C, Levitzki A (1989) Tyrphostins I:synthesis and biological activity of protein tyrosine kinase inhibitors. J Med Chem 32:2344–2352

Gennari R, Menard S, Fagnoni F, Ponchio L, Scelsi M, Tagliabue E, Castiglioni F, Villani L, Magalotti C, Gibelli N, Oliviero B, Ballardini B, Da Prada G, Zambelli A, Costa A (2004) Pilot study of the mechanism of action of preoperative trastuzumab in patients with primary operable breast tumors overexpressing HER2. Clin Cancer Res 10:5650–5655

Gorre ME, Mohammed M, Ellwood K, Hsu N, Paquette R, Rao PN, Sawyers CL (2001) Clinical resistance to STI-571 cancer therapy caused by BCR-ABL gene mutation or amplification. Science 293:876–880

Goudar RK, Shi Q, Hjelmeland MD, Keir ST, McLendon RE, Wikstrand CJ, Reese ED, Conrad CA, Traxler P, Lane HA, Reardon DA, Cavenee WK, Wang XF, Bigner DD, Friedman HS, Rich JN (2005) Combination therapy of inhibitors of epidermal growth factor receptor/vascular endothelial growth factor receptor 2 (AEE788) and the mammalian target of rapamycin (RAD001) offers improved glioblastoma tumor growth inhibition. Mol Cancer Ther 4:101–112

Grandis JR, Drenning SD, Zeng Q, Watkins SC, Melhem MF, Endo S, Johnson DE, Huang L, He Y, Kim JD (2000) Constitutive activation of Stat3 signaling abrogates apoptosis in squamous cell carcinogenesis in vivo. Proc Natl Acad Sci USA 97:4227–4232

Graus-Porta D, Beerli RR, Daly JM, Hynes NE (1997) ErbB-2, the preferred heterodimerization partner of all ErbB receptors, is a mediator of lateral signaling. EMBO J 16:1647–1655

Greulich H, Chen TH, Feng W, Janne PA, Alvarez JV, Zappaterra M, Bulmer SE, Frank DA, Hahn WC, Sellers WR, and Meyerson M (2005) Oncogenic transformation by inhibitor-sensitive and -resistant EGFR mutants. PLoS Med 2:e313

Han SW, Kim TY, Hwang PG, Jeong S, Kim J, Choi IS, Oh DY, Kim JH, Kim DW, Chung DH, Im SA, Kim YT, Lee JS, Heo DS, Bang YJ, Kim NK (2005) Predictive and prognostic impact of epidermal growth factor receptor mutation in non-small-cell lung cancer patients treated with gefitinib. J Clin Oncol 23:2493–2501

Harwerth IM, Wels W, Marte BM, Hynes NE (1992) Monoclonal antibodies against the extracellular domain of the erbB-2 receptor function as partial ligand agonists. J Biol Chem 267:15160–15167

Holbro T, Beerli RR, Maurer F, Koziczak M, Barba, CF 3rd, Hynes NE (2003) The ErbB2/ErbB3 heterodimer functions as an oncogenic unit:ErbB2 requires ErbB3 to drive breast tumor cell proliferation. Proc Natl Acad Sci USA 100:8933–8938

Holbro T, Hynes NE (2004) ErbB receptors:directing key signaling networks throughout life. Annu Rev Pharmacol Toxicol 44:195–217

Hortobagyi GN (2005) Trastuzumab in the treatment of breast cancer. N Engl J Med 353:1734–1736

Hudziak RM, Lewis GD, Winget M, Fendly BM, Shepard HM, and Ullrich A (1989) p185HER2 monoclonal antibody has antiproliferative effects in vitro and sensitizes human breast tumor cells to tumor necrosis factor. Mol Cell Biol 9:1165–1172

Hynes NE, Lane HA (2005) ERBB receptors and cancer: the complexity of targeted inhibitors. Nat Rev Cancer 5:341–354

Izumi Y, Xu L, di Tomaso E, Fukumura D and Jain RK (2002) Tumour biology:herceptin acts as an anti-angiogenic cocktail. Nature 416:279–280

Johnson BE, Janne, PA (2005) Selecting patients for epidermal growth factor receptor inhibitor treatment: A FISH story or a tale of mutations? J Clin Oncol 23:6813–6816

Jones RB, Gordus A, Krall JA, MacBeath G (2006) A quantitative protein interaction network for the ErbB receptors using protein microarrays. Nature 439:168–174

Jorissen RN, Walker F, Pouliot N, Garrett TP, Ward CW, Burgess AW (2003) Epidermal growth factor receptor: mechanisms of activation and signalling. Exp Cell Res 284:31–53

Kim HH, Vijapurkar U, Hellyer NJ, Bravo D, Koland JG (1998) Signal transduction by epidermal growth factor and heregulin via the kinase-deficient ErbB3 protein. Biochem J 334:189–195

Klapper LN, Vaisman N, Hurwitz E, Pinkas-Kramarski R, Yarden Y Sela M (1997) A subclass of tumor-inhibitory monoclonal antibodies to ErbB-2/HER2 blocks crosstalk with growth factor receptors. Oncogene 14:2099–2109

Kobayashi S, Boggon TJ, Dayaram T, Janne PA, Kocher O, Meyerson M, Johnson BE, Eck MJ, Tenen DG, Halmos B (2005) EGFR mutation and resistance of non-small-cell lung cancer to gefitinib. N Engl J Med 352:786–792

Kochupurakkal BS, Harari D, Di-Segni A, Maik-Rachline G, Lyass L, Gur G, Kerber G, Citri A, Lavi S, Eilam R, Chalifa-Caspi V, Eshhar Z, Pikarsky E, Pinkas-Kramarski R, Bacus SS, Yarden Y (2005) Epigen, the last ligand of ErbB receptors, reveals intricate relationships between affinity and mitogenicity. J Biol Chem 280:8503–8512

Lane HA, Beuvink I, Motoyama AB, Daly JM, Neve RM, Hynes NE (2000) ErbB2 potentiates breast tumor proliferation through modulation of p27(Kip1)-Cdk2 complex formation: receptor overexpression does not determine growth dependency. Mol Cell Biol 20:3210–3223

Li S, Schmitz KR, Jeffrey PD, Wiltzius JJ, Kussie P, Ferguson KM (2005) Structural basis for inhibition of the epidermal growth factor receptor by cetuximab. Cancer Cell 7:301–311

Lynch TJ, Bell DW, Sordella R, Gurubhagavatula S, Okimoto RA, Brannigan BW, Harris PL, Haserlat SM, Supko JG, Haluska FG, Louis DN, Christiani DC, Settleman J, Haber DA (2004) Activating mutations in the epidermal growth factor receptor underlying responsiveness of non-small-cell lung cancer to gefitinib. N Engl J Med 350:2129–2139

Mellinghoff IK, Wang MY, Vivanco, I, Haas-Kogan DA, Zhu S, Dia EQ, Lu KV, Yoshimoto K, Huang JH, Chute DJ, Riggs BL, Horvath S, Liau LM, Cavenee WK, Rao PN, Beroukhim R, Peck TC, Lee JC, Sellers WR, Stokoe D, Prados M, Cloughesy TF, Sawyers CL, Mischel PS (2005) Molecular determinants of the response of glioblastomas to EGFR kinase inhibitors. N Engl J Med 353:2012–2024

Minna JD, Peyton MJ, Gazdar AF (2005) Gefitinib versus cetuximab in lung cancer: round one. J Natl Cancer Inst 97:1168–1169

Mitsudomi T, Kosaka T, Endoh H, Horio Y, Hida T, Mori S, Hatooka S, Shinoda M, Takahashi T, Yatabe Y (2005) Mutations of the epidermal growth factor receptor gene predict prolonged survival after gefitinib treatment in patients with non-small-cell lung cancer with postoperative recurrence. J Clin Oncol 23:2513–2520

Moghal N, Sternberg PW (2003) The epidermal growth factor system in Caenorhabditis elegans. Exp Cell Res 284:150–159

Mohsin SK, Weiss HL, Gutierrez MC, Chamness GC, Schiff R, Digiovanna MP, Wang CX, Hilsenbeck SG, Osborne CK, Allred DC, Elledge R, Chang JC (2005) Neoadjuvant trastuzumab induces apoptosis in primary breast cancers. J Clin Oncol 23:2460–2468

Molina MA, Codony-Servat J, Albanell J, Rojo F, Arribas J, Baselga J (2001) Trastuzumab (herceptin), a humanized anti-Her2 receptor monoclonal antibody, inhibits basal and activated Her2 ectodomain cleavage in breast cancer cells. Cancer Res 61:4744–4749

Mosesson Y, Yarden Y (2004) Oncogenic growth factor receptors:implications for signal transduction therapy. Semin Cancer Biol 14:262–270

Motoyama AB, Hynes NE, Lane HA (2002) The efficacy of ErbB receptor-targeted anticancer therapeutics is influenced by the availability of epidermal growth factor-related peptides. Cancer Res 62:3151–3158

Mukohara T, Engelman JA, Hanna NH, Yeap BY, Kobayashi S, Lindeman N, Halmos B, Pearlberg J, Tsuchihashi Z, Cantley LC, Tenen DG, Johnson BE, Janne PA (2005) Differential effects of gefitinib and cetuximab on non-small-cell lung cancers bearing epidermal growth factor receptor mutations. J Natl Cancer Inst 97:1185–1194

Nagata Y, Lan KH, Zhou X, Tan M, Esteva FJ, Sahin AA, Klos KS, Li P, Monia BP, Nguyen NT, Hortobagyi GN, Hung MC, Yu D (2004) PTEN activation contributes to tumor inhibition by trastuzumab, and loss of PTEN predicts trastuzumab resistance in patients. Cancer Cell 6:117–127

Nicholson RI, Gee JM, Harper ME (2001) EGFR and cancer prognosis. Eur J Cancer 37 Suppl 4:S9–S15

Oda K, Matsuoka Y, Funahashi A, Kitano H (2005) A comprehensive pathway map of epidermal growth factor receptor signaling. Mol Systems Biol 1:8–24

Ohgaki H, Dessen P, Jourde B, Horstmann S, Nishikawa T, Di Patre PL, Burkhard C, Schuler D, Probst-Hensch NM, Maiorka PC, Baeza N, Pisani P, Yonekawa Y, Yasargil MG, Lutolf UM, Kleihues P (2004) Genetic pathways to glioblastoma:a population-based study. Cancer Res 64:6892–6899

Olayioye MA, Neve RM, Lane HA, Hynes NE (2000) The ErbB signaling network: receptor heterodimerization in development and cancer. EMBO J 19:3159–3167

Paez JG, Janne PA, Lee JC, Tracy S, Greulich H, Gabriel S, Herman P, Kaye FJ, Lindeman N, Boggon TJ, Naoki K, Sasaki H, Fujii Y, Eck MJ, Sellers WR, Johnson BE, Meyerson M (2004) EGFR mutations in lung cancer: correlation with clinical response to gefitinib therapy. Science 304:1497–1500

Pao W, Miller V, Zakowski M, Doherty J, Politi K, Sarkaria I, Singh B, Heelan R, Rusch V, Fulton L, Mardis E, Kupfer D, Wilson R, Kris M, Varmus H (2004) EGF receptor gene mutations are common in lung cancers from "never smokers" and are associated with sensitivity of tumors to gefitinib and erlotinib. Proc Natl Acad Sci USA 101:13306–13311

Pao W, Miller VA, Politi KA, Riely GJ, Somwar R, Zakowski MF, Kris MG, Varmus H (2005) Acquired resistance of lung adenocarcinomas to gefitinib or erlotinib is associated with a second mutation in the EGFR kinase domain. PLoS Med 2:e73

Piccart-Gebhart MJ, Procter M, Leyland-Jones B, Goldhirsch A, Untch M, Smith I, Gianni L, Baselga J, Bell R, Jackisch C, Cameron D, Dowsett M, Barrios CH, Steger G, Huang CS, Andersson M, Inbar M, Lichnitser M, Lang I, Nitz U, Iwata H, Thomssen C, Lohrisch C, Suter TM, Ruschoff J, Suto T, Greatorex V, Ward C, Straehle C, McFadden E, Dolci MS, Gelber RD (2005) Trastuzumab after adjuvant chemotherapy in HER2-positive breast cancer. N Engl J Med 353:1659–1672

Pollard JW (2004) Tumour-educated macrophages promote tumour progression and metastasis. Nat Rev Cancer 4:71–78

Rich JN, Reardon DA, Peery T, Dowell JM, Quinn JA, Penne KL, Wikstrand CJ, Van Duyn LB, Dancey JE, McLendon RE, Kao JC, Stenzel TT, Ahmed Rasheed BK, Tourt-Uhlig SE, Herndon JE 2nd, Vredenburgh JJ, Sampson JH, Friedman AH, Bigner DD, Friedman HS (2004) Phase II trial of gefitinib in recurrent glioblastoma. J Clin Oncol 22:133–142

Riese DJ 2nd, Stern DF (1998) Specificity within the EGF family/ErbB receptor family signaling network. Bioessays 20:41–48

Romond EH, Perez EA, Bryant J, Suman VJ, Geyer CE Jr, Davidson NE, Tan-Chiu E, Martino S, Paik S, Kaufman PA, Swain SM, Pisansky TM, Fehrenbacher L, Kutteh LA, Vogel VG, Visscher DW, Yothers G, Jenkins RB, Brown AM, Dakhil SR, Mamounas EP, Lingle WL, Klein PM, Ingle JN, Wolmark N (2005) Trastuzumab plus adjuvant chemotherapy for operable HER2-positive breast cancer. N Engl J Med 353:1673–1684

Ross JS, Fletcher JA, Linette GP, Stec J, Clark E, Ayers M, Symmans WF, Pusztai L, Bloom KJ (2003) The Her-2/neu gene and protein in breast cancer 2003: biomarker and target of therapy. Oncologist 8:307–325

Rubin Grandis J, Melhem MF, Gooding WE, Day R, Holst VA, Wagener MM, Drenning SD, Tweardy DJ (1998) Levels of TGF-alpha and EGFR protein in head and neck squamous cell carcinoma and patient survival. J Natl Cancer Inst 90:824–832

Salomon, DS, Brandt, R, Ciardiello, F and Normanno, N (1995) Epidermal growth factor-related peptides and their receptors in human malignancies. Crit Rev Oncol Hematol 19:183–232

Samuels, Y, Wang, Z, Bardelli, A, Silliman, N, Ptak, J, Szabo, S, Yan, H, Gazdar, A, Powell, SM, Riggins, GJ, Willson, JK, Markowitz, S, Kinzler, KW, Vogelstein, B

and Velculescu, VE (2004) High frequency of mutations of the PIK3CA gene in human cancers. Science 304:554

Sato JD, Kawamoto T, Le AD, Mendelsohn J, Polikoff J, Sato GH (1983) Biological effects in vitro of monoclonal antibodies to human epidermal growth factor receptors. Mol Biol Med 1:511–529

Schechter AL, Hung MC, Vaidyanathan L, Weinberg RA, Yang-Feng TL, Francke U, Ullrich A, Coussens L (1985) The neu gene:an erbB-homologous gene distinct from and unlinked to the gene encoding the EGF receptor. Science 229:976–978

Schlessinger J (2004) Common and distinct elements in cellular signaling via EGF and FGF receptors. Science 306:1506–1507

Schreiber AB, Lax I, Yarden Y, Eshhar Z, Schlessinger J (1981) Monoclonal antibodies against receptor for epidermal growth factor induce early and delayed effects of epidermal growth factor. Proc Natl Acad Sci USA 78:7535–7539

Semba K, Kamata N, Toyoshima K, Yamamoto T (1985) A v-erbB-related protooncogene, c-erbB-2, is distinct from the c-erbB-1/epidermal growth factor-receptor gene and is amplified in a human salivary gland adenocarcinoma. Proc Natl Acad Sci USA 82:6497–6501

Shepherd FA, Rodrigues Pereira J, Ciuleanu T, Tan EH, Hirsh V, Thongprasert S, Campos D, Maoleekoonpiroj S, Smylie M, Martins R, van Kooten M, Dediu M, Findlay B, Tu D, Johnston D, Bezjak A, Clark G, Santabarbara P, Seymour, L (2005) Erlotinib in previously treated non-small-cell lung cancer. N Engl J Med 353:123–132

Shigematsu H, Gazdar AF (2006) Somatic mutations of epidermal growth factor receptor signaling pathway in lung cancers. Int J Cancer 118:257–262

Shigematsu H, Takahashi T, Nomura M, Majmudar K, Suzuki M, Lee H, Wistuba II, Fong KM, Toyooka S, Shimizu N, Fujisawa T, Minna JD, Gazdar AF (2005) Somatic mutations of the HER2 kinase domain in lung adenocarcinomas. Cancer Res 65:1642–1646

Slamon DJ, Clark GM, Wong SG, Levin WJ, Ullrich A, McGuire WL (1987) Human breast cancer:correlation of relapse and survival with amplification of the HER-2/neu oncogene. Science 235:177–182

Slamon DJ, Leyland-Jones B, Shak S, Fuchs H, Paton V, Bajamonde A, Fleming T, Eiermann W, Wolter J, Pegram M, Baselga J, Norton L (2001) Use of chemotherapy plus a monoclonal antibody against HER2 for metastatic breast cancer that overexpresses HER2. N Engl J Med 344:783–792

Smith JS, Tachibana I, Passe SM, Huntley BK, Borell TJ, Iturria N, O'Fallon JR, Schaefer PL, Scheithauer BW, James CD, Buckner JC, Jenkins RB (2001) PTEN mutation, EGFR amplification, and outcome in patients with anaplastic astrocytoma and glioblastoma multiforme. J Natl Cancer Inst 93:1246–1256

Sordella R, Bell DW, Haber DA, Settleman J (2004) Gefitinib-sensitizing EGFR mutations in lung cancer activate anti-apoptotic pathways. Science 305:1163–1167

Stephens P, Hunter C, Bignell G, Edkins S, Davies H, Teague J, Stevens C, O'Meara S, Smith R, Parker A, Barthorpe A, Blow M, Brackenbury L, Butler A, Clarke O, Cole J, Dicks E, Dike A, Drozd A, Edwards K, Forbes S, Foster R, Gray K, Greenman C, Halliday K, Hills K, Kosmidou V, Lugg R, Menzies A, Perry J, Petty R, Raine K, Ratford L, Shepherd R, Small A, Stephens Y, Tofts C, Varian J, West S, Widaa S, Yates A, Brasseur F, Cooper CS, Flanagan AM, Knowles M, Leung SY, Louis,DN, Looijenga LH, Malkowicz B, Pierotti MA, Teh B, Chenevix-Trench G, Weber BL, Yuen ST, Harris G, Goldstraw P, Nicholson AG, Futreal PA, Wooster R, Stratton, MR (2004) Lung cancer:intragenic ERBB2 kinase mutations in tumours. Nature 431:525–526

Sunpaweravong P, Sunpaweravong S, Puttawibul P, Mitarnun W, Zeng C, Baron AE, Franklin W, Said S, Varella-Garcia M (2005) Epidermal growth factor receptor and cyclin D1 are independently amplified and over-expressed in esophageal squamous cell carcinoma. J Cancer Res Clin Oncol 131:111–119

Takano T, Ohe Y, Sakamoto H, Tsuta K, Matsuno Y, Tateishi U, Yamamoto S, Nokihara H, Yamamoto N, Sekine I, Kunitoh H, Shibata T, Sakiyama T, Yoshida T, Tamura T (2005) Epidermal growth factor receptor gene mutations and increased copy numbers predict gefitinib sensitivity in patients with recurrent non-small-cell lung cancer. J Clin Oncol 23:6829–6837

Thompson JE, Thompson CB (2004) Putting the rap on Akt. J Clin Oncol 22:4217–4226

Traxler P (2003) Tyrosine kinases as targets in cancer therapy – successes and failures. Expert Opin Ther Targets 7:215–234

Tsao MS, Sakurada A, Cutz JC, Zhu CQ, Kamel-Reid S, Squire J, Lorimer I, Zhang T, Liu N, Daneshmand M, Marrano P, da Cunha Santos G, Lagarde A, Richardson F, Seymour L, Whitehead M, Ding K, Pater J, Shepherd FA (2005) Erlotinib in lung cancer – molecular and clinical predictors of outcome. N Engl J Med 353:133–144

von Minckwitz G, Harder S, Hovelmann S, Jager E, Al-Batran SE, Loibl S, Atmaca A, Cimpoiasu C, Neumann A, Abera A, Knuth A, Kaufmann M, Jager D, Maurer AB, Wels WS (2005) Phase I clinical study of the recombinant antibody toxin scFv(FRP5)-ETA specific for the ErbB2/HER2 receptor in patients with advanced solid malignomas. Breast Cancer Res 7: R617–R626

Yakes FM, Chinratanalab W, Ritter CA, King W, Seelig S, Arteaga CL (2002) Herceptin-induced inhibition of phosphatidylinositol-3 kinase and Akt Is required for antibody-mediated effects on p27, cyclin D1, and antitumor action. Cancer Res 62:4132–4141

Yarden Y, Sliwkowski MX (2001) Untangling the ErbB signalling network. Nat Rev Mol Cell Biol 2:127–137

Inhibition of the IGF-I Receptor for Treatment of Cancer. Kinase Inhibitors and Monoclonal Antibodies as Alternative Approaches

Yan Wang, Qun-sheng Ji, Mark Mulvihill, and Jonathan A. Pachter

Recent Results in Cancer Research, Vol. 172
© Springer-Verlag Berlin Heidelberg 2007

5.1 Introduction

Insulin-like growth factor (IGF) signaling plays a critical role in the growth and differentiation of many tissues, particularly in prenatal growth and puberty. The IGF axis is also implicated in various pathophysiological conditions, and is believed to play a crucial role in tumorigenesis (Pollak et al. 2004).

The IGF system is composed of two peptide ligands (IGF-I and IGF-II); a signaling receptor, the insulin-like growth factor receptor (IGF-IR); a "decoy" receptor for IGF-II, IGF-IIR; and six IGF-binding proteins (IGFBPs). The IGF ligands are 7-kDa polypeptides that act as potent growth stimulators for a wide variety of cells, working in either an autocrine or an endocrine fashion. IGF expression often occurs in specific tissues at developmental stages in which these tissues are undergoing rapid growth. In vitro, IGFs not only promote cell growth but also affect cell differentiation and have antiapoptotic effects. Both IGF-I and IGF-II bind with high affinity to the IGF-IR to initiate signaling. IGF-I is produced largely by the liver in response to growth hormone, while IGF-II is often produced locally, especially by tumor cells.

The human IGF-IR gene is located on chromosome 15 q25/26. Its coding region has 4,101 nucleotides coding for a 1,367-amino acid precursor protein that is proteolytically cleaved into two subunits, α and β (Sepp-Lorenzino 1998). The mature α- and β-subunits are linked by disulfide bonds to form α–β dimers, which in turn dimerize to form $\alpha 2\beta 2$ receptors (IGF-IR). The α-subunits are extracellular and responsible for ligand binding, whereas the β-subunits contain a transmembrane domain and an intracellular tyrosine kinase domain. Binding of an IGF to the α-subunit transmits a signal through the transmembrane domain to the β-subunit, which undergoes a conformational change resulting in autophosphorylation (i.e. activation) of the receptor. Activated IGF-IR in turn phosphorylates tyrosine residues on two major substrates, IRS-1 and Shc, which subsequently signal through the Ras/MAPK and PI3-kinase/AKT pathways.

IGF-IIR is also known as the mannose 6-phosphate receptor and binds IGF-II and other ligands containing a mannose 6-phosphate recognition marker (Okamoto et al. 1990). IGF-IIR binds to IGF-II with high affinity and mediates internalization and degradation of the IGF-II ligand. IGF-IIR has no signaling role but can act as a sink to decrease IGF-II signaling through the IGF-IR.

Insulin receptor (IR) is a closely related receptor tyrosine kinase, and it shares high sequence homology with the IGF-IR. Both the IGF-IR and the IR are tetrameric complexes consisting of two extracellular α-subunits that bind their respective ligands and two β-subunits that mediate ligand-dependent tyrosine kinase activity. In cells that coexpress IGF-IR and IR, heterodimeric receptors can form consisting of one IGF-IR α- and one IGF-IR β-

subunit together with one IR α- and one IR β-subunit. The IGF-IR:IR heterodimeric receptor behaves more like IGF-IR than IR, exhibiting an affinity for IGF-II similar to that of the IGF-IR homodimer. The heterodimeric receptor binds insulin with lower affinity (Siddle et al. 1994).

Most IGFs in circulation bind to members of a family of high-affinity IGF binding proteins (IGFBPs) that are found in the circulation and in extracellular compartments and are produced by most tissues. Six IGFBPs have been identified. The IGFBPs have been proposed to prolong the half-lives of the IGFs and to modulate the interaction of IGFs with their receptors. IGFBPs can also have IGF-independent functions that may include direct nuclear interactions. The overall impact of IGFBP binding is complex and remains an active area of research (Firth and Baxter 2002).

Several decades of research have demonstrated that there is an association between the IGF system and cancer. This review will focus on the role of IGF-IR in cancer and therapeutic approaches targeting the IGF-IR that have been developed for the treatment of cancer.

5.2 Normal Physiology of IGF Action

IGF-I has characteristics of both a circulating hormone and a tissue growth factor. Most IGF-I found in the circulation is produced by the liver. IGF-II is usually produced by local tissues. Both IGF-I and IGF-II signal through IGF-IR.

Studies of knockout mice in which various IGF system components have been ablated have established the roles of the IGF ligands and the IGF-IR in normal physiology, with particularly important roles in prenatal and postnatal growth. Mice with complete ablation of IGF-I expression exhibit marked growth retardation. Birth weights of IGF-I knockout mice are reduced by 40% relative to wild-type mice. The major histological findings in IGF-I knockout mice are delayed ossification, mus-

cular dystrophy, and brain abnormalities. In contrast, heterozygous mice exhibit little to no growth retardation, indicating that a single normal IGF-I allele is sufficient for normal or near-normal growth (Baker et al. 1993; Powell-Braxton et al. 1993).

Birth weights of IGF-II knockout mice are approximately 60% that of wild-type mice. However, the postnatal growth rate of IGF-II knockout mice is normal. But adult IGF-II knockout mice remain approximately 60% of normal size since no postnatal catch-up growth occurs. Fertility of the IGF-II knockout mice is not affected, and the mice live a normal life span. Histologically, IGF-II knockout mice display no apparent abnormalities, suggesting that, with the exception of lower gross body weight, normal functions of IGF-II may be compensated by IGF-I or other factors during development (DeChiara et al. 1990).

Disruption of the gene for IGF-IR results in profound growth retardation. Homozygous knockout mice are approximately 45% of normal size, suggesting that the IGF-IR mediates most of the growth-promoting actions of IGFs (Liu et al. 1993). The histological findings in IGF-IR knockout mice are similar to that of IGF-I knockout mice although more severe, including delayed ossification, muscle hypoplasia, and brain abnormalities. The severe growth retardation occurs during the second half of gestation and is predominantly a deficit in cellular proliferation (hypoplasia). Mice heterozygous for IGF-IR knockout are normal, indicating that a single functional allele is sufficient for normal growth.

Disruption of the IGF-IIR does not result in growth retardation (Lau et al. 1994). Rather, it results in moderate fetal and placental overgrowth. Birth weight of IGF-IIR knockout mice is ~130% of normal. The serum concentration of IGF-II is increased twofold in IGF-IIR knockout mice, consistent with the hypothesis that the overgrowth is due to enhanced IGF-II stimulation. These mouse studies have indicated that IGF-IIR is not part of the IGF growth signaling system, but a "decoy" receptor for IGF-II.

Overexpression studies in mice have also contributed to our understanding of IGF functions. Overexpression of IGF-I or IGF-II induced rather different phenotypes. Mice overexpressing IGF-I are significantly larger and weigh approximately 30% more than normal. Overgrowth is observed in multiple organs including brain, kidney, pancreas, and spleen (Mathews et al. 1988). In contrast, transgenic mice overexpressing IGF-II displayed no overgrowth (Van Buul-Offers et al. 1995; Ward et al. 1994). However, when expressed locally, IGF-II has clearly been shown to stimulate growth (Rogler et al. 1994).

5.3 IGF Signaling in Cancer

IGF ligands and the IGF-IR have been shown to play a critical role in the development and progression of human cancer. Fibroblasts derived from IGF-IR knockout mice are resistant to transformation by Ras, SV40, large T antigen, or EGFR overexpression (Sell et al. 1994). Overexpression of the IGF-IR in NIH-3T3 cells transforms cells as indicated by ligand-dependent mitogenesis under serum-free conditions, anchorage-independent growth, and tumor formation in nude mice (Butler et al. 1998). The IGF-IR is expressed by various cancer cells. Immunohistochemical analysis of IGF-IR protein expression revealed highest levels of receptor expression in epithelial cells of the ovary, prostate, and uterus. Solid tumors are mostly of epithelial origin. Positive IGF-IR staining is associated with poor survival in patients with clear cell renal cell carcinoma (Parker et al. 2002). Recent literature has also suggested that IGF-IR overexpression can confer resistance to both anti-EGFR and anti-Her2 therapies, suggesting potential therapeutic utility for IGF-1R inhibition in combination with inhibitors of EGFR and/or Her2 (Lu et al. 2001; Chakravarti et al. 2002).

In addition to proliferation, IGF-IR activation promotes cellular survival in the presence of a variety of apoptotic stimuli including hypoxia, growth factor depletion, TNF-α, and chemotherapeutic agents. This antiapoptotic activity of the IGF-IR is believed to be mediated predominantly through activation of the PI3-kinase/AKT pathways (Rodriguez-Tarduchy et al. 1992; Wu et al. 1996; Sell et al. 1995; Kulik et al. 1997; Singleton et al. 1996).

In mouse models, constitutive expression of IGF-I in epidermal basal cells resulted in epidermal hyperplasia and hyperkeratosis. IGF-I transgenic mice developed sevenfold more papillomas than their wild-type littermates after application of a tumor initiator and tumor promoter (DiGiovanni et al. 2000a). When IGF-I was constitutively expressed in prostate epithelium, mice developed prostatic hyperplasia by 2–3 months of age and intraepithelial neoplasia by 6–7 months of age (DiGiovanni et al., 2000b).

Epidemiological studies implicate the IGF-I axis as a predisposing factor in the pathogenesis of human breast, prostate, and colorectal cancers (Pollak et al. 2004). One study using prospectively collected plasma samples revealed that men whose IGF-I levels fell into the upper quartile had a greater than twofold increased risk of developing prostate cancer compared with those in the lowest quartile (Chan et al. 1998).

Overexpression of IGF-II in transgenic mouse models also leads to an increased incidence of various malignancies. Overexpression of IGF-II and IGF-IR are important in the pathogenesis of Wilms tumor, a common childhood kidney tumor (Reeve et al. 1985; Werner et al. 1993). When mutated, the tumor suppressor gene WT1 cannot exert its normal repression of IGF-II and IGF-IR transcription. The resulting increase in autocrine IGF-II-induced IGF-IR signaling stimulates uncontrolled tumor growth.

5.4 Targeting the IGF-IR for Treatment of Human Cancer

Since the IGF-IR is the major signaling receptor for both IGF-I and IGF-II, blockade of the IGF-IR is the most direct approach to shut down the tumorigenic effects of the IGF axis. Accordingly, extensive literature has indicated that inhibition of IGF-IR function by antisense, dominant-negative truncation, small-molecule kinase inhibitors, or neutralizing antibodies inhibits transformation and tumor growth in mice.

Two types of dominant-negative mutants of IGF-IR have been documented. One is the soluble receptor truncated at residue 486 (486/STOP), and the other is the truncated receptor at residue 952 (952/STOP). In vitro, both can inhibit IGF-IR signaling and tumor cell growth in soft agar. In vivo, both abrogate tumor growth in mice. Interestingly, neither 486/STOP nor 952/STOP effectively inhibits the monolayer growth of tumor cells (Reiss et al. 1998; D'Ambrosio et al. 1996). Similar to dominant-negative truncations, IGF-IR antisense reverses the transformed phenotype or inhibits tumorigenesis (Burfeind et al. 1996). Although these approaches provided early preclinical proof-of-concept for inhibition of IGF-1R as a means to reduce tumor growth, these approaches may have limited clinical utility. Accordingly, the remainder of this review focuses on IGF-IR kinase inhibitors and human anti-IGF-IR neutralizing antibodies as two promising approaches for the treatment of human cancers. To illustrate these approaches in more depth, one IGF-IR kinase inhibitor (PQIP, OSI Pharmaceuticals) and one human anti-IGF-IR antibody (19D12, Schering-Plough) will be described in some detail.

5.5 IGF-IR: A Target for Treatment of Cancer

5.5.1 Kinase Inhibitors

The protein tyrosine kinase activity of the IGF-IR is essential for its biological function, and inhibition of the kinase activity by small molecules is therefore a direct approach to block the functional role of IGF-IR in cancer (Prager et al. 1994; Kalebic et al. 1998; Scotlandi et al. 2002). One major advantage of small-molecule kinase inhibitors is the potential for oral bioavailability. However, a major challenge in developing a small-molecule IGF-IR kinase inhibitor is building in selectivity over the highly

homologous insulin receptor (IR). The ATP binding sites of IGF-IR and IR are identical, whereas the entire kinase domains share 84% sequence identity. However, the insulin receptor has a distinct biological function in the regulation of glucose transport and biosynthesis of glycogen and fat (De Meyts et al. 2002). X-ray crystal structures have also revealed high structural similarity between these two kinase domains (Favelyukis et al. 2001). Since the IGF-IR can form heterodimeric receptors with IR in many mammalian cells including tumor cells (Frasca et al. 1999; Pandini, et al. 1999), and the insulin receptor-A form of the IR might also mediate tumor cell responses to IGF-II (Sciacca et al. 1999; Denley et al. 2003), there are pros and cons to including some degree of insulin receptor kinase inhibitory activity in an IGF-IR kinase inhibitor designed for the treatment of cancer.

5.5.1.1 Small-Molecule IGF-IR Kinase Inhibitors with Selectivity vs. IR

A number of small-molecule IGF-IR kinase inhibitors including PQIP (OSI Pharmaceuticals), NVP-AEW541 (Novartis), PPP (Karolinska Cancer Institute), and INSM-18 (Insmed) have been reported to demonstrate cellular selectivity relative to the human IR and appear to show a corresponding therapeutic window to induce antitumor efficacy without substantial hyperglycemia in animal models. However, it remains unclear whether this cellular selectivity is partially dependent on cellular background in IGF-1R and IR autophosphorylation assays, and whether the therapeutic window observed in preclinical models is due mainly to cellular selectivity, insulin-mediated homeostatic processes, or both.

PQIP,cis-3-[3-(4-methyl-piperazin-l-yl) cyclobutyl]-(2-phenyl-quinolin-7-yl)-imidazo [1,5-a] pyrazin-8-ylamine (Table 5.1, compound 1), an analog of the phenyl-quinolinyl-imidazo[1,5-a]pyrazine series, has demonstrated potent IGF-IR inhibitory activity with selectivity over human insulin receptor in cellular assays (Ji et al. 2006). PQIP displayed a cellular IC50 of 0.019 µM for inhibition of ligand-dependent autophosphorylation of hu-

Table 5.1 Summary of small-molecule IGF-IR inhibitors

Structure	Name	Comments	Reference
	Compound 1 (PQIP) Imidazo[1,5-a] pyrazine analog	OSI Pharmaceuticals, Inc Reversible ATP-competitive Cellular IC_{50}: IGF-IR=0.019 μM and IR=0.27 μM (14-fold selective) Selective toward panel of 32 kinases Demonstrated in vivo antitumor efficacy No substantial hyperglycemia at maximally efficacious dose in mice Status: preclinical	Ji et al. 2007
	Compound 2 (NVP-AEW541) Pyrrolopyrimidine analog	Novartis Co Reversible ATP-competitive Cellular IC_{50}: IGF-IR=0.086 μM and IR=1.38 μM (16-fold selective) Demonstrated in vivo antitumor efficacy No hyperglycemia in mice Status: preclinical	Garcia-Echeverria et al. 2004
	Compound 3 (PPP)	Karolinska Cancer Institute and Bovitrum Non-ATP-competitive Cellular IC_{50}: IGF-IR^{Tyr1136}=0.4 μM No inhibition of IR phosphorylation Demonstrated in vivo antitumor efficacy No hyperglycemia in mice Status: preclinical	Girnita et al. 2004
Not Disclosed	Compound 4 (INSM18)	Insmed, Inc Dual IGF-IR/Her2 inhibitor Biochemical IC_{50}: IGF-IR=0.3 μM Cellular IC_{50}: IGF-IR=22 μM Demonstrated in vivo antitumor efficacy No hyperglycemia in mice Status: phase II clinical studies for prostate cancer	Hofmann, et. al. 2005
	Compound 5 (BMS-554417) Benzimidazole analog	Bristol-Myers Squibb Co Reversible ATP-competitive Biochemical IC_{50}: IGF-IR=0.068 μM; IR=0.051 μM; FAK=0.090 μM Similar cell activity for inhibiting IGF-IR and IR (nonselective toward IR) CYP3A4-BFC IC_{50}=0.5 μM Demonstrated in vivo antitumor efficacy Hyperglycemia in mice Status: preclinical	Haluska et al. 2006
Not Disclosed	Compound 6 (XL-228)	Exelixis, Inc Dual IGF-IR/Src inhibitor Status: IND track candidate	

Structure	Name	Comments	Reference
Not Disclosed	Compound 7 (OSI-906)	OSI Pharmaceuticals, Inc. Reversible ATP competitive Status: IND track candidate phase I clinical	
	Compound 8 Pyrrole analog	Merck Co Reversible ATP-competitive covalent binder Sixfold selective toward IR Status: research	Bell et al. 2005
	Compound 9 (AG-10240) Tyrphostin analog	Pfizer Co Non-ATP-competitive Cellular IC_{50}: IGF-IR=7 µM and IR=57 µM (8-fold selective) Status: research	Parrizas et al. 1997
	Compound 10 Pyrrolopyrimidine analog	SUNY Stony Brook & Duquesne University Non-ATP-competitive 3× selective toward IR in biochemical assay Status: research	Li et al. 2004
	Compound 11 2,4-Diaminopyrimidine analog	Amgen, Inc Example from patent literature Status: unknown	Harmange et al. 2003
	Compound 12 3,4-Dihydro-1H-pyrrolo[1,2-a]pyrazine analog	Aventis Co Example from patent literature Status: unknown	Ratcliffe et al., 2003

man IGF-IR in 3T3/huIGF1R cells (NIH-3T3 line stably overexpressing full-length human IGF-IR) with 14-fold cellular selectivity relative to the highly homologous human insulin receptor in HepG2 cells. Among a panel of 34 protein kinases tested at 100 µM ATP, this compound was extremely selective, with only IGF-IR and IR showing IC50 values less than 10 µM. When tested in 3T3/huIGF1R cells, PQIP effectively blocked IGF-I-stimulated receptor autophosphorylation and downstream pathway effectors including phospho-ERK, phospho-AKT, and phospho-p70S6 K (Fig. 5.1). In cell-based functional assays, PQIP inhibited proliferation of tumor cells including a human GEO colorectal cancer cell line (Table 5.2).

Further studies revealed that GEO human colorectal cancer cells have an active IGF-II/IGF-IR autocrine loop, as supported by sustained basal phosphorylation of IGF-IR under serum-free conditions without ligand stimulation and significant IGF-II expression (Fig. 5.2a and b). In addition, depleting IGF-II in the conditioned culture medium by a neutralizing antibody diminished the activation of IGF-IR (Fig. 5.2c and d). PQIP fully blocked the active IGF-II autocrine loop, as indicated by the complete inhibition of basal phosphorylation of IGF-IR in the presence of 10% FCS without IGF addition. Furthermore, PQIP effectively inhibited AKT activation but not Erk1/2 activation in the presence of 10% FCS (Fig. 5.2e), suggesting that pAKT is IGF-

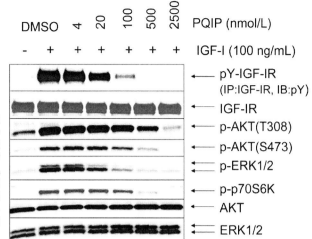

Fig. 5.1 Inhibition of ligand-stimulated pIGF-IR, *pAKT*, *pErk1/2* and *p-p70S6K* by *PQIP* in 3T3/huIGFIR cells. Serum-starved 3T3/huIGFIR cells were incubated with *PQIP* at indicated concentrations for 2 h at 37°C, followed by stimulation with IGF-I ligand for 15 min. Cell lysates were then analyzed by immunoprecipitation and immunoblotting for both total and phosphorylated target protein content

Table 5.2 Antiproliferative effects of PQIP

Tumor type	Cell line	IC$_{50}$ (µM)
Colorectal	SW620	0.023
	Colo205	0.470
	SW480	0.098
	GEO	0.600
	HT29	0.099
	HCT116	0.500
	HCT8	>10.0
Breast	MCF-7	0.040
	DU4475	0.124
Pancreatic	BxPC3	0.220
	MiaPaca2	0.063
	HPAC	0.052
	Panc1	>10.0
	A1165	>10.0

IR dependent and ERK1/2 can be activated by non-IGF-IR-dependent mechanisms in GEO cells. Accordingly, PQIP was found to effectively induce apoptosis of GEO cells, as indicated by PARP cleavage in the presence of 10% FCS (Fig. 5.2f). In cell-based functional assays, the antiproliferative potency of PQIP was comparable between 0.5% FCS and 10% FCS (Table 5.3), suggesting that autocrine IGF-II is the main driver for GEO cell proliferation even in the presence of additional growth factors from serum. Furthermore, anchorage-independent growth of GEO cells was quite sensitive to inhibition by PQIP. When GEO cell tumors were grown as xenografts in nude mice, IGF-IR tyrosine phosphorylation was also detected, and the inhibition of activated IGF-IR in GEO tumors correlated with strong antitumor efficacy of PQIP as a single oral agent in this xenograft model (Figs. 5.3 and 5.4). These data clearly demonstrated that PQIP effectively blocks the active IGF-II/IGF-IR autocrine loop essential for GEO cell growth and survival in vitro and in vivo. Preclinical observations that tumors with an IGF-II/IGF-IR autocrine loop are especially sensitive to IGF-IR inhibition suggest that tumor IGF-II overexpression and basal IGF-IR phosphorylation may be useful as biomarkers to predict clinical efficacy.

The cellular IGF-IR/IR selectivity of PQIP correlated with an in vivo therapeutic window in which antitumor efficacy was achieved with-

Table 5.3 Inhibition of GEO cell proliferation and colony formation by PQIP

Cell	GEO cells		
Assay	Proliferation		Soft agar
Conditions	0.5% FCS	10% FCS	10% FCS
IC$_{50}$ (µM)	0.81	0.60	0.08

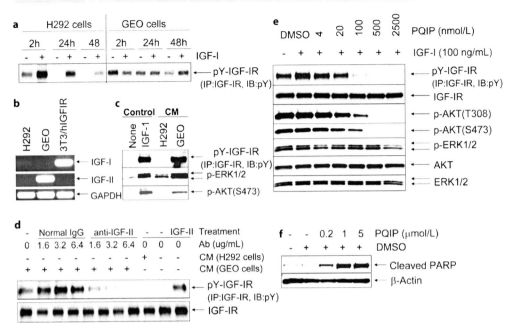

Fig. 5.2a–f. Active IGF-II/IGF-IR autocrine loop in GEO cells and inhibition of the autocrine activation of IGF-IR by PQIP. **a** NCI-H292 and GEO cells were cultured in serum-free DMEM medium for indicated time periods and then stimulated with or without IGF-I (100 ng/ml) for 15 min. Cell lysates were analyzed with immunoprecipitation and immunoblotting for both total and phosphorylated target protein content. **b** mRNA expression of IGF-I or IGF-II was detected by RT-PCR in NCI-H292, GEO, and 3T3/huIGFIR cells. **c** Phosphorylated IGF-IR, AKT, and Erk1/2 were assessed by immunoprecipitation and immunoblotting in serum-starved NCI-H292 cells stimulated with GEO or NCI-H292 conditioned medium (CM). **d** Phosphorylated IGF-IR was assessed in serum-starved NCI-H292 cells stimulated with GEO conditioned culture medium that was preincubated with a neutralizing IGF-II antibody or nonspecific IgG at indicated concentrations. **e** GEO cells cultured in normal growth medium (containing 10% FCS) were treated with PQIP at indicated concentrations for 2 h at 37oC with or without IGF-I (100 ng/ml) stimulation. Cell lysates were then analyzed by immunoprecipitation and immunoblotting for both total and phosphorylated target protein content. **f** Cleaved PARP in GEO cells treated with PQIP was assessed by immunoblotting

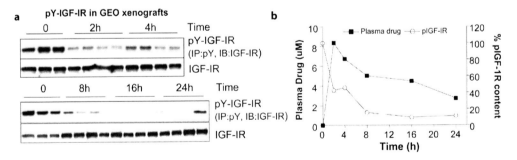

Fig. 5.3a,b. Pharmacokinetic/pharmacodynamic relationship of orally dosed PQIP in GEO tumor xenograft models. **a** Effect on IGF-IR phosphotyrosine content in GEO tumor xenografts for 24 h after a single oral dose of 100 mg/kg PQIP. **b** Quantitation of the extent of inhibition of IGF-IR phosphorylation (*open circles*) in GEO tumor xenografts and the relationship with plasma levels of PQIP (*filled squares*) after a single oral dose of 100 mg/kg PQIP

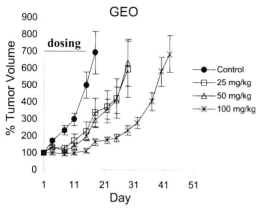

Fig. 5.4 Antitumor activity of orally dosed PQIP in GEO xenograft model. Dose-dependent inhibition of GEO tumor xenograft growth by once daily oral dosing of PQIP for 14 days, followed by outgrowth of tumors in the absence of dosing

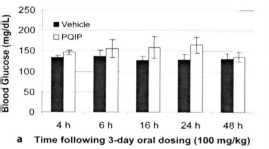

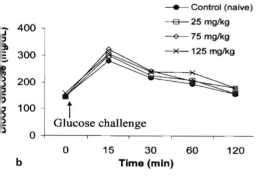

Fig. 5.5a,b. Effect of PQIP on blood glucose in CD-1 mice. **a** Effect on nonfasting blood glucose at indicated times in CD-1 mice after 3-day dosing of PQIP at 100 mg/kg. **b** Effect on glucose clearance in fasted CD-1 mice after 3-day dosing at 25, 75, or 125 mg/kg PQIP. Blood glucose was measured at indicated time points after the glucose challenge

out substantial hyperglycemia. When tested in nonfasted mice, less than 30% blood glucose elevation was observed in the PQIP-treated mice at a maximally efficacious oral dose of 100 mg/kg (Fig. 5.5a) for three consecutive days. This minimal effect on glucose uptake was further confirmed in a glucose tolerance test in which oral doses of PQIP up to 125 mg/kg induced no significant increase in fasting blood glucose (Fig. 5.5b).

Pyrrolo[2,3-d]pyrimidine derivatives, such as NVP-AEW541, represent another class of IGF-IR small-molecule kinase inhibitors targeting the ATP binding pocket. NVP-AEW541 (Table 5.1, compound 2) (IGF-IR cell IC50=0.086 μM) and NVP-ADW742 (IGF-IR cell IC50=0.17 μM) have both been reported to display greater than 16-fold cellular selectivity for IGF-IR relative to the human IR (LeRoith et al. 2004; Garcia-Echeverria et al. 2004; Scotlandi et al. 2005; Mitsiades et al. 2004). In an orthotopic multiple myeloma model, NVP-ADW742 suppressed tumor growth and prolonged survival without significant toxicity when administered alone (10 mg/kg i.p. twice daily) or in combination with the cytotoxic agent melphalan. NVP-ADW541 also induced significant antitumor activity in combination with vincristine in a TC-71 Ewing sarcoma xenograft model. Although blood glucose data were not reported in these xenograft models, a separate study revealed that antitumor efficacy was observed in a fibrosarcoma xenograft model (NIH-3T3 cells stably transfected with human IGF-IR) without blood glucose and insulin alterations when NVP-AEW541 was administered orally at 50 mg/kg for 10 consecutive days.

Although cellular selectivity for IGF-IR over IR has been observed with PQIP and NVP-AEW541 in intact cell systems, neither compound has demonstrated appreciable selectivity between IGF-IR and IR in biochemical assays in which recombinant kinase domains have been used. This suggests that these kinase domains may exist in different conformations in the context of the intact full-length receptors or in the cellular environment. Accordingly, cellular selectivity between these highly homologous receptors may be influenced by cellular proteins associated with the receptors, or by other factors unique to the cellular backgrounds in which selectivity is measured.

Picropodophyllin (PPP) (Table 5.1, compound 3), a cyclolignan-derivative, is a non-ATP-competitive IGF-IR antagonist (Vasilcanu et al. 2005; Girnita et al. 2004; Stromberg et al. 2006). It was reported that PPP inhibited phosphorylation of IGF-IR in cells (IC50=0.04 µM) without interfering with insulin receptor activity. Kinetic studies showed that PPP did not compete with ATP biochemically. Further studies revealed that PPP interfered with phosphorylation in the activation loop of the kinase domain specifically blocking phosphorylation of the tyrosine 1136 residue without affecting phosphorylation of the other two tyrosine residues, 1131 and 1135. PPP has been shown to reduce phosphorylated AKT and ERK1/2 and inhibit cell proliferation and survival of a number of tumor cell lines. Administration of PPP at 20 mg/kg i.p. twice daily led to tumor regression in xenograft models derived from primary human uveal melanoma OCM-1. In vivo antitumor efficacy with prolonged survival was also observed in a 5T33 MM mouse model in which PPP reduced bone marrow burden by 77% and serum paraprotein concentration by 90%. PPP appeared to be tolerated, with no changes in blood glucose and insulin in mouse xenograft models during the dosing period. Recently, it was disclosed that IGF-IR underwent rapid downregulation in cells treated with PPP. It is unclear whether the downregulation of IGF-IR protein by PPP is a consequence of inhibition of Tyr1136 phosphorylation or an alternative mechanism.

INSM-18 (Table 5.1, compound 4) has been reported to inhibit both IGF-IR and Her2 in cells and is currently in phase II clinical trials in patients with prostate cancer (Hofmann et. al. 2005). The inhibitory activity of INSM-18 against the IGF-IR was identified in a cell-based screen that monitored ligand-stimulated phosphorylation of IGF-IR in MCF-7 breast cancer cells. INSM-18 inhibits cellular IGF-IR autophosphorylation with an IC50 value of 22 µM. In vivo efficacy was observed in a prostate cancer xenograft model without apparent effects on blood glucose levels. It was disclosed that in a phase I study patients tolerated a dose of 1.5 g of INSM-18 per day, although additional clinical data have not yet been reported.

5.5.1.2 Small-Molecule IGF-IR Kinase Inhibitors with Comparable Potency Against IR

Benzimidazole derivatives BMS-554417 (Table 5.1, compound 5) and BMS-536924 (Bristol-Myers Squibb) have been disclosed as ATP-competitive small-molecule IGF-IR kinase inhibitors with comparable potency against IR (Haluska et al. 2006; Wittman et al. 2005). In biochemical assays, BMS-554417 displayed IC50 values of 0.068 µM, 0.051 µM, and 0.090 µM for IGF-IR, IR, and focal adhesion kinase (FAK), respectively. In intact MCF-7 cells, this compound inhibited IGF-IR and IR autophosphorylation to a similar degree; however, it did not appear to affect the phosphorylation of FAK at the tyrosine-397 autophosphorylation site. BMS-554417 induced antiproliferative and proapoptotic effects in several cell types that appeared to depend on inhibition of both IGF-IR and IR, and downstream AKT and ERK phosphorylation were inhibited. In a mouse allograft model (IGF-IR Sal) that expressed a constitutively active IGF-IR kinase activity, oral administration of BMS-554417 at 200 mg/kg once daily showed significant antitumor efficacy. A single oral dose of this compound at 200 mg/kg caused transient hyperglycemia and supraphysiologic elevation of insulin in mice. As with BMS-554417, antitumor efficacy and hyperglycemia were also observed in mice treated with BMS-536924.

5.5.1.3 Other Small-Molecule IGF-IR Kinase Inhibitors

There are several small-molecule IGF-IR kinase inhibitors, which have served as probe compounds (pyrrole-5-carboxaldehydes), are examples from the patent literature representing diverse classes of compounds, or are IND-track candidates with limited disclosed information such as XL-228 (Table 5.1, compound 6) and OSI-906 (Table 5.1, compound 7).

Pyrrole-5-carboxaldehyde (Table 5.1, compound 8) is ATP-competitive and a reversible covalent binder to both IR and IGF-IR (Bell et al. 2005). X-ray cocrystal structures were used to determine that the aldehyde moiety of compound 8 reacts chemically with Lys1003 to form an imine or Schiff base with unphosphorylated forms of both IR and IGF-IR. Pyrrole-5-carboxaldehyde showed only modest selectivity against IR kinase (6-fold). No in vivo antitumor activity has been disclosed, suggesting that compound 8 may have served mainly as a probe compound to facilitate the development of more in vivo metabolically stable inhibitors of IGF-IR.

Tyrphostin analogs AG-1024 (Table 5.1, compound 9) and AG-1034 are other examples of non-ATP competitors (Parrizas et al. 1997). These compounds inhibited IGF-IR kinase biochemical activity and had weak cellular activity, inhibiting IGF-IR autophosphorylation with IC50 values of 7–13 µM. They exhibited approximately four- to eightfold selectivity over IR. It was shown that, in combination with an EGFR inhibitor, AG-1024 significantly enhanced both spontaneous and radiation-induced apoptosis in glioblastoma cells.

A pyrrolopyrimidine analog, compound 10 (Table 5.1) was identified in a continuous coupled spectroscopic assay focused on identification of an inhibitor of the unphosphorylated form of IGF-IR, attempting to take advantage of proposed conformational differences between IGF-IR and IR in the unphosphorylated state (Li et al. 2004). Compound 10 was determined to be only modestly selective toward IR (3-fold) biochemically. In competition studies with a non-ATP-competitive analog 5'-(β,γ-imido) triphosphate, it was determined to not be a pure ATP-competitive inhibitor, suggesting a complex binding mode of action. No additional studies with this class of pyrrolopyrimidines have been reported.

Several diverse small-molecule IGF-IR inhibitors are exemplified in the patent literature, and representative examples include 2,4-diaminopyrimidine 11 (Harmange et al. 2003) and 1,2,3,4-tetrahydro-pyrrolo[1,2-a]pyrazine 12 (Ratcliffe et al. 2003) (Table 5.1). In many cases, IGF-IR potency or selectivity toward IR or other targets is not disclosed.

5.5.2 Monoclonal Antibodies

Two early studies showed that a mouse anti-IGF-IR neutralizing antibody was able to inhibit human breast cancer cell growth and Wilms tumor growth in xenograft models (Arteaga et al. 1989; Gansler et al. 1989). A study with a murine anti-IGF-IR neutralizing antibody showed that the antibody not only inhibits IGF signaling but also downmodulates the IGF-IR protein level (Hailey et al. 2002). More recent work using human or humanized antibodies has enabled clinical testing of anti-IGF-IR antibodies.

5.5.2.1 Full-Length Therapeutic Antibodies with Effector Functions

Several humanized or fully human neutralizing monoclonal antibodies against IGF-IR with effector functions have been reported, including the IgG1 monoclonals EM164 (Immunogen/Aventis), A12 (ImClone), 19D12 (Schering-Plough), and h7C10 (Pierre-Fabre/Merck). All have been shown to inhibit proliferation of various tumor cell lines and inhibit growth of various tumor xenograft models representing breast, prostate, ovarian, lung, pancreatic, renal, colorectal, and other tumor types (Maloney et al. 2003; Burtrum et al. 2003; Wang et al. 2005; Goetsch et al. 2005a, 2005b).

19D12 is a fully human anti-IGF-IR monoclonal antibody that inhibits IGF-I binding and autophosphorylation of both IGF-IR:IGF-IR homodimers and IGF-IR:insulin receptor (IR) heterodimers. The upper panel of Fig. 5.6 shows the inhibition of IGF-IR autophosphorylation by 19D12, and the bottom panel shows the inhibition of IGF-IR:IR heterodimer autophosphorylation by 19D12. A single Fab fragment of 19D12 is also able to inhibit receptor autophosphorylation. The binding affinity of the Fab fragment to IGF-IR is similar to that of the full-length antibody, which is consistent with the hypothesis that the epitope that 19D12 binds on IGF-IR resides on a single arm of the receptor dimer. 19D12 does not recognize insulin receptor homodimers. In addition to inhibiting IGF-IR autophosphorylation, 19D12 also inhibits IRS-1 phosphorylation and activation

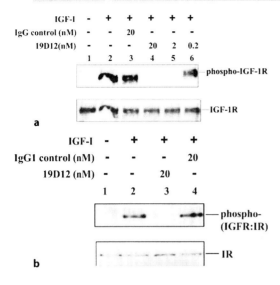

Fig. 5.6a,b. Inhibition of autophosphorylation of IGf-1R:IGF-1R homodimers and IGF-1R:IR heterodimers. **a** A2780 cells were treated with various concentrations of 19D12 antibody (lane 4: 20 nM, lane 5: 2 nM, lane 6: 0.2 nM) or control IgG (lane 3: 20 nM) for 0.5 h before stimulation with IGF-I (20 ng/ml); 400 µg of each cell lysate was subjected to immunoprecipitation with an IGF-1R-specific antibody. The precipitated cell lysates were separated on 10% SDS-PAGE and transferred to a nitrocellulose blot. The filter was probed with anti-phosphotyrosine antibody 4G10. Lane 1 is untreated cells. Lanes 2–6 are IGF-I (20 ng/ml)-treated cells. The blot was then stripped and reprobed with anti-IGF-1R antibody (bottom panel). **b** A2780 cells were treated with 20 nM of 19D12 (lane 3) or control IgG antibody (lane 4) for 0.5 h before stimulation with IGF-I (20 ng/ml) for 5 min; 400 µg of each cell lysate was subjected to immunoprecipitation with an IR-specific antibody. The precipitated cell lysates were separated on 10% SDS-PAGE and transferred to a nitrocellulose blot. The filter was probed with the anti-phosphotyrosine antibody, 4G10. Lane 1 is untreated cells. Lane 2 is IGF-I (20 ng/ml)- only-treated cells. The blot was stripped and reprobed with anti-IR antibody

of the major downstream signaling molecules AKT and ERK1/2, as shown in Fig. 5.7.

Furthermore, 19D12 downregulates the total IGF-IR protein level (Fig. 5.8). The downregulation was observed starting at 1 h of incubation, and the extent of downregulation was maximal at 4 h. An isotype control antibody or IGF-I ligand did not affect the IGF-IR level with up to overnight incubation.

As an IgG1 molecule, 19D12 exhibits antibody-dependent cellular cytotoxicity (ADCC) activity against a non-small cell lung carcinoma cell line in vitro in the presence of isolated human natural killer cells (Fig. 5.9). These three activities, inhibition of IGF signaling, downregulation of the IGF-IR protein level, and ADCC, could all contribute to the antitumor activity of 19D12 in vivo.

19D12 binds tightly to the receptor, with an affinity of 3.8 pM as measured by KinExA. In cell culture, 19D12 inhibits proliferation and soft agar growth of various tumor cell lines. In mice, 19D12 inhibits the growth of various xenograft tumors. Inhibition of a human lung tumor xenograft model H322 by 19D12 is shown as an example in Fig. 5.10.

Other human or humanized neutralizing IgG1 antibodies against the IGF-IR have shown similar cellular activities to those shown for 19D12. A12 antibody (ImClone) is in early-stage clinical testing and has been shown to in-

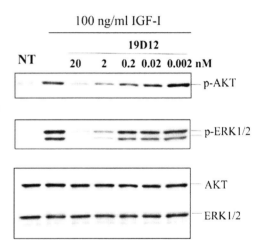

Fig. 5.7 Inhibition of IGF-1R signaling. MCF7 cells were treated with various concentrations of 19D12 antibody (lane 3: 20 nM, lane 4: 2 nM, lane 5: 0.2 nM, lane 6: 0.02 nM, lane 7: 0.002 nM) for 4 h; 50 µg of each cell lysate was separated by a 10% SDS-PAGE and transferred to a nitrocellulose blot. The blot was probed with anti-phospho-AKT antibody first (top panel) and then reprobed with anti-phospho-ERK1/2 antibody (middle panel). The blot was subsequently stripped and probed with anti-AKT and anti-ERk1/2 antibodies (bottom panel). Lane 1 is untreated cells. Lanes 2–7 are IGF-I (20 ng/ml)-treated cells

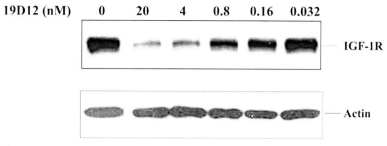

Fig. 5.8 Downmodulation of IGF-1R. A2780 cells were treated with various concentrations of 19D12 antibody (lane 2: 20 nM, lane 3: 4 nM, lane 4: 0.8 nM, lane 5: 0.16 nM, lane 6: 0.032 nM) for 4 h; 50 μg of each cell lysate was separated by a 10% SDS-PAGE and transferred to a nitrocellulose blot. The blot was probed with anti-IGF-1R antibody (top panel), stripped, and reprobed with anti-actin antibody (bottom panel)

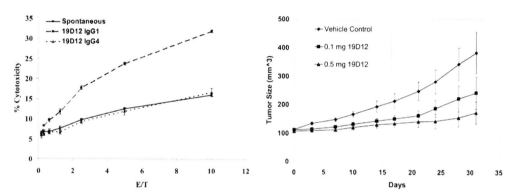

Fig. 5.9 Induction of ADCC by 19D12. NCI-H322 cells and various antibodies were added to a 96-well plate and were opsonized with 100 ng/ml of 19D12 for 30 min at room temperature. Purified human NK cells were then added at various ratios to numbers of target H322 cells. Cells were incubated at 37°C for 9 h. LDH released was then measured as an indicator of cell cytotoxicity. Each data point was assayed in quadruple in the experiment

Fig. 5.10 Inhibition of NCI-H322 tumor growth in mice. Four million NCI-H322 human NSCLC carcinoma cells in 50% growth factor-reduced Matrigel were inoculated subcutaneously into nude mice. 19D12 treatment was initiated when the tumor size reached ~100 mm3 (day 0). 19D12 was administered i.p. twice per week. Tumor volumes were measured by Labcat

hibit both androgen-dependent and androgen-independent prostate tumors. Interestingly, in androgen-dependent tumors, A12 induces apoptosis or G1 arrest; and in androgen-independent prostate tumors, A12 induces G2-M arrest (Wu et al. 2005). An anti-IGF-IR antibody, h7C10 from Pierre-Fabre/Merck, has been shown to bind and inhibit IGF-IR:IR heterodimers in addition to IGF-IR homodimers (Goetsch et al. 2005a, 2005b). Another IgG1 isotype of anti-IGF-IR monoclonal antibody, EM164 (Immunogen/Aventis), has been shown to completely inhibit the growth of BxPC-3 human pancreatic tumors in SCID mice. In combination with gemcitabine, tumor regressions were observed. Indeed, in xenograft models, several anti-IGF-IR antibodies have been shown to enhance the antitumor efficacy of molecular targeted therapies such as EGFR inhibitors or cytotoxic agents such as vinorelbine and taxanes.

Some clinically efficacious therapeutic monoclonal antibodies, such as rituximab and trastuzumab, may owe part of their antitumor efficacy to their ability to induce ADCC. A single-nucleotide polymorphism in the FcγRIIIa gene results in higher affinity for the IgG1 Fc domain and therefore more potent ADCC activity. Non-Hodgkin lymphoma patients with this polymorphism (FcγRIIIa-158V) have shown better response to rituximab treatment. This observation provides strong evidence that ADCC contributes to the antitumor efficacy of rituximab. Thus (e.g. IgG1) anti-IGF-IR neutralizing antibodies with effector functions could potentially confer additional antitumor activity through induction of ADCC.

5.5.2.2 Full-Length Antibodies Without Effector Functions

CP-751,871 (Pfizer) is a fully human anti-IGF-IR neutralizing antibody of the IgG2 isotype, currently in phase II clinical trials. The antibody blocks binding of IGF-I to the IGF-IR (IC50=1.8 nmol/l) and IGF-1-induced receptor autophosphorylation (IC50=0.42 nmol/L) and induces downregulation of IGF-IR. As with other neutralizing anti-IGF-IR antibodies described above, CP-751,871 showed significant antitumor activity both as a single agent and in combination with doxorubicin, 5-fluorouracil, or tamoxifen in multiple tumor models. A linear increase in plasma exposure was observed when CP-751,871 was dosed in the range of 3 to 100 mg/kg i.v. in cynomolgus monkeys, suggesting that all IGF-IR binding sites were saturated at 3 mg/kg. An ex vivo pharmacodynamic assay detected reduced IGF-IR expression in peripheral blood cells after treatment with CP-751,871 (Melvin et al. 2004).

Since an IgG2 antibody is unlikely to induce significant ADCC activity, the antitumor activity of CP-751,871 would be expected to result predominantly from inhibition of IGF signaling and receptor downregulation. This lack of ADCC could result in improved safety and/or reduced efficacy relative to IgG1 anti-IGF-IR antibodies. Initial phase I clinical data reported at the 2006 ASCO meeting indicated that CP-751,871 was tolerated when administered to multiple myeloma patients, and provided preliminary evidence of clinical activity. As early clinical data continue to emerge, it will be of tremendous interest to determine whether IgG1 and IgG2 anti-IGF-IR antibodies show differences in safety and/or efficacy in various clinical settings.

5.5.2.3 Other Antibody-Based Agents

There are several other reported antibody-based anti-IGF-IR agents, notably scFv-Fc-1H7 and a bispecific antibody against both IGF-IR and EGFR. The scfv-Fc-1H7 antibody is not a neutralizing antibody. It has agonist activity, in stimulating both receptor activation and signaling downstream of the IGF-IR receptor. However, this dimeric antibody downregulates the IGF-IR and has been shown to partially inhibit tumor growth in an MCF7 xenograft tumor model (Sachdev et al. 2003), demonstrating that downregulation of the IGF-IR protein level alone can result in antitumor activity.

A novel Di-diabody described by ImClone binds both IGF-IR and EGFR and blocks receptor activation stimulated by both IGF and EGF (Lu et al. 2005). The Di-diabody retained biological activities of its parent monospecific antibodies, including downregulation of the IGF-IR protein level and ADCC activity. When tested in vivo, the Di-diabody showed similar or improved antitumor activity relative to either parent antibody alone. Considering the complex and heterogeneous nature of human solid tumors, the concept of a Di-diabody that targets multiple targets simultaneously is attractive, although technical issues remain with this unique approach.

5.6 Summary and Perspective

Therapeutics targeting the IGF-IR for the treatment of cancer have clearly come of age. As these agents progress through clinical trials, antibodies and small-molecule tyrosine kinase inhibitors are each expected to confer a unique set of potential advantages and liabilities.

Several potential advantages of anti-IGF-IR antibodies may be envisioned. Efficacy may be derived from mechanisms beyond direct inhibition of IGF signaling, including downregulation of IGF-IR expression and induction of tumor cell killing through antibody-directed cellular cytotoxicity (ADCC) and complement-directed cytotoxicity (CDC). Antibodies may also allow for less frequent dosing, perhaps on the order of one parenteral dose per week or once every 3 weeks. In addition, the selectivity of anti-IGF-IR antibodies for IGF-IR homodimers relative to IR homodimers will likely translate to reduced need to monitor and manage hyperglycemia that may result from IR inhibition by IGF-IR kinase inhibitors.

In contrast, several potential advantages of IGF-IR kinase inhibitors may also be envisioned relative to anti-IGF-IR neutralizing antibodies. One obvious advantage is the potential for oral dosing. Direct inhibition of the kinase domain may also yield greater direct inhibition of IGF-IR signaling, without the possibility of partial agonist activity that has been described for some anti-IGF-IR monoclonal antibodies. Some inhibition of the insulin receptor, particularly the exon 11-IR-A isoform that has been reported to respond to IGF-II autocrine stimulation in some human cancers such as breast and thyroid cancer (Sciacca et al. 1999; Denley et al. 2003), may also confer additional antitumor efficacy for IGF-IR kinase inhibitors relative to IGF-IR-selective monoclonal antibodies. While the long half-lives of antibodies may offer advantages of less frequent dosing, the finer temporal control of IGF-IR inhibition with daily dosing of IGF-IR kinase inhibitors might allow for careful control of scheduling of combinations such that IGF-IR can specifically be inhibited before or after exposure to a cytotoxic agent (Yee 2006). A final potential advantage for IGF-IR kinase inhibitors may be greater likelihood of generating small molecules that may cross the blood-brain barrier to allow treatment of IGF-dependent CNS tumors or metastatic lesions.

As one anticipates the clinical utility of anti-IGF-IR therapeutics, several lessons are worth considering from observations of small-molecule inhibitors and monoclonal antibodies directed against the epidermal growth factor receptor (EGFR). The finding that small-molecule inhibitors of the EGFR, such as erlotinib or gefitinib, give greater than additive antitumor efficacy in preclinical xenograft models when combined with the anti-EGFR antibody cetuximab suggests that a kinase inhibitor and antibody directed against the same target may have different but complementary activities (Huang et al. 2004). Differences in the mechanisms of small-molecule inhibitors and antibodies are further apparent from the observation that erlotinib and gefitinib were able to inhibit the growth of head and neck tumor cells that were selected for resistance to cetuximab (Huang et al. 2004). Thus small-molecule kinase inhibitors and antibodies directed against the same target might both be worthwhile to develop as they may find clinical utility in different cancer indications or even in combination with each other.

It is expected that over the next several years, abundant clinical information will emerge on safety and tolerability as well as clinical efficacy of anti-IGF-IR antibodies and small-molecule IGF-IR kinase inhibitors. Perhaps most exciting will be the elucidation of the specific cancer indications in which these treatment modalities will impart the greatest clinical benefit.

References

Arteaga CL, Kitten LJ, Coronado EB, Jacobs S, Kull Jr FC, Alired DC, Osborne CK. (1989) Blockade of the type I somatomedin receptor inhibits growth of human breast cancer cells in athymic mice. J Clin Invest 84:1418–1423

Baker J, Liu J, Robertson EJ et al. (1993) Role of insulin-like growth factors in embryonic and postnatal growth. Cell 75:73

Bell IM, Stirdivant SM, Ahern J, Culberson JC, Darke PL, Dinsmore CJ, Drakas RA, Gallicchio SN, Graham SL, Heimbrook DC, Hall DL et al. (2005) Biochemical and structural characterization of a novel class of inhibitors of the type I insulin-like growth factor and insulin receptor kinases. Biochemistry 44:9430–9440

Burfeind P, Chernicky CL, Rininsland F, Ilan J (1996) Antisense RNA to the type I insulin-like growth factor receptor suppresses tumor growth and prevents invasion by rat prostate cancer cells in vivo. Proc Natl Acad Sci USA 93:7263–7268

Burtrum D, Zhu Z, Lu D et al. (2003) A fully human monoclonal antibody to the insulin-like growth factor I receptor blocks ligand-dependent signaling and inhibits human tumor growth in vivo. Cancer Res 63:8912–8921

Butler AA, Blakesley VA, Tsokos M, Pouliki V, Wood TL, LeRoith D. (1998) Stimulation of tumor growth by recombinant human insulin-like growth factor 1 (IGF-I) is dependent on the dose and the level of IGF-I receptor expression. Cancer Res 58:3021–3027

Chan JM, Stampfer MJ, Giovannucci E et al. (1998) Plasma insulin-like growth factor-I and prostate cancer risk: A prospective study. Science 279:563–566

Chakravarti A, Loeffler JS, Dyson NJ (2002) Insulin-like growth factor reeptor I mediates resistance to anti-EGFR therapy in primary human glioblastoma cells through continued activation of phosphoinositide 3-kinase signaling. Cancer Res 62:200–207

D'Ambrosio C, Ferber A, Resnicoff M, Baserga RA (1996) Soluble insulin-like growth factor I receptor that induces apoptosis of tumor cells in vivo and inhibits tumorigenesis. Cancer Res 56:4013–4020

DeChiara TM, Efstratiadis A, Robertson EJ et al. (1990) A growth-deficiency phenotype in heterozygous mice carrying an insulin-like growth factors II gene disrupted by targeting. Nature 345:78

De Myets P, Whittaker J (2002) Structural biology of insulin and IGF1 receptors:implications for drug design. Nat Rev Drug Disc 1:769–785

Denley A, Wallace, JC, Cosgrove LJ, Forbes BE (2003) The insulin receptor isoform exon 11- (IR-A) in cancer and other diseases:a review. Horm Metab Res 35:778–785

DiGiovanni J, Bol DK, Wilker E, Beltran L, Carbajal S, Moats S, Ramirez A, Jorcano J, Kiguchi K (2000a) Constitutive expression of insulin-like growth factor-i in epidermal basal cells of transgenic mice leads to spontaneous tumor promotion. Cancer Res 60:1561–1570

DiGiovanni J, Kiguchi K, Frijhoff A, Wilker E, Bol DK, Beltran L, Moats S, Ramirez A, Jorcano J, Cludio C (2000b) Deregulated expression of insulin-like growth factor 1 in prostate epithelium leads to neoplasia in transgenic mice. Proc Natl Acad Sci USA 97:3455–3460

Favelyukis S, Till JH, Hubbard SR, Miller WT (2001) Structure and autoregulation of the insulin-like growth factor 1 receptor kinase. Nat Struct Biol 8:1058–1063

Firth SM, Baxter RC (2002) Cellular actions of the insulin-like growth factor binding proteins. Endocr Rev 23:824–854

Frasca F, Pandini G, Psalia P, Sciacca L, Mineo R, Costantino A, Goldfine ID, Belfiore A, Vigneri R (1999) Insulin receptor isoform A, a newly recognized, high-affinity insulin-like growth factor II receptor in fetal and cancer cells. Mol Cell Biol 19:3278–3288

Garcia-Echeverria C, Pearson MA, Marti A, Meyer T, Mestan J, Zimmermann J, Gao J, Brueggen J, Capraro HG, Cozens R, Evans DB, Fabbro D, Furet P, Porta DG, Liebetanz J, Martiny-Baron G, Ruetz S, Holmann F (2004) In vivo antitumor activity of NVP-AEW541 – A novel, potent, and selective inhibitor of the IGF-IR kinase. Cancer Cell 3:231–239

Gansler T, Furlanetto R, Grambling TS et al. (1989) Antibody to type 1 insulin-like growth factor inhibits

growth of Wilms' tumor in culture and in athymic mice. Am J Pathol 135:961–966

Girnita A, Girnita L, Prete FD, Bartolazzi A, Larsson O, Axelson M (2004) Cyclolignans as inhibitors of the insulin-like growth factor receptor and malignant cell growth. Cancer Res 64:236–242

Goetsch L, Gonzalez A, Leger O, Beck A, Pauwels PJ, Haeuw JF, Corvaia N (2005a) A recombinant humanized anti-insulin-like growth factor receptor type I antibody (h7C10) enhances the antitumor activity of vinorelbine and anti-epidermal growth factor receptor therapy against human cancer xenografts. Int J Cancer 113(2):316–328

Goetsch L, Corvaia N, Duflos A, Haeuw JF, Leger O, Beck A (2005b) Novel anti-IGF-1R and/or anti-insulin/IGF-I hybrid receptor antibodies and uses thereof. US 2005/0249730

Hailey J, Maxwell E, Koukouras K, Bishop WR, Pachter JA, Wang Y (2002) Neutralizing anti-insulin-like growth factor receptor 1 antibodies inhibit receptor function and induce receptor degradation in tumor cells. Mol Cancer Therapeut 1:1349–1353

Haluska P, Carboni JM, Loegering DA, Lee FY, Wittman M, Saulnier MG, Frennesson DB, Kalli KR, Conover CA, Attar, RM, Kaufmann SH, Gottardis M, Erlichman C (2006) In vitro and in vivo antitumor effects of the dual insulin-like growth factor-I/insulin receptor inhibitor, BMS-554417. Cancer Res 66:362–371

Harmange J-C, Booker S, Buchanan JL, Chaffee S, Novak PM, Van Der Plas S, Zhu X (2003) 2,4-Disubstituted pyrimidinyl derivatives for use as anticancer agents. WO03/018021A1

Hofmann F, Garcia-Echeverria C (2005) Blocking insulin-like growth factor-I receptor as a strategy for targeting cancer. Drug Discovery Today 10(15):1041–1047

Huang S, Armstrong EA, Benavente S, Chinnaiyan P, Harari PM (2004) Dual-agent molecular targeting of the epidermal growth factor receptor (EGFR):Combining anti-EGFR antibody with tyrosine kinase inhibitor. Cancer Res 64:5355–5362

Ji QS, Mulvihill MJ, Rosenfeld-Franklin M,Cooke A, Feng L, Mak G, O'Connor M, Yao Y, Pirritt C, Buck E, Eyzaguirre A, Arnold LD, Gibson NW, Pachter JA (2007) A novel, potent and selective Insulin-like growth factor-I receptor (IGF-IR) kinase inhibitor blocks IGF-IR signaling in vitro and inhibits IGF-IR dependent tumor growth in vivo. Submitted to Mol Cancer Therapeutics

Kalebic T, Blakesley V, Slade C, Plasschaert S, Leroith D, Helman LJ (1998) Expression of a kinase-deficient IGF-I-R suppresses tumorigenicity of rhabdomyosarcoma cells constitutively expressing a wild type IGF-I-R. Int J Cancer 76:223–227

Kulik G, Klippel A, Weber MJ (1997) Anti-apoptotic signaling by the insulin-like growth factor I receptor, phosphatidylinositol 3-kinase and Akt. Mol Cell Biol 17:1595–1606.

Lau MM, Stewart CE, Liu Z et al. (1994) Loss of the imprinting IGF2/cation-independent mannose 6-

phosphate receptor results in fetal overgrowth and perinatal lethality Genes Dev 8:2953

LeRoith D, Helman L (2004) The new kid on the block(ade) of the IGF-1 receptor. Cancer Cell 5:201–202

Li W, Favelyukis S, Yang J, Zeng Y, Yu J, Gangjee A, Miller WT (2004) Biochem Pharmacol 68:145

Liu J, Baker J, Perkins AS et al. (1993) Mice carrying null mutations of the genes encoding insulin-like growth factor I (IGF-1) and type 1 IGF receptor. Cell 75:59

Lu D, Zhang H, Koo H, Tonra J, Balderes P, Prewett M, Corcoran E, Maggalampalli V, Bassi R, Anselma D, Patel D, Kang X, Ludwig DL, Hicklin DJ, Bohlen P, Witte L, Zhu Z (2005) A fully human recombinant IgG-like bispecific antibody to both the epidermal growth factor receptor and the insulin-like growth factor receptor for enhanced antitumor activity. J Biol Chem 280:19665–19672

Lu Y, Zi X, Zhao Y, Mascarenhas D, Pollark M (2001) Insulin-like growth factor-I receptor signaling and resistance to trastuzumab (Herceptin). J Natl Cancer Inst 93:1852

Mathews LS, Hammer RE, Behringger RR et al. (1988) Growth enhancement of transgenic mice expressing human insulin-like growth factor I. Endocrinology123:2827

Melvin C, Paterson J, Gehard D, Littman B, Gualberto A (2004) Inhibition of the insulin-like growth factor 1 receptor by a specific monoclonal antibody in multiple myeloma. Poster at AACR

Mitsiades CS, Mitsiades NS, McMullan CJ et al. (2004) Inhibition of the insulin-like growth factor receptor-1 tyrosine kinase activity as a therapeutic strategy for multiple myeloma, other hematologic malignancies, and solid tumors. Cancer Cell 5:221–230

Maloney EK, McLaughlin JL, Dagdigian NE, Garrett LM, Connors KM, Zhou X, Blattler WA, Chittenden T, Singh R (2003) An anti-insulin-like growth factor receptor antibody that is a potent inhibitor of cancer cell proliferation. Cancer Res 63:5073–5083

Okamoto T, Nishimoto I, Murayama Y, Ohkuni Y, Ogata E (1990) Insulin-like growth factor-II/mannose-6-phosphate receptor is incapable of activating GTP-binding proteins in response to mannose-6-phosphate, but capable in response to insulin-like growth factor-II. Biochem Biophys Res Commun 168:1201–1210

Pandini G, Vigneri R, Costantino A, Frasca F, Ippolito A, Fujita-Uamaguchi Y, Siddle K, Goldfine ID, Belfiore A (1999) Insulin and insulin-like growth factor-I (IGF-I) receptor overexpression in breast cancers leads to insulin/IGF-I hybrid receptor overexpression:evidence for a second mechanism of IGF-I signaling. Clin Cancer Res 5:1935–1944

Parker AS, Cheville JC, Janney CA, Cerhan JR (2002) High expression levels of insulin-like growth factor-I receptor predict poor survival among women with clear-cell renal cell carcinoma. Human Path 33:801–805

Parrizas M, Gazit A, Levitzki A, Wertheimer E, LeRoith D (1997) Specific inhibition of insulin-like growth factor-I and insulin receptor tyrosine kinase activity

and biological function of tyrphostins. Endocrinology 138(4):1427–1433

Pollak MN, Schernhammer ES, Hankinson SE (2004) Insulin-like growth factors and neoplasia. Nat Rev Cancer 4:505–518

Powell-Braxton L, Hollingshead P, Warburton C et al. (1993) IGF-I is required for normal embryonic growth in mice Genes Dev 7:2609

Prager D, Li HL, Asa S, Melmed S (1994) Dominant negative inhibition of tumourogenesis in vivo by human insulin-like growth factor I receptor mutant. Proc Natl Acad Sci USA 91:2181–2185

Ratcliffe AJ, Walsh RJA, Majid TN, Thurairatnam S, Amendola, S, Aldous DJ (2003). Chemical Compounds, WO03/024967A2

Reeve AE, Eccles MR, Wilkins RJ, Bell GI, Millow LJ (1985) Expression of insulin-like growth factor-II transcripts in Wilms' tumour. Nature 317:258–262

Reiss K, D'Ambrosio C, Tu X, Tu C, Baserga R (1998) Inhibition of tumor growth by a dominant negative mutant of the insulin-like growth factor I receptor with a bystander effect. Clin Cancer Res 4:2647–2655

Rodriguez-Tarduchy G, Collins MK, Garcia I., Lopez-Rivas A (1992) Insulin-like growth factor I inhibits apoptosis in IL3 dependent hemopoietic cells. J Immunol 149:535–540

Rogler CE, Yang D, Rosetti L et al. (1994) Altered body composition and increased frequency of diverse malignancies insulin-like growth factor transgenic mice. J Biol Chem 269:13779

Sachdev D, Li S, Hartell JS, Fujita-Yamaguchi Y, Miller JS, Yee D (2003) A chimeric humanized single-chain antibody against the type i insulin-like growth factor (IGF) receptor renders breast cancer cells refractory to the mitogenic effects of IGF-I. Cancer Res 63(3):627–635

Sciacca L, Costantino A, Pandini G, Mineo R, Frasca F, Scalia P, Sbraccia P, Goldfine ID, Vigneri R, Belfiore A (1999) Insulin receptor activation by IGF-II in breast cancers:evidence for a new autocrine/paracrine mechanism. Oncogene 18:2471–2479

Scotlandi K, Avnet S, Benini S et al. (2002) Expression of an IGF-I receptor dominant negative mutant induces apoptosis, inhibits tumourogenesis and enhances chemosensitivity in Ewing's sarcoma cells. Int J Cancer 101:11–16

Scotlandi K, Manara MC, Nicoletti G, Lollini P–L, Lukas S, Benini S, Croci S, Perdichizzi S, Zambelli D, Serra M, Garcia-Echeverria C, Hofman F, Picci P (2005) Antitumor activity of the insulin-like growth factor-i receptor kinase inhibitor NVP-AEW541 in musculoskeletal tumors. Cancer Res 65(9):3868–3876

Sell C, Baserga R, Rubin R (1995) Insulin-like growth factor I (IGF-I) and the IGF-I receptor prevent etoposide induced apoptosis. Cancer Res 55:303–306

Sell C, Dumenil G, Deveaud C, Miura M, Coppola D, DeAngelis T, Rubin R, Efstratiadis A, Baserga R (1994) Effect of a null mutation of the type 1 IGF receptor gene on growth and transformation of mouse embryo fibroblasts. Mol Cell Biol 14:3604

Sepp-Lorenzino L (1998) Structure and function of the insulin-like growth factor I receptor. Breast Cancer Res Treatment 47:235–253

Siddle K, Soos MA, Field CE, Nave BT (1994) Hybrid and atypical insulin/insulin-like growth factor I receptors. Horm Res 41:56–65

Singleton JR, Dixit VM, Feldman EL (1996) Type I insulin-like growth factor receptor activation regulates apoptotic proteins. J Biol Chem 271:31791–31794

Stromberg T, Ekman S, Girnita L, Dimberg, LY, Larsson O, Axelson M, Lennartsson J, Hellman U, Carlson K, Osterborg A, Vanderkerken K, Nilsson K, Jernberg-Wiklund H (2006) IGF-1 receptor tyrosine kinase inhibition by the cyclolignan PPP induces G2/M-phase accumulation and apoptosis in multiple myeloma cells. Blood 107:669–678

Van Buul-Offers SC, de Haan K, Reijnen-Gresnigt MG et al. (1995) Overexpression of human insulin-like growth factor-II in transgenic mice causes increased growth of the thymus. J Endocrinol 144:491

Vasilcanu D, Girnita A, Girnita L, Vasilcanu R, Axelson M, Larsson O (2005) The cyclolignan PPP induces activation loop-specific inhibition of tyrosine phosphorylation of the insulin-like growth factor-1 receptor. Link to the phosphatidyl inositol-3 kinase/Akt apoptotic pathway. Oncogene 23(47):7854–7862

Wang Y, Hailey J, Williams D, Wang X, Lipari P, Malkowski M, Wang Y, Xie L, Li G, Saha D, Ling WLW, Cannon-Carlson S, Greenberg R, Ramos RA, Shields R, Presta L, Brams P, Bishop WR, Pachter JA (2005) Inhibition of insulin-like growth factor-I receptor (IGF-IR) signaling and tumor cell growth by a fully human neutralizing anti-IGF-1R antibody. Mol Cancer Ther 4:1214–1221

Ward A, Bate P, Fisher R et al. (1994) Disproportionate growth in mice with igf-2 transgenes. Proc Natl Acad Sci USA 91:10365

Werner H, Re GG, Drummond IA et al. (1993) Increased expression of the insulin-like growth factor I receptor gene, IGF1R, in Wilms tumor is correlated with modulation of IGF1R promoter activity by the WT1 Wilms tumor gene product. Proc Natl Acad Sci USA 90:5828–5832

Wittman M, Carboni J, Attar R, Balasubramanian B, Balimane P, Brassil P, Beaulieu F, Chang C, Clarke W, Dell J, Eummer J, Frennesson D, Gottardis M, Greer A, Hansel S, Hurlburt W, Jacobson B, Krishnananthan S, Lee FY, Li A, Lin T-A, Liu P, Ouellet C, Sang X, Saulnier MG, Stoffan K, Sun Y, Velaparthi U, Wong H, Yang Z, Zimmermann K, Zoeckler M, Vyas D (2005) Discovery of a 1H-benzoimidazol-2-yl)-1H-pyridin-2-one (BMS-536924) inhibitor of insulin-like growth factor I receptor kinase with in vivo antitumor activity. J Med Chem 48(18):5639–5643

Wu JD, Odman A, Higgins LM, Haugk K, Vessella R, Ludwig DL, Plymate SR (2005) In vivo effects of the human type I insulin-like growth factor receptor antibody A12 on androgen-dependent and androgen-independent xenograft human prostate tumors. Clin Cancer Res 11:3065–3074

Wu Y, Tewari M, Cui S, Rubin R (1996) Activation of the insulin-like growth factor I receptor inhibits tumor necrosis factor induced cell death. J Cell Physiol 168:499–509

Yee D (2006) Targeting insulin-like growth factor pathways. Br J Cancer 94:465–468

Inhibition of the TGF–β Signaling Pathway in Tumor Cells

Klaus Podar, Noopur Raje, and Kenneth C. Anderson

Recent Results in Cancer Research, Vol. 172
© Springer-Verlag Berlin Heidelberg 2007

6.1 Introduction

Transforming growth factor–β (TGF–β) plays an important physiologic role in the regulation of cell proliferation, motility, and apoptosis as well as extracellular matrix (ECM) production. It therefore modulates physiologic functions such as embryonic development, wound healing, vasculogenesis and angiogenesis, as well as immune surveillance. Moreover, TGF–β has been associated with a wide variety of diseases: atherosclerosis; fibrotic diseases of the lung, kidney, and liver; Alzheimer disease; developmental defects; hereditary hemorrhagic teleangiectasia; as well as both solid tumors and hematologic malignancies. Importantly, TGF–β signaling pathways mediate both early-stage tumor- suppressing, as well as late-stage tumor-promoting, effects. In addition, TGF–β can synergize with oncogenes in transformation and tumor progression. Recent therapeutic approaches in cancer target TGF–β signaling, either alone or in combination with conventional or novel targeted therapy, to improve patient outcome.

6.2 Structure and Biochemical Function of TGF–β

6.2.1 Structure of TGF–β, TGF–β Receptors, and Smad Proteins

The cytokine TGF–β belongs to a superfamily of dimeric polypeptide ligands characterized by six conserved cysteine residues, which also includes activin/nodal, as well as the bone morphogenetic protein (BMP)/growth and differentiation factor (GDF)/Muellerian inhibiting substance (MIS) subfamily. The TGF–β family is highly conserved among different species including Caenorhabditits elegans, Drosophila melanogaster, mouse, Xenopus, and other vertebrates. Each TGF–β ligand has several type I and/or type II receptors, including TβR-I [activin receptor-like kinase (ALK)5], ALK3 (BMPR-IA), ALK4 (ActR-IB), and ALK6 (BMPR-IB); or TβR-I, BMPR-II, and AMHR, which selectively bind TGF–β, BMPs, and MIS, respectively. The expression of distinct type I and type II receptors is cell type specific (Massague et al. 2000).

The mammalian cytokine isoforms TGF–β1, TGF–β2, and TGF–β3 (25 kDa) are encoded by distinct genes located at different chromosomes within 42 open reading frames, differ in their TGF–β receptor binding affinity, and are expressed in a tissue- and development-specific manner. TGF–β1 is the most abundant isoform, as it is expressed in endothelial, hematopoietic, and connective tissue cells. TGF–β is transcribed as a large precursor consisting of TGF–β and a propeptide. After cleavage, both the propeptide and TGF–β are secreted and stored attached to the extracellular matrix (ECM) (de Martin et al. 1987; Derynck et al. 1985, 1988; Madisen et al. 1988, 1989; ten Dijke et al. 1988a, 1988b; Webb et al. 1988).

TGF–β ligands including TGF–β1, TGF–β2, and TGF–β3 form dimers that are stabilized by hydrophobic interactions and intersubunit disulfide bridges. The monomers have "cystine knot" structures formed by extended β-strands connected by three conserved disulfide bonds, and TGF–β ligands are therefore also called the cystine-knot growth-factor superfamily. Each monomer has contact sites for both the type I and the type II receptors (Kirsch et al. 2000).

Type I and type II receptors consist of the extracellular region, which forms a globular domain, and the cytoplasmic region consisting of a short juxtamembrane segment, the protein kinase domain, and alternatively spliced extensions in both the extracellular and the cytoplasmic region. For example, a mutation within the extension of the BMP type II receptor causes familial primary hypertension in humans.

Orthologs of the first mediators of TGF–β signaling, mothers against decapentaplegic (dpp) function (MAD) were first discovered in Drosophila and subsequently described in the worm and vertebrates and named "Smads" (Attisano and Wrana 2000; Derynck and Zhang 1996; S. A. Hahn et al. 1996; Moustakas et al. 2001; Wrana and Attisano 2000).

Smads are divided into three groups: (1) Smads that serve as receptor substrates (R-Smads); (2) the only human co-mediator Smad (Co-Smad), Smad4 [located at 18q21 and previously named deleted in pancreatic carcinoma locus 4 (DPC4)], which is shared by all R-Smads and is essential for the assembly of transcriptional complexes; and (3) the inhibitory Smads (I-Smads), regulators of Smad complex formation. There are two groups of R-Smads, each serving one branch of the TGF–β family. Specifically, Smad2 (located at 18q21)/Smad3 mediates TGF–β/activin/nodal-initiated signals and Smad1/Smad5/Smad8 mediates bone morphogenetic protein (BMP)/growth and differentiation factor (GDF)/anti-Muellerian hormone/Muellerian inhibiting substance (AMH/MIS)-induced signaling (Massague et al. 2000).

Co-Smads contain two conserved globular domains, the N-terminal MAD-homology1 (MH1) and the C-terminal MH2 domain. R-Smads additionally contain a characteristic SXS domain within the MH2 domain, which drives the activation of the R-Smad. The MH1 domains of Smad4 and the R-Smads exhibit sequence-specific DNA-binding activity. The highly conserved MH2 domain mediates receptor interaction, Smad complex formation, and nuclear transport. In the absence of TGF–β, a nuclear export signal (NES) keeps Smad4 in the cytoplasm (Massague and Wotton 2000).

6.2.2 Signal Transduction

6.2.2.1 TGF–β Signaling Pathways: Smad-Dependent and Smad-Independent Signaling Pathways

TGF–β is stored in the ECM complexed with latent TGF–β binding proteins, which are expressed in a tissue-specific manner (Sinha et al. 1998). The exact mechanism of TGF–β activation is unknown; however, thrombospondin-1 has been identified as a major factor mediating this effect (Crawford et al. 1998).

TGF–β initiates signals by binding to a heteromeric receptor complex consisting of the serine/threonine kinases, type I and type II receptors. The ligand-receptor complex consists of two TβRI and TβRII molecules and the TGF–β dimer (P. D. Sun and Davies 1995). The function of type II receptors is to activate type I receptors, which mediate their activity by phosphorylation of Smads and/or activation of Smad-independent molecules.

Specifically, TGF–β isoforms bind to three high-affinity receptors, TβRI, TβRII, and TβRIII (β-glycan). β-Glycan is abundant on most cells and functions to present the ligand to the TGF–β receptor II (Lopez-Casillas et al. 1993). Constitutively active TβRII triggers recruitment and activation of TβRI via transphosphorylation of the GS domain (for the GSGS sequence) within the cytoplasmic receptor I kinase domain (Massague 1998). Phosphorylated TβRI then binds and phosphorylates the receptor-activated Smad (R-Smad) proteins, Smad2 and Smad3 at a characteristic SXS domain. The phosphorylated R-Smad proteins are then released from the receptor complex and associate with a co-mediator Smad (Co-Smad), Smad4. This activated heterotrimeric Smad complex then translocates through nucleoporins into the nucleus, where it binds with low affinity to DNA via Smad cognate CAGAC sequences in TGF–β-responsive promoters. Dependent on their lineage, developmental stage, and microenvironment, cells contain a distinct repertoire of Smad cofactors, which markedly increase DNA binding affinity and thereby modulate specific gene responses. The first cofactor identified for Smad2 was the forkhead family member FOXH1/FAST1 (X. Chen et al. 1996), and the first for Smad1 was the zinc- finger protein OAZ (Hata et al. 2000). Several more proteins have since been identified: Coactivators include p300, CBP, or SMIF (Massague and Wotton 2000); corepressors include p107 (C.R. Chen et al. 2002), SKI, SNON, TGIF, EVI1, and SIP1 (Ten Dijke et al. 2002).

Target genes of TGF–β include those encoding cyclin kinase inhibitors p21 and p15. Moreover, TGF–β-induced cell growth suppression is also mediated via downregulation of c-Myc expression (Derynck et al. 2001; Siegel and Massague 2003; Shi and Massague 2003).

In addition to the Smad-dependent pathways, TGF–β also induces Smad-independent signaling: MAPK signaling pathways including p38 and extracellular signal-regulated kinase (ERK); c-Jun NH2-terminal kinase (JNK); phosphatidylinositol-3 kinase (PI3K); Rho guanosine triphosphatases; and protein phosphatase 2A (Bakin et al. 2000; Bhowmick et al. 2001; Engel et al. 1999; Hocevar et al. 1999; Petritsch et al. 2000; Yu et al. 2002). The biochemical link between TGF–β receptors and the MAPK pathways is represented by TGF–β-activated kinase 1 (TAK1) (Yamaguchi et al. 1995). Activation of some of these molecules, e.g., Ras (Lo et al. 2001; B. J. Park et al. 2000; Saha et al. 2001), can positively or negatively regulate SMAD signaling (Fig. 6.1).

6.2.2.2 Regulation of the TGF–β Signaling Pathway

TGF–β signaling is regulated by a variety of mechanisms including TGF–β receptor internalization, receptor activity modulation, I-Smads, and associated proteins (e.g., SARA and HSR).

TGF–β internalization is equally mediated through both the clathrin endosome and the lipid raft pathways. Specifically, early endosome antigen-1 (EEA-1)-containing early endosomes, but not late p62-positive endosomes, upregulate TGF–β signal transduction. In contrast, lipid raft/caveolin-1-associated receptor internalization downregulates TGF–β signaling by triggering TGF–β degradation (Di Guglielmo et al. 2003; Hayes et al. 2002; Le Roy and Wrana 2005a, 2005b; Penheiter et al. 2002).

Receptor activation is regulated by three distinct mechanisms: (1) soluble proteins acting as ligand binding traps including the "latency-associated polypepetide" (LAP), the small proteoglycan decorin, the circulating α2-macroglobulin, follistatin, as well as three protein families – noggin, chordin/SOG, and DAN/Cerberus; (2) membrane-anchored proteins (including β-glycan/TβRIII and endoglin); and (3) intracellular proteins (e.g., FKBP12 and FKBP12.6). Specifically, the immunophils FKBP12 and FKBP12.6 bind to the GS domain, thereby stabilizing the type I receptor in an inactive state.

In the basal state, Smad2 and Smad3 are retained in the cytoplasm by several proteins, including the Smad anchor for receptor activation (SARA). On TGF–β binding SARA, which is enriched in the EEA-1-containing early endosomes, presents R-Smads to the activated receptor complex, thereby mediating phosphorylation of Smad2. Smad2 phosphorylation in turn releases SARA and enables the binding of Smad2/3 to Smad4. Moreover, hepatocyte growth factor-regulated tyrosine kinase substrate (HRS) cooperates with SARA in receptor-mediated activation of Smad2 (Miura et al. 2000; Tsukazaki et al. 1998; L. Xu et al. 2000).

I-Smads have weak sequence homology to the MH1 domain, but do not bind to DNA. The I-Smads Smad7 and Smad 6, downregulate TGF–β-triggered signaling by inducing degradation of the receptors or by competing with R-Smads for Co-Smad interaction. Specifically, Smad7 forms a complex with the homologous to E6AP COOH-terminus (HECT)-domain containing E3 ubiquitin ligases Smad ubiquitination-related factor (Smurf) 1 and 2. Smurfs

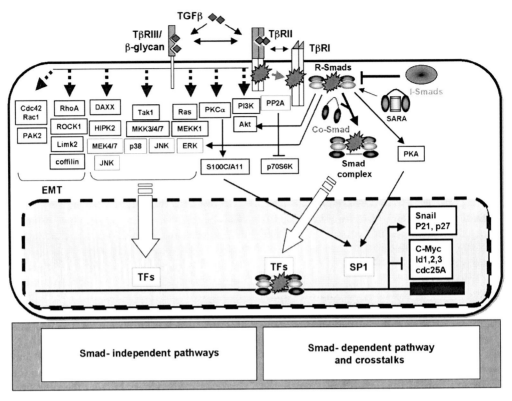

Fig. 6.1 TGF–β- signaling via Smad-dependent and Smad-independent pathways. TGF–β binds either to TβRIII, thereby inducing association with TβRII, or directly to TβRII. After phosphorylation of TβRII, TβRI is transphosphorylated and induces phosphorylation of the regulatory Smads (R-Smads), Smad2 and Smad3. Smad2/Smad3 complex then associates with the Co-Smad Smad4 after release from SARA. The Smad complex then translocates into the nucleus, binds to a variety of transcription factors (TFs), and induces transcription of cell- and tissue-specific target genes. I-Smads Smad6 and Smad7 inhibit TGF–β signaling by preventing phosphorylation of the Smad2/Smad3 complex. In addition to the Smad-dependent pathways, TGF–β also induces Smad-independent signaling pathways. Moreover, cross talk between these pathways is conferred by a multitude of proteins (e.g., JNK, ERK)

ubiquitinate and degrade R-Smads within the nucleus (Izzi and Attisano 2004). Moreover, the Smad-Smurf complex recognizes activated TGF–β receptor complex and induces receptor ubiquitination, caveolin-associated receptor internalization, and subsequent degradation (Di Guglielmo et al. 2003; Ebisawa et al. 2001; Kavsak et al. 2000). Other E3 ubiquitin ligases implicated in Smad degradation include Jun-activating domain binding protein 1(Jab1) and SCF/Roc1 (Fukuchi et al. 2001; Wan et al. 2002). Moreover, a recent study demonstrated that Smad7 inactivates RB and derepresses E2F without blocking the activation of βRI and the nuclear translocation of Smad2/3. Smad7 therefore allows TGF–β1 to exert effects in cancer cells resistant to TGF–β1-mediated growth inhibition (Boyer Arnold and Korc 2005).

The second I-Smad, Smad6, blocks TGF–β signaling via preventing Smad2 interaction with Smad4 (Imamura et al. 1997).

The linker sequences between Smad MH1 and MH2 domains contain multiple phosphorylation sites that confer binding with a multitude of proteins, thereby allowing cross talk with other signaling pathways. For example, Smads interact with the JNK and p38 substrates c-Jun/c-fos and ATF2, respectively (Hanafusa et al. 1999; Sano et al. 1999; Wong et al. 1999; Zhang et al. 1998).

6.3 Role of TGF–β In Vivo and Its Importance in Tumorigenesis and Other Human Diseases

6.3.1 Physiologic Functions of TGF–β

Although initially identified as a proliferation factor for fibroblasts (Moses et al. 1981; Roberts et al. 1980), TGF–β is predominantly known for its cytostatic and apoptotic as well as migratory functions in epithelial cells of the skin, lung, and mammary gland; endothelial cells; neuronal cells; and hematopoietic cells. TGF–β therefore modulates physiologic functions including embryonic development (e.g., of the heart and lung as well as the palate), wound healing, vasculogenesis and angiogenesis, as well as hematopoiesis and immune surveillance. Importantly, TGF–β exerts both cell type-specific and tissue-specific effects dependent on the microenvironment, thereby maintaining homeostasis in many organ systems (Attisano and Wrana 2002; Derynck et al. 2001; Fortunel et al. 2000; Massagué 1998; Moustakas et al. 2001; Shi and Massague 2003; Siegel and Massague 2003; Whitman 1998). For example, TGF–β plays a crucial role in osteoblastic differentiation and TGF–β/activin/nodal signaling is necessary for the maintainance of pluripotency in human embryonic stem cells (James et al. 2005; Maeda et al. 2004).

TGF–β-mediated growth arrest is mediated by at least two different mechanisms, one involving cyclin-dependent kinases and the other c-Myc. Specifically, TGF–β enhances transcription of cyclin-dependent kinase inhibitors (CDKI) INK4B/p15 (CDKN2B) and CDKN1A/p21 (WAF1, CIP1), as well as KIP1/p27, which induce hypophosphorylation of the retinoblastoma protein (Rb) and subsequent sequestration of the transcription factor E2F (Datto et al. 1995; Hannon and Beach 1994; Polyak et al. 1994). TGF–β also induces repression of c-Myc. Specifically, E2F4/5 and p107 can serve as Smad cofactors linking TGF–β-triggered signals to rapid and cell cycle-independent downregulation of c-Myc.

Several signaling molecules have additionally been demonstrated to mediate the proapoptotic effects of TGF–β. For example, TGF–β inhibits the expression of the inhibitors of differentiation (Id) proteins (Id1, Id2, and Id3), which function as negative regulators of basic helix-loop-helix (bHLH) transcription factors (C. R. Chen et al. 2002; Kang et al. 2003a; Norton 2000; Siegel et al. 2003b). In addition, TGF–β inhibits p70S6 kinase via protein phosphatase 2A (PP2A), thereby inducing G1 arrest (Petritsch et al. 2000). Cell cycle arrest is also achieved by TGF–β-induced inhibition of Cdc25A via RhoA and ROCK1 (Bhowmick et al. 2001). Interaction of the type II receptor for TGF–β and the proapoptotic adapter protein Daxx leads to homeodomain-interacting protein kinase 2 (HIPK2)-dependent activation of MEKK4 and MEKK7 and ultimately JNK (Hofmann et al. 2003). Other downstream targets include the phospholipid phosphatase SHIP, death-associated protein kinase (DAPK), and TGF–β-inducible early response gene 1 (TIEG1) (Siegel and Massague 2003).

6.3.2 TGF–β and Tumorigenesis

Functions of TGF–β seem to follow a biphasic mode during tumorigenesis, acting as tumor suppressors in early-stage disease and as potent stimulators of tumor progression in late-stage disease.

Although TGF–β was first identified as a factor that induces transformation in rat fibroblasts (de Larco and Todaro 1978; Frolik et al. 1983), subsequent studies predominantly focused on the autocrine tumor-suppressive properties of TGF–β. Signaling pathways mediating this inhibitory impact of TGF–β on tumor growth have been delineated. Loss-of-function mutations of TGF–β, its receptors, and Smad proteins, as well as decreased TGF–β sensitivity due to decreased TβRII expression, have been associated with early stages of tumorigenesis.

Recent data demonstrate that many tumors overexpress TGF–β, also implicating TGF–β in late tumor stages defined by tumor invasion, metastasis, and lack of immune surveillance.

Therefore the optimal time for treatment with TGF–β inhibitors is when the tumor is

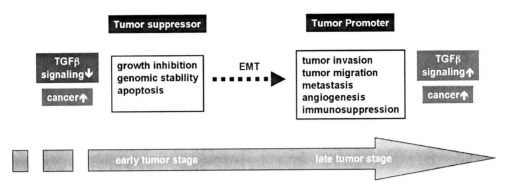

Fig. 6.2 Biphasic functions of TGF–β during tumorigenesis. In tumorigenesis, early-stage disease is associated with tumor cells that are refractory to TGF–β stimulation; in contrast, late-stage disease is associated with increased TGF–β stimulation leading to enhanced epithelial-mesenchymal transdifferentiation (EMT), tumor invasiveness, tumor cell migration, angiogenesis, and immunosuppression

refractory to TGF–β-induced growth suppression, but still responsive to tumor-promoting TGF–β effects including tumor invasion, angiogenesis, and metastasis (Fig. 6.2).

6.3.2.1 TGF–β and Tumor Suppression

TGF–β is a potent growth inhibitor and inducer of apoptosis (Coffey et al. 1988; Perlman et al. 2001). Conversely, hereditary and somatic mutations of TGF–β receptors (predominantly TβRII) and Smad proteins abrogate the growth-inhibitory effects of TGF–β, thereby leading to enhanced tumor development in certain forms of cancer (Derynck et al. 2001; Massague et al. 2000; Wakefield and Roberts 2002). Additional potential mechanisms leading to TGF–β resistance in tumor cells include decreased receptor expression; increased expression of the I-Smad Smad7; repression of TGF–β signaling by oncoproteins (i.e., p53, c-Myc, E1A, Ras, Ski/SnoN, and Evi-1); reduced expression of tumor suppressors [i.e., menin, disabled-2, and runx3 (Bae and Choi 2004)]; activation of telomerase; and activation of PKC (Alexandrow et al. 1995; Y. R. Chen et al. 1996b; Datto et al. 1997; Ewen et al. 1995; W. C. Hahn 2003; Hocevar et al. 2001; Kaji et al. 2001; Katakura et al. 1999; Kim et al. 1999; Kleeff et al. 199, 2000; Kretzschmar et al. 1999; Kurokawa et al. 1998; Q. L. Li et al. 2002; Nicolas and Hill 2003; Stroschein et al. 1999; Y. Sun et al. 1999; Yakymovych et al. 2001).

Moreover, a recent study demonstrated that PI3K modulates Foxo transcription factor, thereby attenuating the Smad-dependent antimitogenic effect on neuroepithelium and glioblastoma cell proliferation (Seoane et al. 2004).

Mutations of the TGF–β Receptors

TβRII Microsatellite Instability and Missense Mutations
Microsatellite instability (MSI), which causes DNA mismatch repair defects, is common in a variety of both sporadic and hereditary tumors. Inactivating TβRII mutations associated with MSI (e.g., BAT-RII inactivating mutations in the polyadenine repeat of the extracellular domain) occur in gliomas, sporadic gastrointestinal cancers, as well as hereditary nonpolyposis colon cancer (HNPCC). In contrast, TβRII mutations are uncommon in endometrial, breast, pancreas, and liver cancer (Izumoto et al. 1997; Lu et al. 1996; Markowitz et al. 1995; Myeroff et al. 1995; Parsons et al. 1995; J. Wang et al. 1995).

The SNU-638 human gastric cancer cell line encodes a truncated, inactive TβRII protein. Retroviral infection with a wild-type TβRII leads to significant reduction of proliferation; conversely, addition of TGF–β-neutralizing antibodies leads to increased proliferation of SNU-638 cells carrying the wild-type TβRII, without effects on control cells (Chang et al. 1997). Furthermore, TβRII mutations inactivate tumor suppressor activity in replication error-positive colon carcinoma cells (J. Wang et al. 1995).

In addition to MSI cancers with TβRII mutations, TβRII missense mutations in the TβRII kinase domain occur in 15% of MS-stable colon cancers (Grady et al. 1999).

TβRI Mutations and Polymorphism

Inactivating TβRI mutations occur in ovarian cancer; missense mutations in the TβRI kinase domain occur in metastatic breast cancer; and deletions of TβRI occur in pancreatic and biliary carcinomas as well as cutaneous T-cell lymphoma (T. Chen et al. 1998; Goggins et al. 1998; Schiemann et al. 1999; D. Wang et al. 1999, 2000). Moreover, the homozygous presence of the attenuated TβRI(6A) gene causes increased risk of colon cancer (Pasche et al. 1999).

Importantly, a recently performed meta-analysis of 12 case-control studies shows increased cancer risk in individuals carrying TGFBRI*6A, a somatically acquired polymorphism in colon and head and neck cancer. It impairs TGF–β-mediated antiproliferative response and increases cell proliferation of breast and colon cancer cells (Bian et al. 2005; Pasche et al. 2004, 2005).

The association of tumorigenesis and the impairment of TGF–β signaling is also supported in animal models. For example, mammary tumor development in a mouse mammary tumor virus (MMTV)-TGF-α murine model was markedly suppressed by coexpression with activated TGF–β1 (Pierce et al. 1995). Moreover, transgenic mice overexpressing a dominant-negative mutant TβRII show enhanced tumorigenesis in the mammary gland and lung in response to carcinogen 7,12-dimethylbenz-[a]-anthracene (Bottinger et al. 1997).

Mutations of the Smads

Deletions of Smad4 have been reported in pancreatic cancer, metastatic colon cancer, and the autosomal dominant juvenile polyposis syndrome (S. A. Hahn et al. 1996; Howe et al. 1998; Miyaki et al. 1999). Moreover, biliary cancer and colon cancer show Smad4 mutations together with TβRI and TβRII mutations, respectively (Goggins et al. 1998; Grady et al. 1999). Mutations of Smad 2 have been reported

in human colorectal and lung cancer (Eppert et al. 1996; Uchida et al. 1996).

Mice with homozygous deletions of both Smad2 and Smad4 die in utero. In contrast, mice with haploid deletions are viable but have a high incidence of gastrointestinal polyps (Takaku et al. 1998; X. Xu et al. 2000). In Smad 4-deficient pancreatic cancer cells, TGF–β triggers increased cell motility and invasiveness due to autocrine production and activation of TGF–β (Subramanian et al. 2004). Compound mutant APC+/- Smad4+/- mice develop several polyps that progress to invasive adenocarcinoma on loss of the remaining APC and Smad4 genes (Takaku et al. 1998). Compound disruption of smad2 accelerates malignant progression of intestinal tumors in APC-knockout mice (Hamamoto et al. 2002). Finally, Smad 3-mutant mice develop metastatic colorectal cancer (Zhu et al. 1998).

6.3.2.2 TGF–β and Tumor Progression

Recent data show that many tumors overexpress TGF–β, suggesting a strong positive role for TGF–β in tumor invasion and metastasis (Elliott and Blobe 2005). However, we are just beginning to understand the precise pathophysiologic mechanisms. For example, in addition to directly affecting tumor cells, TGF–β promotes effects on nontumor stromal cells. Specifically, TGF–β induces enhanced production and secretion of mitogenic growth factors including platelet-derived growth factor (PDGF), fibroblast growth factor (FGF), and IL-6, as well as the PDGF and EGF receptors.

Cui et al. were among the first to show a bimodal role of TGF–β1 in tumorigenesis. Specifically, they demonstrated that TGF–β1 inhibits formation of benign skin tumors, but also enhances progression to invasive spindle carcinomas, in transgenic mice (Cui et al. 1996). Other studies have shown similar results, for example, in breast cancer (Tang et al. 2003) and skin cancer (Oft et al. 2002).

These studies show that TGF–β follows a biphasic mode during tumorigenesis, acting early as a tumor suppressor and later as a potent stimulator of tumor progression (Dumont and Arteaga 2003; Wakefield and Roberts 2002). Moreover, recent studies demonstrate that TGF–β modulates (1) epithelial-to-mesenchymal-transition (EMT); (2) tumor immune suppression; (3) tumor angiogenesis; and (4) tissue-specific metastasis. Recent data also demonstrate that TGF–β decreases Rad51 expression, thereby promoting DNA instability and inhibition of DNA repair. These effects contribute to tumor progression by increasing the rate of tumor-promoting mutations in malignant cells (Kanamoto et al. 2002).

TGF–β and Epithelial-Mesenchymal Transdifferentiation

EMT frequently occurs in late tumor stages of carcinoma and correlates with increased rates of metastasis (Thiery 2002). TGF–β induces Smad-dependent EMT and enhances tumor cell invasiveness (i.e., squamous mammary, lung, as well as head and neck cancer) in synergy with other signaling pathways, for example, the Ras/Raf signaling pathway (Derynck et al. 2001; Itoh et al. 2003; Janda et al. 2002; Johansson et al. 2000; Leivonen et al. 2006; Oft et al. 1996, 1998, 2002; Yu et al. 2002). Furthermore, a recent study demonstrates that both MAPKAPK2 and HSP27 are necessary for TGF–β-mediated increases in MMP-2 and cell invasion in human prostate cancer (L. Xu et al. 2006). Importantly, TGF–β also activates Rho GTPases, followed by downstream activation of ROCK1 and Limk2, which leads to inhibition of cofilin depolymerization and thereby to actin polymerization (Vardouli et al. 2005).

TGF–β also positively regulates the zinc finger proteins SIP1, SNAIL, and SLUG, which downregulate the calcium-dependent cell adhesion receptor E-cadherin and thereby induce EMT. Specifically, TGF–β increases the expression of SIP1, SNAIL, and SLUG, which downregulate E-cadherin (Comijn et al. 2001; Hajra et al. 2002; Peinado et al. 2003, 2004; Savagner et al. 1997). Conversely, overexpression of E-cadherin markedly suppresses tumor cell invasion (Miettinen et al. 1994; Oft et al. 1996; Thiery 2002).

TGF–β and Immune Suppression

Given the negative regulatory role of TGF–β on hematopoiesis, one of the obvious consequences of TGF–β-associated tumorigenesis is immunosuppression. Targets of TGF–β include T-lymphocytes, dendritic cells, and major histocompatibility complex class II (MHC II).

Specifically, studies in transgenic mice show that TGF–β negatively regulates T (CD4+ as well as CD8+) lymphocytes. Consequently, abrogation of TGF–β leads to spontaneous T cell differentiation and autoimmune disease (Gorelik et al. 2002; Gorelik and Flavell 2000, 2002). Blockade of TGF–β signaling generates an immune response capable of eradicating tumors in mice challenged with live tumor cells (Gorelik and Flavell 2001). T cells carrying dominant-negative TβRII promote the rapid and complete eradication of both injected thymoma and melanoma cells (Gorelik and Flavell 2001; Torre-Amione et al. 1990).

TGF–β also blocks the noncognate maturation of human dendritic Langerhans cells, macrophage activation, as well as the expression of the MHC II complex, thereby negatively affecting T cell activation (J.J. Chen et al. 1998; Geiser et al. 1993; Geissmann et al. 1999; Mustafa et al. 1993; Reimold et al. 1993; Wallick et al. 1990).

Finally, TGF–β-mediated suppression of antitumor immunity may also be mediated via its effects on natural killer cells and neutrophils (Arteaga et al. 1993b; J.J. Chen et al. 1998; Wallick et al. 1990).

TGF–β and Angiogenesis

TGF–β is a strong mediator of angiogenesis (Dickson et al. 1995; Goumans et al. 1999; Larsson et al. 2001; Martin et al. 1995; Oshima et al. 1996). Increased levels of TGF–β1 have been correlated with increased microvessel density in invasive breast cancer and non-small lung cancer (de Jong et al. 1998; Hasegawa et al. 2001). TGF–β1 induces the expression of angiogenic growth factors including vascular endothelial growth factor (VEGF) and the hypertrophic chondrocyte-specific connective tissue growth factor (CTGF) in fibroblastic and endothelial cells (Kang et al. 2003b; Pertovaara et al. 1994; Shimo et al. 2001). In addition, TGF–β inhibits angiopoietin1 (Ang1) expression, which confers vessel integrity (Enholm et al. 1997) as well as inducing the expression and secretion of matrix metalloproteinases, thereby leading to tissue remodeling and tumor metastasis (Hagedorn et al. 2001).

Endoglin is an endothelium-specific TGF–β receptor pivotal for angiogenesis (Johnson et al. 1996; McAllister et al. 1994). Importantly, the expression of endoglin is markedly increased during tumor-associated angiogenesis, therefore providing a potential antitumor target (Burrows et al. 1995).

The importance of TGF–β signaling in tumor angiogenesis has also been supported in animal models. For example, increased angiogenesis associated with metastasis has been demonstrated in a xenograft mouse model of prostate cancer; in this setting, angiogenesis is decreased on inhibition of TGF–β1 (Stearns et al. 1999; Tuxhorn et al. 2002).

TGF–β and Tissue-Specific Metastasis

Tumor metastasis is a major cause of cancer-related death (Sporn 1996). Besides its indirect effects via enhancing EMT and angiogenesis while suppressing antitumor immunity, TGF–β also directly triggers metastasis. Specifically, Siegel et al. demonstrated that TGF–β impairs Neu-induced mammary tumorigenesis while promoting pulmonary metastasis (Siegel et al. 2003a). Moreover, TGF–β stimulates the expression of the osteoclast-activating factor parathyroid hormone-related peptide (PTHrP), CTGF, and the osteoclast differentiation factor IL-11, thereby promoting bone metastasis (Kang et al. 2003b; Yin et al. 1999). Conversely, lifetime exposure to a soluble TGF–β antagonist, expressed as a transgene in the mammary glands of transgenic mice, protects against metastasis without affecting tumor growth or inflammatory side effects (Muraoka et al. 2002; Yang et al. 2002). Furthermore, TGF–β blockade-induced inhibition of PTHrP secretion abrogates bone metastasis in a murine breast cancer model (Kang et al. 2003b).

6.3.3 TGF–β and Hematopoietic Malignancies

To date the complex role of TGF–β in tumorigenesis has been predominantly stud-

ied in solid tumors. However, recently a role of TGF–β has also been reported in hematologic malignancies. Specifically, Imai et al. reported two mutations of Smad4 gene in acute myelogenous leukemia, which block the antiproliferative effect of TGF–β (Imai et al. 2001). Moreover, mutations of TβRI and TβRII expression have been reported in myelofibrosis with myeloid metaplasia (MMM), malignant progression of cutaneous T-cell lymphoma and other lymphomas, as well as chronic lymphocytic leukemia (DeCoteau et al. 1997; Knaus et al. 1996; Le Bousse-Kerdiles et al. 1996; Lowsky et al. 2000). Furthermore, AML1/ETO and AML1/EVI-1 fusion proteins in AML with t(8;21) translocation bind to Smad3 and inhibit TGF–β1-induced effects, thereby contributing to leukemogenesis (Jakubowiak et al. 2000; Mitani 2004). Wolfraim et al. reported that the loss of Smad3, coupled with the loss of p27, causes T-lineage acute lymphoblastic leukemia (T-cell ALL), indicating that TGF–β participates in blocking the development of T-cell ALL by suppressing T cell proliferation (Wolfraim et al. 2004). In acute promyelocytic leukemia (APL) cytoplasmic PML physically interacts with Smad2/3 and SARA, thereby regulating internalization of the TβRI/II/SARA/Smad2/3 complex into the early endosome. Importantly, the PML-RARα oncoprotein of APL antagonizes cytoplasmic PML function, causing defects in TGF–β signaling similar to those observed in Pml-/- cells. These studies therefore identified cytoplasmic PML as a critical TGF–β regulator and implicate deregulated TGF–β signaling in leukemogensis (Lin et al. 2004). Finally, in multiple myeloma (MM) high levels of TGF–β1 are produced and secreted by tumor cells, which trigger IL-6 secretion by bone marrow stromal cells (BMSCs), with related MM cell proliferation (Portier et al. 1993; Urashima et al. 1996). Moreover, increased TGF–β levels are correlated with the incidence of osteolytic lesions as well as the degree of immunoparesis (Brown et al. 2001; Jiang et al. 1995; Kyrtsonis et al. 1998; Otsuki et al. 2001).

6.4 Validation of TGF-β and Its Drugability

TGF-β plasma levels as well as TGF-β receptor mutations are used as diagnostic, prognostic, and predictive tools in cancer detection and treatment (Elliott and Blobe 2005). Specifically, TGF-β serum levels are elevated in a variety of progressive tumors. For example, elevated urinary TGF-β1 levels serve as a tumor marker that predicts poor survival in cirrhotic hepatocellular carcinoma. They are more sensitive tumor markers in hepatocellular carcinomas than AFP (Tsai et al. 1997a, 1997b, 1997c). Increased TGF-β1 levels correlate with tumor recurrence after prior surgery and/or conventional chemotherapy for cancers including colon cancer, prostate cancer, bladder cancer, gastric cancer, and breast cancer (C. Li et al. 1999; Saito et al. 2000; Shariat et al. 2001a, 2001b; Tsushima et al. 2001). Importantly, TGF-β also serves as a predictor of liver and lung fibrosis after autologous bone marrow transplantation for advanced breast cancer (Anscher et al. 1993). An example of the therapy predicated upon the value of plasma TGF-β levels is their use during radiotherapy to select patients with NSCLC for dose escalation (Anscher et al. 2003). Moreover, favorable outcome of adjuvant fluorouracil was observed in patients both with MS-stable colon cancer and retention of the 18q alleles and with MSI colon cancer with a mutation of the TβRII (Watanabe et al. 2001).

Another potential biomarker for TGF-β inhibitor therapy is the TGFBRI*6A polymorphism in colon and head and neck cancers (Pasche et al. 2005).

As described above, TGF-β plays a complex role in tumorigenesis since TGF-β acts as a tumor suppressor early and as a potent stimulator of tumor progression later in tumor development (Dumont and Arteaga 2003; Wakefield and Roberts 2002). Therefore therapeutic strategies aim to enhance TGF-β signaling effects in early, and to inhibit TGF-β signaling effects in late, tumor development.

Specifically, enhancement of TGF-β signaling (e.g., by inducing TβRII expression) can be achieved by a variety of agents including the histone deacetylase inhibitor MS-275, the angiotensin-converting enzyme (ACE) inhibitor captopril, the farnesyltransferase inhibitor FTI-277, interferon alpha (Castilla et al. 1991), prednisone (Ziesche et al. 1999), and the DNA methyltransferase inhibitor 5-aza-2'-deoxycytidine (Adnane et al. 2000; Kavsak et al. 2000; Miyajima et al. 2001; S. H. Park et al. 2002; Venkatasubbarao et al. 2001). Moreover, anticancerogen effects of both tamoxifen and retinoids may be at least in part be caused by increased TGF-β levels (Comerci et al. 1997; Grainger and Metcalfe 1996; Grainger et al. 1995; McDonald et al. 1995).

In contrast, there are several different approaches to inhibit TGF-β signaling: inhibition of TGF-β binding (using soluble receptors); inhibition of TGF-β receptor activation and intracellular signaling (using large-molecule inhibitors, i.e., monoclonal antibodies, as well as small-molecule inhibitors); and TGF-β antisense approaches (Yingling et al. 2004). Moreover, anti-endoglin antibodies have been shown to inhibit tumor angiogenesis (Matsuno et al. 1999).

The ideal time point for initiation of treatment with TGF-β inhibitors would be when tumor cells are refractory to TGF-β-induced growth suppression but still responsive to tumor-promoting TGF-β effects including tumor invasion, angiogenesis, and metastasis (Arteaga 2006; Elliott and Blobe 2005). Treatment regimens with TGF-β inhibitors also benefit from T cell-specific blockade of TGF-β signaling, thereby augmenting antitumor immunity (Gorelik and Flavell 2001). Furthermore, TGF-β can synergize with transforming oncogenes in transformation and tumor progression. Recent therapeutic approaches in cancer treatment are aimed to target TGF-β signaling in late-stage tumors, alone or in combination with conventional or novel targeted therapy. However, care must be taken in treatment planning and timing, because of the potential risk of TGF-β antagonists to accelerate preneoplastic lesions or to induce autoimmune diseases and inflammation.

6.5 Compounds and Leads

6.5.1 Inhibition of TGF–β Binding

TGF–β is a cytokine with a myriad of functions on tumor biology. One approach to target this pathway would be to inhibit TGF binding to endogenous receptors. An example of such an agent is the soluble chimeric protein Fc:TβRII, which is comprised of the extracellular domain of TβRII and the Fc portion of the murine IgG1 heavy chain. This soluble receptor protein has been tested by Muraoka et al. (Muraoka et al. 2002) in transgenic and transplantable models of breast cancer metastasis, in which systemic administration of this soluble receptor protein resulted in increased apoptosis of primary tumors, accompanied by decreased tumor motility and metastatic potential associated with inhibition of AKT and further downstream inhibition of phosphorylation of FKHRL1. This chimera interferes with TGF–β binding to its receptors and blocks TGF–β-induced in vivo fibrosis (George et al. 1999). Another TGF–β soluble receptor antagonist in preclinical testing is the recombinant soluble betaglycan (sBG) (Bandyopadhyay et al. 1999). Systemic administration of sBG inhibits breast and prostate cancer xenograft growth, as well as angiogenesis (Bandyopadhyay et al. 2002, 2005). A potential advantage of the sBG compared to the soluble fusion protein is its greater affinity for TGF–β2 (Fig. 6.3).

6.5.2 Inhibition of TGF–β Receptor Activation and Intracellular Signaling

6.5.2.1 Large-Molecule TGF–β Inhibitors

Another approach to target TGF–β is the use of monoclonal antibodies (mAb) that act by blocking the ligand interaction with its receptors. Several monoclonal antibodies against TGF–β are in preclinical and clinical development.

Lerdelimumab (CAT-152/Trabio) is a humanized TGF–β2 mAb developed for clinical use by Cambridge Antibody Technologies (Cordeiro 2003). It is a recombinant human immunoglobulin G4 anti-TGF–β2 mAb that has been produced with phage display technology. To date, it has mainly been used in ophthalmic indications including glaucoma and cataract surgery, primarily for the prevention of postoperative scarring (Mead et al. 2003; Siriwardena et al. 2002; Wormstone et al. 2002). Ledelimumab has been administered in a phase I clinical trial to 56 patients undergoing surgery for glaucoma, without significant adverse effects at a 6-month follow-up (Bayes et al. 2003). Metelimumab (CAT-192) is a humanized anti-TGF–β1 mAb that has been studied with in vivo models of diabetic nephropathy. When given in combination with the ACE inhibitor lisinopril in a rat model CAT-192 arrests the development of proteinuria and renal

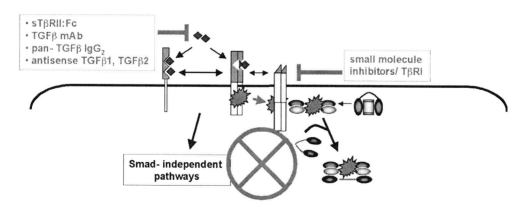

Fig. 6.3 Sites of actions of TGF–β inhibitors

injury and prevents the development of diabetic nephropathy (Benigni et al. 2003). Both antibodies have been awarded orphan status in Europe, and CAT-192 is currently undergoing phase I/II evaluation in the treatment of scleroderma.

Several panspecific anti-TGF–β antibodies that target all three TGF–β receptors are also being developed. The murine 1D11 mAb is a panspecific TGF–β mAb in preclinical development, which has shown antineoplastic potential inhibiting angiogenesis in renal cell cancer (Ananth et al. 1999). More recently, this mAb has also demonstrated protection against renal injury and attenuation of hypertension in uremic rats (Lavoie et al. 2005). 2G7 is another panspecific anti-TGF–β mAb that has shown antitumor potential in a variety of cancers including breast cancer and melanoma (Arteaga et al. 1993a; Wojtowicz-Praga et al. 1996). Its mechanism of action is mainly immunomodulation via its effects on dendritic cells, T cells, and NK cells (Arteaga et al. 1993b; Verdaguer et al. 1999). GC-1008 is also a human anti-TGF–β mAb about to enter phase I clinical testing for the treatment of idiopathic pulmonary fibrosis (Yingling et al. 2004) (Fig. 6.3).

6.5.2.2 TGF–β Antisense Approaches

Another exciting area of TGF–β targeting is the development of antisense oligonucleotides. Antisense TGF–β2 vaccine is currently being tested in phase I/II trials. These studies are based on preclinical data generated in rats with established intracranial gliomas. Animals were immunized with genetically modified 9L gliosarcoma cells containing antisense plasmid vector that inhibits TGF–β2 expression. Treated animals survived the duration of the study period, as compared to controls. Similar results have been obtained in a c6 rat glioma model (Fakhrai et al. 1996; Liau et al. 1998). Several other immunotherapy strategies have tested antisense approaches to TGF–β in bladder caner, liver cancer, and ovarian teratoma models (Dorigo et al. 1998; Maggard et al. 2001; Tzai et al. 1998, 2000).

AP-12009 is an example of a large-molecule antisense oligonucleotide being developed for treatment of gliomas (Bayes et al. 2004). Since it is being developed for intratumoral therapy, it has been injected intrathecally and within brain parenchyma in rabbits and monkeys without any evidence of local toxicity (Schlingensiepen et al. 2006). The safety and efficacy of AP-12009 have been tested in a phase I/II open-label dose escalation study in high-grade glioma patients. The drug was well tolerated and showed an increase in median survival time compared to historical controls. Based on these data, a phase I/II study in pancreatic carcinoma and malignant melanoma is currently ongoing. (Schlingensiepen et al. 2006). AP-11014 is another TGF–β1 specific phosphothioate antisense oligonucleotide in preclinical development for lung, colorectal, and prostate cancers (Yingling et al. 2004) (Fig. 6.3).

6.5.2.3 Small-Molecule TGF–β RI Kinase Inhibitors

Compared to large-molecule TGF–β inhibitors, small-molecule inhibitors have better tissue delivery and cell penetration. However, they are pharmacologically unstable and require more frequent administration. In addition, they are more likely to cross-react with other serine-threonine receptor kinases. These small-molecule inhibitors are all ATP-competitive inhibitors of TβRI that spare TβRII receptors and therefore do not completely inhibit TGF–β function. This could result in decreased antitumor activity, but adverse side effects including inflammatory effects could also be ameliorated (Fig. 6.3).

LY580276 and LY364947 (Lilly Research Laboratories)

LY580276 and LY364947 are highly selective TβRI inhibitors that potently inhibit EMT (Peng et al. 2005; Sawyer et al. 2004). Structurally similarly to this inhibitor, A-83-01 was found to be more potent in the inhibition of TβRI than LY364947, also preventing phosphorylation of Smad2/3 (Tojo et al. 2005).

SB-431542 and SB-505124 (GlaxoSmithKline)

SB-431542 is a potent and specific inhibitor of the TGF–β superfamily type I activin receptor-like kinase receptors Alk4, Alk5, and Alk7, but it has no effect on BMP-binding receptors (Inman et al. 2002; Laping et al. 2002). SB-431542 attenuates tumor-promoting effects of TGF–β including EMT, cell motility, migration and invasion, as well as angiogenesis (Halder et al. 2005). Specifically, in human glioma cell lines SB-431542 inhibits cell proliferation, motility, and secretion of VEGF and Ang-1 (Hjelmeland et al. 2004). In esophageal squamous cell carcinoma, trastuzumab-mediated ADCC is enhanced by treatment with SB-431542 (Mimura et al. 2005). In human osteosarcoma cells, SB-431542 and Gleevec inhibit TGF–β-induced proliferation (Matsuyama et al. 2003). SB-505124 is a three to five times more potent and selective inhibitor of TGF–β type I receptors Alk4, Alk5, and Alk7 (but not Alk1–3 or Alk6) than SB-431542 (Byfield et al. 2004).

SD-093, SD-908, SD-208

The TβRI inhibitor SD-093 markedly inhibits both in vitro motility and invasiveness of pancreatic cancer cells but does not affect their growth or cell morphology. It therefore represents a potential new therapeutic approach to treat patients with advanced pancreatic cancer (Subramanian et al. 2004).

SD-208, similar to SB-505124, inhibits Alk4, Alk5, and Alk7. As shown by in vitro and in vivo experiments, SD-208 inhibits growth and invasiveness and enhances immunogenicity of murine and human cells (Uhl et al. 2004). In MM, SD-208 inhibits production of IL-6 and VEGF and associated MM cell growth, survival, drug resistance, and migration in the BM milieu, thereby providing the preclinical rationale for clinical evaluation of SD-208 to improve patient outcome in MM (Hayashi et al. 2004).

Other Small-Molecule Inhibitors

Other prototypical preclinical small-molecule inhibitors include LY550410 (Sawyer et al. 2004) and NPC 30345 (Ge et al. 2004).

6.6 Conclusion

TGF–β has a multitude of opposing effects, dependent on the specific cell, the tissue environment and microenvironment, as well as the developmental stage. These effects are mediated via a complex network of Smad-dependent and Smad-independent TGF–β signaling pathways, as well as cross talk with other signaling pathways. In tumorigenesis, early-stage disease is associated with tumor cells that are refractory to TGF–β stimulation; and late-stage disease is associated with increased TGF–β stimulation leading to enhanced EMT, tumor invasiveness, angiogenesis, and immunosuppression. In addition, TGF–β can synergize with oncogenes in transformation and tumor progression.

Based on preclinical data, blocking TGF–β signaling represents a potentially powerful and novel approach to treat patients with advanced cancer. However, because of the dual role of TGF–β, care must be taken to avoid potential acceleration of preneoplastic lesions or cancers caused by the inhibition of a still tumor-suppressive TGF–β. Biomarkers for the selection of patients to be recruited to clinical TGF–β-inhibitor trials must therefore be identified. Potential markers include TGF–β, mutations of TGF–β receptors, as well as TGFBR polymorphisms.

Ongoing preclinical and clinical studies will help to further delineate complex TGF–β-triggered signaling pathways; to evaluate existing and design new more effective TGF–β inhibitors; and to determine the appropriate patient populations in whom to evaluate novel therapies inhibiting TGF–β signaling.

Acknowledgements

This work was supported by The Multiple Myeloma Research Foundation (MMRF) Senior Research Grant Award (to N.R. and K.P.); National Institutes of Health Grants RO 50947, PO-1 78378, SPORE P50 CA100707 and the Doris Duke Distinguished Clinical Research Scientist Award (to K.C.A.).

References

Adnane J et al. (2000) Inhibition of farnesyltransferase increases TGFbeta type II receptor expression and enhances the responsiveness of human cancer cells to TGFbeta. Oncogene 19:5525–5533

Alexandrow MG et al. (1995) Overexpression of the c-Myc oncoprotein blocks the growth-inhibitory response but is required for the mitogenic effects of transforming growth factor beta 1. Proc Natl Acad Sci USA 92:3239–3243

Ananth S et al. (1999) Transforming growth factor beta1 is a target for the von Hippel-Lindau tumor suppressor and a critical growth factor for clear cell renal carcinoma. Cancer Res 59:2210–2216

Anscher MS et al. (1993) Transforming growth factor beta as a predictor of liver and lung fibrosis after autologous bone marrow transplantation for advanced breast cancer. N Engl J Med 328:1592–1598

Anscher MS et al. (2003) Risk of long-term complications after TFG-beta1-guided very-high-dose thoracic radiotherapy. Int J Radiat Oncol Biol Phys 56:988–995

Arteaga CL et al. (1993a) Evidence for a positive role of transforming growth factor-beta in human breast cancer cell tumorigenesis. J Cell Biochem Suppl 17G:187–193

Arteaga CL et al. (1993b) Anti-transforming growth factor (TGF)-beta antibodies inhibit breast cancer cell tumorigenicity and increase mouse spleen natural killer cell activity. Implications for a possible role of tumor cell/host TGF-beta interactions in human breast cancer progression. J Clin Invest 92:2569–2576

Arteaga CL (2006) Inhibition of TGFbeta signaling in cancer therapy. Curr Opin Genet Dev 16:30–37

Attisano L, Wrana JL (2000) Smads as transcriptional comodulators. Curr Opin Cell Biol 12:235–243

Attisano L, Wrana JL (2002) Signal transduction by the TGF-beta superfamily. Science 296:1646–1647

Bae SC, Choi JK (2004) Tumor suppressor activity of RUNX3. Oncogene 23:4336–4340

Bakin AV et al. (2000) Phosphatidylinositol 3-kinase function is required for transforming growth factor beta-mediated epithelial to mesenchymal transition and cell migration. J Biol Chem 275:36803–36810

Bandyopadhyay A et al. (1999) A soluble transforming growth factor beta type III receptor suppresses tumorigenicity and metastasis of human breast cancer MDA-MB-231 cells. Cancer Res 59:5041–5046

Bandyopadhyay A et al. (2002) Antitumor activity of a recombinant soluble betaglycan in human breast cancer xenograft. Cancer Res 62:4690–4695

Bandyopadhyay A et al. (2005) Systemic administration of a soluble betaglycan suppresses tumor growth, angiogenesis, and matrix metalloproteinase-9 expression in a human xenograft model of prostate cancer. Prostate 63:81–90

Bayes M et al. (2003) Gateways to clinical trials. Methods Find Exp Clin Pharmacol 25:317–340

Bayes M et al. (2004) Gateways to clinical trials. Methods Find Exp Clin Pharmacol 26:587–612

Benigni A et al. (2003) Add-on anti-TGF-beta antibody to ACE inhibitor arrests progressive diabetic nephropathy in the rat. J Am Soc Nephrol 14:1816–1824

Bhowmick NA et al. (2001) Transforming growth factor-beta1 mediates epithelial to mesenchymal transdifferentiation through a RhoA-dependent mechanism. Mol Biol Cell 12:27–36

Bian Y et al. (2005) TGFBR1*6A may contribute to hereditary colorectal cancer. J Clin Oncol 23:3074–3078

Bottinger EP et al. (1997) Transgenic mice overexpressing a dominant-negative mutant type II transforming growth factor beta receptor show enhanced tumorigenesis in the mammary gland and lung in response to the carcinogen 7,12-dimethylbenz-[a]-anthracene. Cancer Res 57:5564–5570

Boyer Arnold N, Korc M (2005) Smad7 abrogates transforming growth factor-beta1-mediated growth inhibition in COLO-357 cells through functional inactivation of the retinoblastoma protein. J Biol Chem 280:21858–21866

Brown RD et al. (2001) Dendritic cells from patients with myeloma are numerically normal but functionally defective as they fail to up-regulate CD80 (B7-1) expression after huCD40LT stimulation because of inhibition by transforming growth factor-beta1 and interleukin-10. Blood 98:2992–2998

Burrows FJ et al. (1995) Up-regulation of endoglin on vascular endothelial cells in human solid tumors: implications for diagnosis and therapy. Clin Cancer Res 1:1623–1634

Byfield SD et al. (2004) SB-505124 is a selective inhibitor of transforming growth factor-beta type I receptors ALK4, ALK5, and ALK7. Mol Pharmacol 65:744–752

Castilla A et al. (1991) Transforming growth factors beta 1 and alpha in chronic liver disease. Effects of interferon alfa therapy. N Engl J Med 324:933–940

Chang J et al. (1997) Expression of transforming growth factor beta type II receptor reduces tumorigenicity in human gastric cancer cells. Cancer Res 57:2856–2859

Chen CR et al. (2002) E2F4/5 and p107 as Smad cofactors linking the TGFbeta receptor to c-myc repression. Cell 110:19–32

Chen JJ et al. (1998) Regulation of the proinflammatory effects of Fas ligand (CD95L). Science 282:1714–1717

Chen T et al. (1998) Transforming growth factor beta type I receptor kinase mutant associated with metastatic breast cancer. Cancer Res 58:4805–4810

Chen X et al. (1996) A transcriptional partner for MAD proteins in TGF-beta signalling. Nature 383:691–696

Chen YR et al. (1996) The role of c-Jun N-terminal kinase (JNK) in apoptosis induced by ultraviolet C and gamma radiation. Duration of JNK activation may determine cell death and proliferation. J Biol Chem 271:31929–31936

Coffey RJ, Jr. et al. (1988) Selective inhibition of growth-related gene expression in murine keratinocytes by transforming growth factor beta. Mol Cell Biol 8:3088–3093

Comerci JT, Jr. et al. (1997) Induction of transforming growth factor beta-1 in cervical intraepithelial neoplasia in vivo after treatment with beta-carotene. Clin Cancer Res 3:157–160

Comijn J et al. (2001) The two-handed E box binding zinc finger protein SIP1 downregulates E-cadherin and induces invasion. Mol Cell 7:1267–1278

Cordeiro MF (2003) Technology evaluation:lerdelimumab, Cambridge Antibody Technology. Curr Opin Mol Ther 5:199–203

Crawford SE et al. (1998) Thrombospondin-1 is a major activator of TGF-beta1 in vivo. Cell 93:1159–1170

Cui W et al. (1996) TGFbeta1 inhibits the formation of benign skin tumors, but enhances progression to invasive spindle carcinomas in transgenic mice. Cell 86:531–542

Datto MB et al. (1995) Transforming growth factor beta induces the cyclin-dependent kinase inhibitor p21 through a p53-independent mechanism. Proc Natl Acad Sci USA 92:5545–5549

Datto MB et al. (1997) The viral oncoprotein E1A blocks transforming growth factor beta-mediated induction of p21/WAF1/Cip1 and p15/INK4B. Mol Cell Biol 17:2030–2037

de Jong JS et al. (1998) Expression of growth factors, growth-inhibiting factors, and their receptors in invasive breast cancer. II:Correlations with proliferation and angiogenesis. J Pathol 184:53–57

de Larco JE, Todaro GJ (1978) Growth factors from murine sarcoma virus-transformed cells. Proc Natl Acad Sci USA 75:4001–4005

de Martin R et al. (1987) Complementary DNA for human glioblastoma-derived T cell suppressor factor, a novel member of the transforming growth factor-beta gene family. EMBO J 6:3673–3677

DeCoteau JF et al. (1997) Loss of functional cell surface transforming growth factor beta (TGF-beta) type 1 receptor correlates with insensitivity to TGF-beta in chronic lymphocytic leukemia. Proc Natl Acad Sci USA 94:5877–5881

Derynck R et al. (1985) Human transforming growth factor-beta complementary DNA sequence and expression in normal and transformed cells. Nature 316:701–705

Derynck R et al. (1988) A new type of transforming growth factor-beta, TGF-beta 3. EMBO J 7:3737–3743

Derynck R, Zhang Y (1996) Intracellular signalling:the mad way to do it. Curr Biol 6:1226–1229

Derynck R et al. (2001) TGF-beta signaling in tumor suppression and cancer progression. Nat Genet 29:117–129

Di Guglielmo GM et al. (2003) Distinct endocytic pathways regulate TGF-beta receptor signalling and turnover. Nat Cell Biol 5:410–421

Dickson MC et al. (1995) Defective haematopoiesis and vasculogenesis in transforming growth factor-beta 1 knock out mice. Development 121:1845–1854

Dorigo O et al. (1998) Combination of transforming growth factor beta antisense and interleukin-2 gene therapy in the murine ovarian teratoma model. Gynecol Oncol 71:204–210

Dumont N, Arteaga CL (2003) Targeting the TGF beta signaling network in human neoplasia. Cancer Cell 3:531–536

Ebisawa T et al. (2001) Smurf1 interacts with transforming growth factor-beta type I receptor through Smad7 and induces receptor degradation. J Biol Chem 276:12477–12480

Elliott RL, Blobe GC (2005) Role of transforming growth factor beta in human cancer. J Clin Oncol 23:2078–2093

Engel ME et al. (1999) Interdependent SMAD and JNK signaling in transforming growth factor-beta-mediated transcription. J Biol Chem 274:37413–37420

Enholm B et al. (1997) Comparison of VEGF, VEGF-B, VEGF-C and Ang-1 mRNA regulation by serum, growth factors, oncoproteins and hypoxia. Oncogene 14:2475–2483

Eppert K et al. (1996) MADR2 maps to 18q21 and encodes a TGFbeta-regulated MAD-related protein that is functionally mutated in colorectal carcinoma. Cell 86:543–552

Ewen ME et al. (1995) p53-dependent repression of CDK4 translation in TGF-beta-induced G1 cell-cycle arrest. Genes Dev 9:204–217

Fakhrai H et al. (1996) Eradication of established intracranial rat gliomas by transforming growth factor beta antisense gene therapy. Proc Natl Acad Sci USA 93:2909–2914

Fortunel NO et al. (2000) Transforming growth factor-beta:pleiotropic role in the regulation of hematopoiesis. Blood 96:2022–2036

Frolik CA et al. (1983) Purification and initial characterization of a type beta transforming growth factor from human placenta. Proc Natl Acad Sci USA 80:3676–3680

Fukuchi M et al. (2001) Ligand-dependent degradation of Smad3 by a ubiquitin ligase complex of ROC1 and associated proteins. Mol Biol Cell 12:1431–1443

Ge R et al. (2004) Selective inhibitors of type I receptor kinase block cellular transforming growth factor-beta signaling. Biochem Pharmacol 68:41–50

Geiser AG et al. (1993) Transforming growth factor beta 1 (TGF-beta 1) controls expression of major histocompatibility genes in the postnatal mouse:aberrant histocompatibility antigen expression in the pathogenesis of the TGF-beta 1 null mouse phenotype. Proc Natl Acad Sci USA 90:9944–9948

Geissmann F et al. (1999) TGF-beta 1 prevents the noncognate maturation of human dendritic Langerhans cells. J Immunol 162:4567–4575

George J et al. (1999) In vivo inhibition of rat stellate cell activation by soluble transforming growth factor beta type II receptor:a potential new therapy for hepatic fibrosis. Proc Natl Acad Sci USA 96:12719–12724

Goggins M et al. (1998) Genetic alterations of the transforming growth factor beta receptor genes in pancreatic and biliary adenocarcinomas. Cancer Res 58:5329–5332

Gorelik L, Flavell RA (2000) Abrogation of TGFbeta signaling in T cells leads to spontaneous T cell differentiation and autoimmune disease. Immunity 12:171–181

Gorelik L, Flavell RA (2001) Immune-mediated eradication of tumors through the blockade of transforming growth factor-beta signaling in T cells. Nat Med 7:1118–1122

Gorelik L et al. (2002) Mechanism of transforming growth factor beta-induced inhibition of T helper type 1 differentiation. J Exp Med 195:1499–1505

Gorelik L, Flavell RA (2002) Transforming growth factor-beta in T-cell biology. Nat Rev Immunol 2:46–53

Goumans MJ et al. (1999) Transforming growth factor-beta signalling in extraembryonic mesoderm is required for yolk sac vasculogenesis in mice. Development 126:3473–3483

Grady WM et al. (1999) Mutational inactivation of transforming growth factor beta receptor type II in microsatellite stable colon cancers. Cancer Res 59:320–324

Grainger DJ et al. (1995) Tamoxifen elevates transforming growth factor-beta and suppresses diet-induced formation of lipid lesions in mouse aorta. Nat Med 1:1067–1073

Grainger DJ, Metcalfe JC (1996) Tamoxifen:teaching an old drug new tricks? Nat Med 2:381–385

Hagedorn HG et al. (2001) Synthesis and degradation of basement membranes and extracellular matrix and their regulation by TGF-beta in invasive carcinomas (Review). Int J Oncol 18:669–681

Hahn SA et al. (1996) DPC4, a candidate tumor suppressor gene at human chromosome 18q21.1. Science 271:350–353

Hahn WC (2003) Role of telomeres and telomerase in the pathogenesis of human cancer. J Clin Oncol 21:2034–2043

Hajra KM et al. (2002) The SLUG zinc-finger protein represses E-cadherin in breast cancer. Cancer Res 62:1613–1618

Halder SK et al. (2005) A specific inhibitor of TGF-beta receptor kinase, SB-431542, as a potent antitumor agent for human cancers. Neoplasia 7:509–521

Hamamoto T et al. (2002) Compound disruption of smad2 accelerates malignant progression of intestinal tumors in apc knockout mice. Cancer Res 62:5955–5961

Hanafusa H et al. (1999) Involvement of the p38 mitogen-activated protein kinase pathway in transforming growth factor-beta-induced gene expression. J Biol Chem 274:27161–27167

Hannon GJ, Beach D (1994) p15INK4B is a potential effector of TGF-beta-induced cell cycle arrest. Nature 371:257–261

Hasegawa Y et al. (2001) Transforming growth factor-beta1 level correlates with angiogenesis, tumor progression, and prognosis in patients with nonsmall cell lung carcinoma. Cancer 91:964–971

Hata A et al. (2000) OAZ uses distinct DNA- and protein-binding zinc fingers in separate BMP-Smad and Olf signaling pathways. Cell 100:229–240

Hayashi T et al. (2004) Transforming growth factor beta receptor I kinase inhibitor down-regulates cytokine secretion and multiple myeloma cell growth in the bone marrow microenvironment. Clin Cancer Res 10:7540–7546

Hayes S et al. (2002) TGF beta receptor internalization into EEA1-enriched early endosomes:role in signaling to Smad2. J Cell Biol 158:1239–1249

Hjelmeland MD et al. (2004) SB-431542, a small molecule transforming growth factor-beta-receptor antagonist, inhibits human glioma cell line proliferation and motility. Mol Cancer Ther 3:737–745

Hocevar BA et al. (1999) TGF-beta induces fibronectin synthesis through a c-Jun N-terminal kinase-dependent, Smad4-independent pathway. EMBO J 18:1345–1356

Hocevar BA et al. (2001) The adaptor molecule Disabled-2 links the transforming growth factor beta receptors to the Smad pathway. EMBO J 20:2789–2801

Hofmann TG et al. (2003) HIPK2 regulates transforming growth factor-beta-induced c-Jun NH(2)-terminal kinase activation and apoptosis in human hepatoma cells. Cancer Res 63:8271–8277

Howe JR et al. (1998) Mutations in the SMAD4/DPC4 gene in juvenile polyposis. Science 280:1086–1088

Imai Y et al. (2001) Mutations of the Smad4 gene in acute myelogeneous leukemia and their functional implications in leukemogenesis. Oncogene 20:88–96

Imamura T et al. (1997) Smad6 inhibits signalling by the TGF-beta superfamily. Nature 389:622–626

Inman GJ et al. (2002) SB-431542 is a potent and specific inhibitor of transforming growth factor-beta superfamily type I activin receptor-like kinase (ALK) receptors ALK4, ALK5, and ALK7. Mol Pharmacol 62:65–74

Itoh S et al. (2003) Elucidation of Smad requirement in transforming growth factor-beta type I receptor-induced responses. J Biol Chem 278:3751–3761

Izumoto S et al. (1997) Microsatellite instability and mutated type II transforming growth factor-beta receptor gene in gliomas. Cancer Lett 112:251–256

Izzi L, Attisano L (2004) Regulation of the TGFbeta signalling pathway by ubiquitin-mediated degradation. Oncogene 23:2071–2078

Jakubowiak A et al. (2000) Inhibition of the transforming growth factor beta 1 signaling pathway by the AML1/ETO leukemia-associated fusion protein. J Biol Chem 275:40282–40287

James D et al. (2005) TGFbeta/activin/nodal signaling is necessary for the maintenance of pluripotency in human embryonic stem cells. Development 132:1273–1282

Janda E et al. (2002) Ras and TGF[beta] cooperatively regulate epithelial cell plasticity and metastasis:

dissection of Ras signaling pathways. J Cell Biol 156:299–313

Jiang X et al. (1995) Increased intraplatelet and urinary transforming growth factor-beta in patients with multiple myeloma. Acta Haematol 94:1–6

Johansson N et al. (2000) Expression of collagenase-3 (MMP-13) and collagenase-1 (MMP-1) by transformed keratinocytes is dependent on the activity of p38 mitogen-activated protein kinase. J Cell Sci 113 Pt 2:227–235

Johnson DW et al. (1996) Mutations in the activin receptor-like kinase 1 gene in hereditary haemorrhagic telangiectasia type 2. Nat Genet 13:189–195

Kaji H et al. (2001) Inactivation of menin, a Smad3-interacting protein, blocks transforming growth factor type beta signaling. Proc Natl Acad Sci USA 98:3837–3842

Kanamoto T et al. (2002) Functional proteomics of transforming growth factor-beta1-stimulated Mv1Lu epithelial cells:Rad51 as a target of TGFbeta1-dependent regulation of DNA repair. EMBO J 21:1219–1230

Kang Y et al. (2003a) A self-enabling TGFbeta response coupled to stress signaling:Smad engages stress response factor ATF3 for Id1 repression in epithelial cells. Mol Cell 11:915–926

Kang Y et al. (2003b) A multigenic program mediating breast cancer metastasis to bone. Cancer Cell 3:537–549

Katakura Y et al. (1999) Transforming growth factor beta triggers two independent-senescence programs in cancer cells. Biochem Biophys Res Commun 255:110–115

Kavsak P et al. (2000) Smad7 binds to Smurf2 to form an E3 ubiquitin ligase that targets the TGF beta receptor for degradation. Mol Cell 6:1365–1375

Kim WS et al. (1999) Reduced transforming growth factor-beta type II receptor (TGF-beta RII) expression in adenocarcinoma of the lung. Anticancer Res 19:301–306

Kirsch T et al. (2000) BMP-2 antagonists emerge from alterations in the low-affinity binding epitope for receptor BMPR-II. EMBO J 19:3314–3324

Kleeff J et al. (1999) The TGF-beta signaling inhibitor Smad7 enhances tumorigenicity in pancreatic cancer. Oncogene 18:5363–5372

Kleeff J et al. (2000) Pancreatic cancer–new aspects of molecular biology research. Swiss Surg 6:231–234

Knaus PI et al. (1996) A dominant inhibitory mutant of the type II transforming growth factor beta receptor in the malignant progression of a cutaneous T-cell lymphoma. Mol Cell Biol 16:3480–3489

Kretzschmar M et al. (1999) A mechanism of repression of TGFbeta/ Smad signaling by oncogenic Ras. Genes Dev 13:804–816

Kurokawa M et al. (1998) The oncoprotein Evi-1 represses TGF-beta signalling by inhibiting Smad3. Nature 394:92–96

Kyrtsonis MC et al. (1998) Serum transforming growth factor-beta 1 is related to the degree of immunopa-resis in patients with multiple myeloma. Med Oncol 15:124–128

Laping NJ et al. (2002) Inhibition of transforming growth factor (TGF)-beta1-induced extracellular matrix with a novel inhibitor of the TGF-beta type I receptor kinase activity:SB-431542. Mol Pharmacol 62:58–64

Larsson J et al. (2001) Abnormal angiogenesis but intact hematopoietic potential in TGF-beta type I receptor-deficient mice. EMBO J 20:1663–1673

Lavoie P et al. (2005) Neutralization of transforming growth factor-beta attenuates hypertension and prevents renal injury in uremic rats. J Hypertens 23:1895–1903

Le Bousse-Kerdiles MC et al. (1996) Differential expression of transforming growth factor-beta, basic fibroblast growth factor, and their receptors in CD34+ hematopoietic progenitor cells from patients with myelofibrosis and myeloid metaplasia. Blood 88:4534–4546

Le Roy C, Wrana JL (2005a) Signaling and endocytosis:a team effort for cell migration. Dev Cell 9:167–168

Le Roy C, Wrana JL (2005b) Clathrin- and non-clathrin-mediated endocytic regulation of cell signalling. Nat Rev Mol Cell Biol 6:112–126

Leivonen SK et al. (2006) Activation of Smad signaling enhances collagenase-3 (MMP-13) expression and invasion of head and neck squamous carcinoma cells. Oncogene

Li C et al. (1999) TGF-beta1 levels in pre-treatment plasma identify breast cancer patients at risk of developing post-radiotherapy fibrosis. Int J Cancer 84:155–159

Li QL et al. (2002) Causal relationship between the loss of RUNX3 expression and gastric cancer. Cell 109:113–124

Liau LM et al. (1998) Prolonged survival of rats with intracranial C6 gliomas by treatment with TGF-beta antisense gene. Neurol Res 20:742–747

Lin HK et al. (2004) Cytoplasmic PML function in TGF-beta signalling. Nature 431:205–211

Lo RS et al. (2001) Epidermal growth factor signaling via Ras controls the Smad transcriptional co-repressor TGIF. EMBO J 20:128–136

Lopez-Casillas F et al. (1993) Betaglycan presents ligand to the TGF beta signaling receptor. Cell 73:1435–1444

Lowsky R et al. (2000) MSH2-deficient murine lymphomas harbor insertion/deletion mutations in the transforming growth factor beta receptor type 2 gene and display low but not high frequency microsatellite instability. Blood 95:1767–1772

Lu SL et al. (1996) Genomic structure of the transforming growth factor beta type II receptor gene and its mutations in hereditary nonpolyposis colorectal cancers. Cancer Res 56:4595–4598

Madisen L et al. (1988) Transforming growth factor-beta 2:cDNA cloning and sequence analysis. DNA 7:1–8

Madisen L et al. (1989) Expression and characterization of recombinant TGF-beta 2 proteins produced in mammalian cells. DNA 8:205–212

Maeda S et al. (2004) Endogenous TGF-beta signaling suppresses maturation of osteoblastic mesenchymal cells. EMBO J 23:552–563

Maggard M et al. (2001) Antisense TGF-beta2 immunotherapy for hepatocellular carcinoma:treatment in a rat tumor model. Ann Surg Oncol 8:32–37

Markowitz S et al. (1995) Inactivation of the type II TGF-beta receptor in colon cancer cells with microsatellite instability. Science 268:1336–1338

Martin JS et al. (1995) Analysis of homozygous TGF beta 1 null mouse embryos demonstrates defects in yolk sac vasculogenesis and hematopoiesis. Ann NY Acad Sci 752:300–308

Massague J (1998) TGF-beta signal transduction. Annu Rev Biochem 67:753–791

Massague J et al. (2000) TGFbeta signaling in growth control, cancer, and heritable disorders. Cell 103:295–309

Massague J, Wotton D (2000) Transcriptional control by the TGF-beta/Smad signaling system. EMBO J 19:1745–1754

Matsuno F et al. (1999) Induction of lasting complete regression of preformed distinct solid tumors by targeting the tumor vasculature using two new anti-endoglin monoclonal antibodies. Clin Cancer Res 5:371–382

Matsuyama S et al. (2003) SB-431542 and Gleevec inhibit transforming growth factor-beta-induced proliferation of human osteosarcoma cells. Cancer Res 63:7791–7798

McAllister KA et al. (1994) Endoglin, a TGF-beta binding protein of endothelial cells, is the gene for hereditary haemorrhagic telangiectasia type 1. Nat Genet 8:345–351

McDonald CC et al. (1995) Cardiac and vascular morbidity in women receiving adjuvant tamoxifen for breast cancer in a randomised trial. The Scottish Cancer Trials Breast Group. BMJ 311:977–980

Mead AL et al. (2003) Evaluation of anti-TGF-beta2 antibody as a new postoperative anti-scarring agent in glaucoma surgery. Invest Ophthalmol Vis Sci 44:3394–3401

Miettinen PJ et al. (1994) TGF-beta induced transdifferentiation of mammary epithelial cells to mesenchymal cells:involvement of type I receptors. J Cell Biol 127:2021–2036

Mimura K et al. (2005) Trastuzumab-mediated antibody-dependent cellular cytotoxicity against esophageal squamous cell carcinoma. Clin Cancer Res 11:4898–4904

Mitani K (2004) Molecular mechanisms of leukemogenesis by AML1/EVI-1. Oncogene 23:4263–4269

Miura S et al. (2000) Hgs (Hrs), a FYVE domain protein, is involved in Smad signaling through cooperation with SARA. Mol Cell Biol 20:9346–9355

Miyajima A et al. (2001) Captopril restores transforming growth factor-beta type II receptor and sensitivity to transforming growth factor-beta in murine renal cell cancer cells. J Urol 165:616–620

Miyaki M et al. (1999) Higher frequency of Smad4 gene mutation in human colorectal cancer with distant metastasis. Oncogene 18:3098–3103

Moses HL et al. (1981) Transforming growth factor production by chemically transformed cells. Cancer Res 41:2842–2848

Moustakas A et al. (2001) Smad regulation in TGF-beta signal transduction. J Cell Sci 114:4359–4369

Muraoka RS et al. (2002) Blockade of TGF-beta inhibits mammary tumor cell viability, migration, and metastases. J Clin Invest 109:1551–1559

Mustafa M et al. (1993) The major histocompatibility complex influences myelin basic protein 63–88-induced T cell cytokine profile and experimental autoimmune encephalomyelitis. Eur J Immunol 23:3089–3095

Myeroff LL et al. (1995) A transforming growth factor beta receptor type II gene mutation common in colon and gastric but rare in endometrial cancers with microsatellite instability. Cancer Res 55:5545–5547

Nicolas FJ, Hill CS (2003) Attenuation of the TGF-beta-Smad signaling pathway in pancreatic tumor cells confers resistance to TGF-beta-induced growth arrest. Oncogene 22:3698–3711

Norton JD (2000) ID helix-loop-helix proteins in cell growth, differentiation and tumorigenesis. J Cell Sci 113 (Pt 22):3897–3905

Oft M et al. (1996) TGF-beta1 and Ha-Ras collaborate in modulating the phenotypic plasticity and invasiveness of epithelial tumor cells. Genes Dev 10:2462–2477

Oft M et al. (1998) TGFbeta signaling is necessary for carcinoma cell invasiveness and metastasis. Curr Biol 8:1243–1252

Oft M et al. (2002) Metastasis is driven by sequential elevation of H-ras and Smad2 levels. Nat Cell Biol 4:487–494

Oshima M et al. (1996) TGF-beta receptor type II deficiency results in defects of yolk sac hematopoiesis and vasculogenesis. Dev Biol 179:297–302

Otsuki T et al. (2001) Expression and in vitro modification of parathyroid hormone-related protein (PTHrP) and PTH/PTHrP-receptor in human myeloma cells. Leuk Lymphoma 41:397–409

Park BJ et al. (2000) Mitogenic conversion of transforming growth factor-beta1 effect by oncogenic Ha-Ras-induced activation of the mitogen-activated protein kinase signaling pathway in human prostate cancer. Cancer Res 60:3031–3038

Park SH et al. (2002) Transcriptional regulation of the transforming growth factor beta type II receptor gene by histone acetyltransferase and deacetylase is mediated by NF-Y in human breast cancer cells. J Biol Chem 277:5168–5174

Parsons R et al. (1995) Microsatellite instability and mutations of the transforming growth factor beta type II receptor gene in colorectal cancer. Cancer Res 55:5548–5550

Pasche B et al. (1999) TbetaR-I(6A) is a candidate tumor susceptibility allele. Cancer Res 59:5678–5682

Pasche B et al. (2004) TGFBR1*6A and cancer:a meta-analysis of 12 case-control studies. J Clin Oncol 22:756–758

Pasche B et al. (2005) Somatic acquisition and signaling of TGFBR1*6A in cancer. JAMA 294:1634–1646

Peinado H et al. (2003) Transforming growth factor beta-1 induces snail transcription factor in epithelial cell lines:mechanisms for epithelial mesenchymal transitions. J Biol Chem 278:21113–21123

Peinado H et al. (2004) Snail mediates E-cadherin repression by the recruitment of the Sin3A/histone deacetylase 1 (HDAC1)/HDAC2 complex. Mol Cell Biol 24:306–319

Peng SB et al. (2005) Kinetic characterization of novel pyrazole TGF-beta receptor I kinase inhibitors and their blockade of the epithelial-mesenchymal transition. Biochemistry 44:2293–2304

Penheiter SG et al. (2002) Internalization-dependent and -independent requirements for transforming growth factor beta receptor signaling via the Smad pathway. Mol Cell Biol 22:4750–4759

Perlman R et al. (2001) TGF-beta-induced apoptosis is mediated by the adapter protein Daxx that facilitates JNK activation. Nat Cell Biol 3:708–714

Pertovaara L et al. (1994) Vascular endothelial growth factor is induced in response to transforming growth factor-beta in fibroblastic and epithelial cells. J Biol Chem 269:6271–6274

Petritsch C et al. (2000) TGF-beta inhibits p70 S6 kinase via protein phosphatase 2A to induce G(1) arrest. Genes Dev 14:3093–3101

Pierce DF, Jr. et al. (1995) Mammary tumor suppression by transforming growth factor beta 1 transgene expression. Proc Natl Acad Sci USA 92:4254–4258

Polyak K et al. (1994) p27Kip1, a cyclin-Cdk inhibitor, links transforming growth factor-beta and contact inhibition to cell cycle arrest. Genes Dev 8:9–22

Portier M et al. (1993) Cytokine gene expression in human multiple myeloma. Br J Haematol 85:514–520

Reimold AM et al. (1993) Transforming growth factor beta 1 repression of the HLA-DR alpha gene is mediated by conserved proximal promoter elements. J Immunol 151:4173–4182

Roberts AB et al. (1980) Transforming growth factors: isolation of polypeptides from virally and chemically transformed cells by acid/ethanol extraction. Proc Natl Acad Sci USA 77:3494–3498

Saha D et al. (2001) Oncogenic ras represses transforming growth factor-beta /Smad signaling by degrading tumor suppressor Smad4. J Biol Chem 276:29531–29537

Saito H et al. (2000) An elevated serum level of transforming growth factor-beta 1 (TGF-beta 1) significantly correlated with lymph node metastasis and poor prognosis in patients with gastric carcinoma. Anticancer Res 20:4489–4493

Sano Y et al. (1999) ATF-2 is a common nuclear target of Smad and TAK1 pathways in transforming growth factor-beta signaling. J Biol Chem 274:8949–8957

Savagner P et al. (1997) The zinc-finger protein slug causes desmosome dissociation, an initial and necessary step for growth factor-induced epithelial-mesenchymal transition. J Cell Biol 137:1403–1419

Sawyer JS et al. (2004) Synthesis and activity of new aryl- and heteroaryl-substituted 5,6-dihydro-4H-pyrrolo[1,2-b]pyrazole inhibitors of the transforming growth factor-beta type I receptor kinase domain. Bioorg Med Chem Lett 14:3581–3584

Schiemann WP et al. (1999) A deletion in the gene for transforming growth factor beta type I receptor abolishes growth regulation by transforming growth factor beta in a cutaneous T-cell lymphoma. Blood 94:2854–2861

Schlingensiepen KH et al. (2006) Targeted tumor therapy with the TGF-beta2 antisense compound AP 12009. Cytokine Growth Factor Rev 17:129–139

Seoane J et al. (2004) Integration of Smad and forkhead pathways in the control of neuroepithelial and glioblastoma cell proliferation. Cell 117:211–223

Shariat SF et al. (2001a) Preoperative plasma levels of transforming growth factor beta(1) strongly predict clinical outcome in patients with bladder carcinoma. Cancer 92:2985–2992

Shariat SF et al. (2001b) Preoperative plasma levels of transforming growth factor beta(1) (TGF-beta(1)) strongly predict progression in patients undergoing radical prostatectomy. J Clin Oncol 19:2856–2864

Shi Y, Massague J (2003) Mechanisms of TGF-beta signaling from cell membrane to the nucleus. Cell 113:685–700

Shimo T et al. (2001) Involvement of CTGF, a hypertrophic chondrocyte-specific gene product, in tumor angiogenesis. Oncology 61:315–322

Siegel PM, Massague J (2003) Cytostatic and apoptotic actions of TGF-beta in homeostasis and cancer. Nat Rev Cancer 3:807–821

Siegel PM et al. (2003a) Transforming growth factor beta signaling impairs Neu-induced mammary tumorigenesis while promoting pulmonary metastasis. Proc Natl Acad Sci USA 100:8430–8435

Siegel PM et al. (2003b) Mad upregulation and Id2 repression accompany transforming growth factor (TGF)-beta-mediated epithelial cell growth suppression. J Biol Chem 278:35444–35450

Sinha S et al. (1998) Cellular and extracellular biology of the latent transforming growth factor-beta binding proteins. Matrix Biol 17:529–545

Siriwardena D et al. (2002) Human antitransforming growth factor beta(2) monoclonal antibody–a new modulator of wound healing in trabeculectomy:a randomized placebo controlled clinical study. Ophthalmology 109:427–431

Sporn MB (1996) The war on cancer. Lancet 347:1377–1381

Stearns ME et al. (1999) Role of interleukin 10 and transforming growth factor beta1 in the angiogenesis and metastasis of human prostate primary tumor lines from orthotopic implants in severe combined immunodeficiency mice. Clin Cancer Res 5:711–720

Stroschein SL et al. (1999) Negative feedback regulation of TGF-beta signaling by the SnoN oncoprotein. Science 286:771–774

Subramanian G et al. (2004) Targeting endogenous transforming growth factor beta receptor signaling in SMAD4-deficient human pancreatic carcinoma cells inhibits their invasive phenotype1. Cancer Res 64:5200–5211

Sun PD, Davies DR (1995) The cystine-knot growth-factor superfamily. Annu Rev Biophys Biomol Struct 24:269–291

Sun Y et al. (1999) Interaction of the Ski oncoprotein with Smad3 regulates TGF-beta signaling. Mol Cell 4:499–509

Takaku K et al. (1998) Intestinal tumorigenesis in compound mutant mice of both Dpc4 (Smad4) and Apc genes. Cell 92:645–656

Tang B et al. (2003) TGF-beta switches from tumor suppressor to prometastatic factor in a model of breast cancer progression. J Clin Invest 112:1116–1124

ten Dijke P et al. (1988a) Transforming growth factor type beta 3 maps to human chromosome 14, region q23-q24. Oncogene 3:721–724

ten Dijke P et al. (1988b) Identification of another member of the transforming growth factor type beta gene family. Proc Natl Acad Sci USA 85:4715–4719

Ten Dijke P et al. (2002) Regulation of cell proliferation by Smad proteins. J Cell Physiol 191:1–16

Thiery JP (2002) Epithelial-mesenchymal transitions in tumour progression. Nat Rev Cancer 2:442–454

Tojo M et al. (2005) The ALK-5 inhibitor A-83-01 inhibits Smad signaling and epithelial-to-mesenchymal transition by transforming growth factor-beta. Cancer Sci 96:791–800

Torre-Amione G et al. (1990) A highly immunogenic tumor transfected with a murine transforming growth factor type beta 1 cDNA escapes immune surveillance. Proc Natl Acad Sci USA 87:1486–1490

Tsai JF et al. (1997a) Urinary transforming growth factor-beta 1 in relation to serum alpha-fetoprotein in hepatocellular carcinoma. Scand J Gastroenterol 32:254–260

Tsai JF et al. (1997b) Elevated urinary transforming growth factor-beta1 level as a tumour marker and predictor of poor survival in cirrhotic hepatocellular carcinoma. Br J Cancer 76:244–250

Tsai JF et al. (1997c) Clinical evaluation of urinary transforming growth factor-beta1 and serum alpha-fetoprotein as tumour markers of hepatocellular carcinoma. Br J Cancer 75:1460–1466

Tsukazaki T et al. (1998) SARA, a FYVE domain protein that recruits Smad2 to the TGFbeta receptor. Cell 95:779–791

Tsushima H et al. (2001) Circulating transforming growth factor beta 1 as a predictor of liver metastasis after resection in colorectal cancer. Clin Cancer Res 7:1258–1262

Tuxhorn JA et al. (2002) Inhibition of transforming growth factor-beta activity decreases angiogenesis in a human prostate cancer-reactive stroma xenograft model. Cancer Res 62:6021–6025

Tzai TS et al. (1998) Antisense oligonucleotide specific for transforming growth factor-beta 1 inhibit both in vitro and in vivo growth of MBT-2 murine bladder cancer. Anticancer Res 18:1585–1589

Tzai TS et al. (2000) Immunization with TGF-beta antisense oligonucleotide-modified autologous tumor vaccine enhances the antitumor immunity of MBT-2 tumor-bearing mice through upregulation of MHC class I and Fas expressions. Anticancer Res 20:1557–1562

Uchida K et al. (1996) Somatic in vivo alterations of the JV18-1 gene at 18q21 in human lung cancers. Cancer Res 56:5583–5585

Uhl M et al. (2004) SD-208, a novel transforming growth factor beta receptor I kinase inhibitor, inhibits growth and invasiveness and enhances immunogenicity of murine and human glioma cells in vitro and in vivo. Cancer Res 64:7954–7961

Urashima M et al. (1996) Transforming growth factor-beta1:differential effects on multiple myeloma versus normal B cells. Blood 87:1928–1938

Vardouli L et al. (2005) LIM-kinase 2 and cofilin phosphorylation mediate actin cytoskeleton reorganization induced by transforming growth factor-beta. J Biol Chem 280:11448–11457

Venkatasubbarao K et al. (2001) Reversion of transcriptional repression of Sp1 by 5 aza-2' deoxycytidine restores TGF-beta type II receptor expression in the pancreatic cancer cell line MIA PaCa-2. Cancer Res 61:6239–6247

Verdaguer J et al. (1999) Two mechanisms for the non-MHC-linked resistance to spontaneous autoimmunity. J Immunol 162:4614–4626

Wakefield LM, Roberts AB (2002) TGF-beta signaling: positive and negative effects on tumorigenesis. Curr Opin Genet Dev 12:22–29

Wallick SC et al. (1990) Immunoregulatory role of transforming growth factor beta (TGF-beta) in development of killer cells:comparison of active and latent TGF-beta 1. J Exp Med 172:1777–1784

Wan M et al. (2002) Jab1 antagonizes TGF-beta signaling by inducing Smad4 degradation. EMBO Rep 3:171–176

Wang D et al. (1999) Mutation analysis of the Smad3 gene in human ovarian cancers. Int J Oncol 15:949–953

Wang D et al. (2000) Analysis of specific gene mutations in the transforming growth factor-beta signal transduction pathway in human ovarian cancer. Cancer Res 60:4507–4512

Wang J et al. (1995) Demonstration that mutation of the type II transforming growth factor beta receptor inactivates its tumor suppressor activity in replication error-positive colon carcinoma cells. J Biol Chem 270:22044–22049

Watanabe T et al. (2001) Molecular predictors of survival after adjuvant chemotherapy for colon cancer. N Engl J Med 344:1196–1206

Webb NR et al. (1988) Structural and sequence analysis of TGF-beta 2 cDNA clones predicts two different precursor proteins produced by alternative mRNA splicing. DNA 7:493–497

Whitman M (1998) Smads and early developmental signaling by the TGFbeta superfamily. Genes Dev 12:2445–2462

Wojtowicz-Praga S et al. (1996) Modulation of B16 melanoma growth and metastasis by anti-transforming growth factor beta antibody and interleukin-2. J Immunother Emphasis Tumor Immunol 19:169–175

Wolfraim LA et al. (2004) Loss of Smad3 in acute T-cell lymphoblastic leukemia. N Engl J Med 351:552–559

Wong C et al. (1999) Smad3-Smad4 and AP-1 complexes synergize in transcriptional activation of the c-Jun promoter by transforming growth factor beta. Mol Cell Biol 19:1821–1830

Wormstone IM et al. (2002) TGF-beta2-induced matrix modification and cell transdifferentiation in the human lens capsular bag. Invest Ophthalmol Vis Sci 43:2301–2308

Wrana JL, Attisano L (2000) The Smad pathway. Cytokine Growth Factor Rev 11:5–13

Xu L et al. (2000) The nuclear import function of Smad2 is masked by SARA and unmasked by TGFbeta-dependent phosphorylation. Nat Cell Biol 2:559–562

Xu L et al. (2006) MAPKAPK2 and HSP27 are downstream effectors of p38 MAP kinase-mediated matrix metalloproteinase type 2 activation and cell invasion in human prostate cancer. Oncogene

Xu X et al. (2000) Haploid loss of the tumor suppressor Smad4/Dpc4 initiates gastric polyposis and cancer in mice. Oncogene 19:1868–1874

Yakymovych I et al. (2001) Regulation of Smad signaling by protein kinase C. FASEB J 15:553–555

Yamaguchi K et al. (1995) Identification of a member of the MAPKKK family as a potential mediator of TGF-beta signal transduction. Science 270:2008–2011

Yang YA et al. (2002) Lifetime exposure to a soluble TGF-beta antagonist protects mice against metastasis without adverse side effects. J Clin Invest 109:1607–1615

Yin JJ et al. (1999) TGF-beta signaling blockade inhibits PTHrP secretion by breast cancer cells and bone metastases development. J Clin Invest 103:197–206

Yingling JM et al. (2004) Development of TGF-beta signalling inhibitors for cancer therapy. Nat Rev Drug Discov 3:1011–1022

Yu L et al. (2002) TGF-beta receptor-activated p38 MAP kinase mediates Smad-independent TGF-beta responses. EMBO J 21:3749–3759

Zhang Y et al. (1998) Smad3 and Smad4 cooperate with c-Jun/c-Fos to mediate TGF-beta-induced transcription. Nature 394:909–913

Zhu Y et al. (1998) Smad3 mutant mice develop metastatic colorectal cancer. Cell 94:703–714

Ziesche R et al. (1999) A preliminary study of long-term treatment with interferon gamma-1b and low-dose prednisolone in patients with idiopathic pulmonary fibrosis. N Engl J Med 341:1264–1269

The Mammalian Target of Rapamycin Kinase and Tumor Growth Inhibition

Anne Boulay and Heidi A. Lane

Recent Results in Cancer Research, Vol. 172
© Springer-Verlag Berlin Heidelberg 2007

Human cancer expression profiling studies highlight the important variability in gene expression patterns and signaling pathways activated within tumors of a homogenous pathological group. These observations support the need for marker and molecular signature identification to adapt appropriate treatments to the patient. Increasing evidence indicates that the mammalian target of rapamycin [mTOR; also named rapamycin-associated protein (FRAP) or rapamycin and FKBP12 target (RAFT)] signaling pathway is hyperactive in a number of cancers, suggesting that this pathway may represent an attractive target for cancer therapy. mTOR is a highly conserved, 290-kDa serine-threonine protein kinase that belongs to the phosphoinositide kinase-related kinase (PIKK) family comprising also ataxia-telangiectasia (ATM), ATM and Rad3-related protein kinase (ATR) and DNA-dependent protein kinase (DNA-PK) (Abraham 2004). Besides the catalytic domain, mTOR shares central FAT (for FRAP, ATM, TRAP) and carboxy-terminal FATC (FAT carboxy-terminal) regulatory domains with other PIKK members. These domains are essential for mTOR catalytic activity and might interact to expose the kinase domain. In addition, mTOR contains a series of HEAT (for Huntington, EF3, A subunit of PP2A, TOR) protein-protein interaction repeats in the amino-terminal region and a regulatory region referred to as FKBP/rapamycin-binding (FRB) domain adjacent to the kinase domain. The presence of multiple interaction and regulatory domains supports the assumption that, besides its catalytic kinase activity, mTOR possesses a scaffolding function to recruit an array of partners to integrate various inputs and to exert its functions. Like other PIKK members, mTOR is a sensor for cellular stress; specifically, mTOR functions as a nutrient-, energy-, and mitogen-sensing checkpoint, controlling cell growth.

TOR proteins were initially identified in yeast as the target of rapamycin, a macrolide antibiotic identified in the early 1970s and produced by Streptomyces hygroscopicus (reviewed in Schmelzle and Hall 2000). Rapamycin binds with high affinity to the intracellular receptor FKBP12 (FK506-binding protein 12 kDa) and forms a gain-of-function complex that selectively binds to the FRB domain of mTOR, thereby compromising downstream signaling by a still-elusive mechanism. Therefore, rapamycin is a highly selective inhibitor of mTOR. Interestingly, mTOR is essential in mammals (Murakami et al. 2004; Gangloff et al. 2004); however, rapamycin treatment causes milder phenotypes, generally exhibiting cytostatic activity. These observations raise the possibilities that rapamycin partially inhibits mTOR activity or, alternatively but nonexclusively, particular functions of mTOR. Hence, rapamycin treatment does not recapitulate all aspects of a kinase-dead allele of mTOR in vitro (Edinger et al. 2003), and a rapamycin-insensitive mTOR activity was recently characterized in higher eukaryotes (Loewith et al. 2002; Sarbassov et al. 2004; Jacinto et al. 2004). Nevertheless, on rapamycin exposure, cell growth and proliferation are severely impaired. Consistent with the very potent effects primarily documented on T-cell proliferation, rapamycin and its derivatives have been profiled as immunosuppressants and approved for preventing rejection in patients receiving organ transplants. They also demonstrate potent inhibitory activity against a wide range of cell lines and animal models derived from solid tumors, supporting their development in the cancer indication. In this chapter, we describe recent advances in our understanding of mTOR regulation and function, followed by a description of the importance of the signaling pathway in cancer. Recent progress on the preclinical and clinical development of rapamycin derivatives in oncology will be presented, with specific emphasis on the derivative known as RAD001 (everolimus).

7.1 The mTOR Signaling Pathway

7.1.1 mTOR Complexes

There are two TOR homologs in yeast that have redundant as well as specific functions, some of these being sensitive to rapamycin. In higher eukaryotes, a single protein (mTOR) recapitulates TOR functions. Recently, it has been demonstrated that mTOR exists in at least two distinct complexes: a rapamycin-sensitive and a rapamycin-resistant complex characterized by the presence of the raptor (regulatory-associated protein of mTOR; Kim et al. 2002; Hara et al. 2002; Loewith et al. 2002) and rictor (rapamycin-insensitive companion of mTOR; Loewith et al. 2002; Sarbassov et al. 2004; Jacinto et al. 2004) proteins, respectively (Fig. 7.1). This is an important breakthrough shedding new light on mTOR signaling in higher eukaryotes and begs a careful reevaluation of former biochemical studies.

7.1.1.1 The mTORC1 Complex

mTOR functions as part of a large signaling complex named mTORC1 (Kim et al. 2002; Hara et al. 2002; Loewith et al. 2002). Two subunits have been identified, raptor and GβL (also named mLST8). These proteins are conserved from budding yeast (KOG1 and LST8, respectively) to mammalian cells. Raptor contains HEAT and WD protein-protein interaction domains, and GβL consists entirely of WD motifs, suggesting that they possess scaffolding functions. Several lines of evidence support that raptor has a positive role in maintaining mTOR activity. For instance, siRNA-mediated knockdown of raptor results in reduced mTOR effector phosphorylation (Hara et al. 2002) and decreases cell size, comparable to that triggered by mTOR depletion (Kim et al. 2002). Raptor functions to present mTOR substrates (at least S6K1 and 4E-BP1) for phosphorylation by binding to the TOS (TOR signaling) motif (Hara et al. 2002; Schalm et al. 2002, 2003). Importantly, all studies related to mTORC1 support that this complex mediates rapamycin-sensitive mTOR functions in mammalian cells (see below). The mechanism whereby rapamycin inhibits mTORC1 is still elusive. Sabatini and colleagues suggested that rapamycin might lead to the destabilization of mTORC1 (Kim et al. 2002), although the same authors have recently rediscussed the relevance of this observation (Sarbassov et al. 2004).

There remain a number of uncertainties regarding raptor. Sabatini and coworkers reported that the stability of the endogenous mTORC1 complex increases in amino acid- and energy-starved conditions and suggested that raptor is a bidirectional regulator of mTOR: it inhibits the complex under nutrient-deprived conditions and activates it in nutrient-replete conditions (Kim et al. 2002). Interestingly, they observed that stability regulation is specific to the nutrient-sensor function, as it is not observed in response to growth factor deprivation. This suggests that mTORC1 might be more responsive to acute nutrient modulations than growth factor supply changes, a possibility worthy of further investigation.

GβL, the third known component of the mTORC1 complex, binds constitutively to the kinase domain of mTOR (Kim et al. 2003). Interestingly, although the rapamy-

7 The Mammalian Target of Rapamycin Kinase and Tumor Growth Inhibition

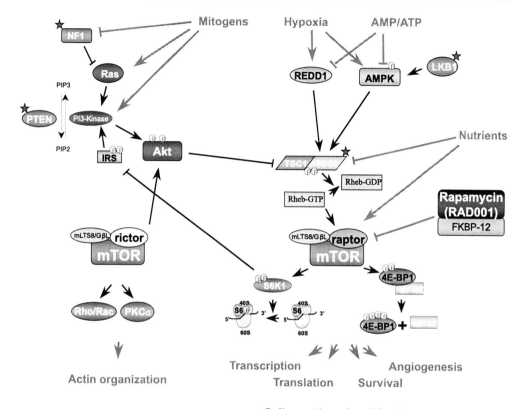

Fig. 7.1 The mTOR pathway, a cellular checkpoint for cell growth and proliferation. mTOR exists in two large complexes, identified as mTORC1 (containing the raptor regulatory protein) and mTORC2 (containing the rictor regulatory protein). These complexes exert specific functions, driving cell growth and proliferation and actin cytoskeleton organization, respectively. mTORC1 is specifically inhibited by rapamycin and rapamycin derivatives, such as RAD001 (everolimus), as a gain of function complex with the immunophilin FKBP12. mTORC1 is a central sensor for growth factors, nutrients, and energy moieties. The various inputs are sensed and mediated by a number of signaling pathways known to be frequently deregulated in various human tumor types; for instance, Ras, PI3K, and Akt are well-defined oncogenes while PTEN, NF1, LKB1, and TSC exert tumor suppressor functions (red stars indicate tumor suppressors whose inactivation leads to hamartomatous proliferative diseases). The linear signaling pathway has recently been challenged by the description of feedback mechanisms involving the mTORC1 effector S6K1 and the mTORC2 complex, as well as cross talk between upstream regulatory pathways feeding into the TSC/Rheb/mTOR module (see text)

cin/FKBP12 and GβL binding sites are closely juxtaposed, there is no evidence for spatial interference. GβL positively regulates the capacity of mTOR to phosphorylate itself as well as S6K1 and 4E-BP1. Moreover, it was proposed that mTOR, raptor, and GβL form the minimal elements needed for the formation of a nutrient-sensitive complex, although this is exclusively based on recombinant protein studies (Kim et al. 2003).

7.1.1.2 The mTORC2 Complex

mTOR has been identified in mammalian cells as part of a second large protein complex termed mTORC2, based on the presence of the specific component rictor (Loewith et al. 2002; Sarbassov et al. 2004; Jacinto et al. 2004). In addition to mTOR, this complex shares GβL with mTORC1 but lacks raptor. Rictor, a 200-kDa protein with no obvious functional domain, is homologous to the AVO3 subunit of the TORC2 complex in S. cerevisiae. Molecular characterization of the yeast TORC2 complex allowed for the identification of additional components (AVO1, AVO2, and BIT61; Loewith et al. 2002), but orthologs have not yet been identified or functionally implicated in mTORC2 function in mammalian cells. Rictor binds to the amino-terminal HEAT repeats of mTOR and appears essential for complex integrity. Furthermore, mTORC2 phosphorylates rictor, but this event seems not to be required for the integrity of the complex (Jacinto et al. 2004; Wullschleger et al. 2005).

In contrast to the mTORC1 complex, mTORC2 is insensitive to acute rapamycin treatment (Sarbassov et al. 2004; Jacinto et al. 2004), as previously described for TORC2 in budding yeast (Loewith et al. 2002). It is not known how rictor or another component of the complex hinders rapamycin from binding to the RBD domain of mTOR. Unexpectedly, it was recently suggested that prolonged rapamycin treatment could inhibit mTORC2 signaling by impairing complex formation in certain cell types (Sarbassov et al. 2006), a possibility necessitating further investigation.

It is not clear what cues signal to mTORC2, as contradictory observations were reported regarding responsiveness to growth factors and nutrient stimulation. Importantly, although mTORC2 is catalytically active it seems not to signal to cell growth effectors downstream of mTORC1 (Sarbassov et al. 2004; Jacinto et al. 2004). Therefore, it exhibits specific functions that are not shared with mTORC1. In S. cerevisiae, TORC2 positively signals to RhoI GTPase and activates the RHOI/PKC1/MAPK cascade to regulate actin reorganization. Although little is known in mammals, the mechanism whereby mTORC2 controls the actin cytoskeleton may be conserved as rictor and mTOR downregulation prevents actin polymerization and cell spreading (Sarbassov et al. 2004; Jacinto et al. 2004). Furthermore, activated Rho or Rac suppresses the actin defect caused by the loss of mTORC2 (Jacinto et al. 2004), and PKCα phosphorylation is modulated in response to rictor or mTOR depletion (Sarbassov et al. 2004). However, the role of mTORC2-de-pendent regulation of the actin cytoskeleton remains to be determined.

7.1.2 Downstream Effectors: Mediators of Translational Regulation and Cell Growth

A number of potential effectors of mTORC1 were postulated based on expression and phosphorylation changes that occur in response to rapamycin exposure. In addition, a number of genomic approaches led to the identification of gene sets regulated by mTOR in a rapamycin-sensitive manner (Peng et al. 2002; Gera et al. 2004; Majumder et al. 2004). However, the best-characterized targets are regulators of the translational machinery, consistent with the known role of mTORC1 in translational regulation (Beuvink et al. 2005).

7.1.2.1 S6 Ribosomal Protein Kinases

S6 ribosomal kinases (S6Ks) have homology with the AGC-family kinases and are the major kinases for the ribosomal protein S6. There are two highly related genes encoding S6K1 and S6K2. Activation of both kinases is inhibited by rapamycin, and ablation of both proteins is necessary to reduce S6 phosphorylation to the same extent as rapamycin (Pende et al. 2004, Ohanna et al. 2005). Importantly, S6K1 appears crucial for cell growth (Shima et al. 1998; Ohanna et al. 2005). Considerably less is known about S6K2, but genetic models suggested that S6K1 and S6K2 have redundant as well as distinct functions (Shima et al. 1998; Pende et al. 2004; Ohanna et al. 2005).

Several lines of evidence support mTOR as a major regulator of S6K activation in response to a number of stimuli. Nutrient and mitogenic stimulation increases S6K and S6 phosphorylation in a rapamycin-sensitive manner. Moreover, S6K is directly phosphorylated by mTOR in vitro (Burnett et al. 1998). Notably, the contradictory observation that a truncated rapamycin-resistant form of S6K1 is still phosphorylated on T389 in response to mitogen stimulation was recently related to a non-specific activity of mTORC2 (Ali and Sabatini

2005). Interestingly, two reports suggested that S6K1 also phosphorylates mTOR on a carboxy-terminal site, indicative of a feedback regulatory loop (Holz and Blenis 2005; Chiang and Abraham 2005). However, the functional significance of this event is unknown.

Mammalian cell size is controlled by mTORC1, an effect believed to be mediated at least partly by S6K1 (Fingar et al. 2002; Ohanna et al. 2005; Ruvinsky et al. 2005). Indeed, homozygous deletion of S6K1 in mice demonstrates a small-animal phenotype (Shima et al. 1998). S6Ks were suggested to mediate mTORC1-dependent cell growth regulation by increasing translation of 5'-terminal oligopyrimidine (5'TOP) tract mRNAs, which largely code for ribosomal proteins and other elements of the translational machinery, in a S6 phosphorylation-dependent manner (Jefferies et al. 1997). However, this assumption was recently challenged, as amino acid-induced translation of 5'TOP mRNAs was shown to be partially dependent on mTOR, but independent of S6K and S6 phosphorylation in cells (Tang et al. 2001; Ruvinsky et al. 2005). Additionally, mitogens enhance translation of 5'TOP mRNAs in a rapamycin-sensitive manner in cells derived from S6K1 and S6K2 compound knockout mice, although S6 phosphorylation is dramatically reduced (Pende et al. 2004). Thus, mTOR appears to regulate 5'TOP mRNA translation in a S6K- and S6 phosphorylation-independent manner, at least under certain circumstances. As mTORC1 exerts a global effect on translation (Beuvink et al. 2005), this may indicate that mTOR and S6K regulate cell growth by a mechanism independent of translation. Taken together, these observations still leave open the question of the role of S6K in mTORC1-regulated processes.

7.1.2.2 Eukaryotic Translation Initiation Factor 4E-Binding Proteins

Another well-characterized substrate for mTOR kinase is the eukaryotic initiation factor-4E (eIF-4E)-binding protein 4E-BP1. The mammalian family consists of three members, 4E-BP1 (also named PHAS1), 4E-BP2, and 4E-BP3. 4E-BPs are multisite phosphorylated repressors of the cap-binding protein eIF-4E, the limiting factor for eIF-4F initiation complex formation and cap-dependent translation (reviewed in Gingras et al. 2001). The affinity of 4E-BP1 for eIF-4E is regulated by 4E-BP1 phosphorylation, 4E-BP1 being tightly bound to eIF-4E when hypophosphorylated. Binding of 4E-BP1 and the scaffolding protein eIF-4G to eIF-4E (priming step for a functional eIF-4F complex formation) are mutually exclusive. In the presence of sufficient nutrients and mitogens, mTOR causes 4E-BP1 to become highly phosphorylated, and to dissociate from eIF-4E. This results in increased translation of a subset of capped mRNA that contain highly structured 5'UTRs, and code for key proteins involved in G1 to S progression like cyclin D1, c-myc, or VEGF (reviewed in De Benedetti and Graff 2004).

The importance of 4E-BPs in oncogenesis is exemplified by the observations that 4E-BP1 overexpression results in cell cycle arrest in G1 (Gingras et al. 2001) and reversion of the malignant phenotype induced by eIF-4E (Rousseau et al. 1996; Avdulov et al. 2004). Several observations support the role of 4E-BPs and eIF-4E-regulated cap-dependent translation in mTOR signaling. First, mTOR can directly phosphorylate 4E-BP1 on several residues in vitro (Gingras et al. 1999), which are also phosphorylated in response to mitogenic stimulation. Moreover, phosphorylation of these sites occurs in an ordered fashion (Gingras et al. 1999, Mothe-Satney et al. 2000), the final activation sites being rapamycin-sensitive. Thereby, 4E-BP1 mediates mTOR -effects on cell size (Fingar et al. 2002) and proliferation (Fingar et al. 2004).

7.1.2.3 Eukaryotic Translation Initiation Factor 4E

The initiation of translation might also be regulated at additional levels by mTOR signaling. eIF-4E is phosphorylated on residue S209 (the major in vivo site), presumably by Mnk kinases. The functional importance of this phosphorylation event is still under debate, although the preferred hypothesis suggests that eIF-4E phosphorylation has a positive effect on cap-dependent translation by increasing the affinity for the cap and the mRNA (Scheper and Proud 2002). We and others have shown recently that eIF-4E phosphorylation on S209 is consistently increased on short-term rapamycin treatment in vitro (Boulay et al. 2005; Sun et al. 2005), an event occurring concomitantly with effects on S6Ks and 4E-BPs. These observations are rather contradictory to the general belief. Although it is possible that eIF-4E is phosphorylated to compensate for increased rapamycin-induced sequestration of the cap binding protein by 4E-BPs, it is tempting to speculate that, under certain conditions, eIF-4E phosphorylation on S209 might negatively regulate translation. Indeed, the mechanism whereby rapamycin induces eIF-4E phosphorylation is suggested to involve PI3K signaling, rather than the MEK and p38MAPK pathways that are known to regulate the Mnk kinases (Sun et al. 2005).

7.1.3 mTOR Functions

The limited number of tools has long hindered a deeper understanding of mTOR functions, and the identification of two mTOR complexes has opened new avenues. Little is known yet regarding the role of mTORC2. Therefore, we focus the discussion on rapamycin-sensitive mTORC1 functions.

7.1.3.1 Growth Control Function

Cell growth is a carefully orchestrated process specifying the size of cells, organs, and organisms. Mitogenic stimulation of resting mammalian cells in the presence of sufficient nutrients and energy results in the activation of anabolic processes, in particular protein translation. This allows the cell to reach a threshold size necessary to proceed through the cell cycle, thereby linking translational control and cell growth to cell proliferation.

The first indication that TOR signaling coordinates nutrient availability with cell growth was provided in yeast, where TOR gene depletion or rapamycin treatment triggered a stress response strongly resembling the nutrient star-

vation phenotype (Peng et al. 2002). In mammals, cell and organismal growth is essentially controlled by growth factor and nutrient supply, to help integrate individual cell growth within the environment of a complex organ and organism. This resulted in debates regarding whether mTORC1 is strictly a nutrient-sensing pathway parallel to a mitogenic signal-sensing pathway or whether mTORC1 integrates both nutrient and growth factor cues in higher eukaryotes. Recent progress strongly argues for a convergent nutrient and mitogenic checkpoint function for mTORC1, also integrating energy inputs like ATP and oxygen levels.

Growth Factors Impinge on mTORC1 via PI3K/Akt

Growth factors like insulin enhance mTORC1 function, increasing phosphorylation of S6K1 and 4E-BP1 in a rapamycin-sensitive manner. There is strong evidence that this mitogenic effect is mediated by PI3K (reviewed in Gingras et al. 2001; Shamji et al. 2003; Hay and Sonenberg 2004), as exemplified by the observation that a mutated insulin receptor substrate 1 (IRS1), which only signals to PI3K, is sufficient to promote phosphorylation of 4E-BP1. Furthermore, cells deficient for PTEN, the phosphatase antagonizing PI3K activity (Fig. 7.1), exhibit elevated phospho-4E-BP1 and phospho-S6K1 levels (Neshat et al. 2001; Podsypanina et al. 2001). A major downstream element of the PI3K pathway is the AGC-family kinase Akt. It has been proposed that Akt directly phosphorylates mTOR on residue S2448 in response to insulin stimulation; although there is no evidence that this results in modulation of mTORC1 activity (Scott et al. 1998; Nave et al. 1999; Sekulic et al. 2000). However, mice deficient for Akt1 and Akt2 exhibit decreased phosphorylation of 4E-BP1 and to a lesser extent S6K1 (Peng et al. 2003, Hahn-Windgassen et al. 2005), and rapamycin blocks transformation of chicken embryo fibroblasts induced by PI3K and Akt (Aoki et al. 2001). These data demonstrate that mTORC1 is an essential mediator of the PI3K/Akt pathway.

Mitogens can activate PI3K by various adaptor molecules that are dependent on the receptor engaged. The small GTPase Ras is an upstream activator of PI3K, mutated in a large array of tumors. However, until recently, its possible contribution to mTOR signaling was poorly documented, not to say contradicted, as its oncogenic activity was reported to be independent of mTORC1 (Aoki et al. 2001). Neurofibromatosis type 1 is a familial cancer syndrome characterized by hamartomas in the peripheral and central nervous system, which rarely become malignant (Table 7.1). It is caused by mutation in the tumor suppressor NF1 encoding a GTPase-activating protein (GAP) regulating Ras. mTORC1 is overactivated in NF1-deficient primary cells in a Ras- and PI3K/Akt-dependent manner (Johannessen et al. 2005; Dasgupta et al. 2005). Hence, Ras activation is required for maximal activation of mTORC1 in fibroblasts by growth factors (Johannessen et al. 2005), indicating that Ras mediates mitogenic cues to mTORC1 under certain circumstances. The observation of a positive correlation between increased phospho-S6 and K-Ras-activating alterations in human non-small cell lung cancers (Conde 2006) further supports the molecular link between mTOR and Ras.

Energy Cues Impinge on mTORC1 via LKB1/AMPK and REDD1

Protein translation is a high energy consuming process. It is therefore assumed that lack of appropriate fuel, mitochondrial dysfunction, or decreased ATP levels regulate protein synthesis to maintain homeostasis. It has been proposed that mTOR can sense intracellular ATP levels because of its high Km for ATP (Dennis et al. 2001). However, AMP level is a much more sensitive indicator of energy status, as a small reduction in ATP results in a substantial rise in AMP. AMP level is sensed by the 5'AMP-activated protein kinase (AMPK) (Carling 2004) (Fig. 7.1), which is also regulated by hy-

Table 7.1 PI3K/mTOR pathway components implicated in human disease and tumor development

Marker	Aberrations	Diseases	Tumor/lesion location
PTEN	LOH, mutation	Cowden disease	Various organs (inc. breast, thyroid)
		Lhermitte–Duclos disease	Brain
		Bannayan–Riley–Ruvalcaba syndrome	Various organs (inc. breast, thyroid)
NF1	LOH, mutation	Neurofibromas	Central nervous system
LKB1	LOH, mutation	Peutz–Jeghers syndrome	Gastrointestinal tract
TSC1 and TSC2	LOH, mutation	Tuberous sclerosis syndromeb	Various organs (inc. CNS, kidney, lung)
PTEN	Mutation, silencing	Cancer	Glioma, endometrial, prostate, melanoma, breast
PI3K p110	Amplification, mutation	Cancer	Ovarian, colorectal, glioma, gastric, hepatocellular, breast, lung
PI3K p85	Mutation	Cancer	Colon, ovarian, glioma
Akt	Mutation, amplification	Cancer	Ovarian, gastric, pancreas, colorectal, breast
eIF-4E	Overexpression	Cancer	Breast, head and neck, colon, prostate, bladder, cervix, lung
LKB1	Mutation	Cancer	Lung, colorectal
TSC1 and TSC2	Mutation, ↓expression	Cancer	Bladder, astrocytomas

poxia-induced energy stress (Liu et al. 2006). AMPK controls translation by phosphorylating the eukaryotic elongation factor eIF-2 in a mTORC1-independent manner (Horman et al. 2002). However, expression of activated or dominant-negative forms of AMPK was shown to decrease and increase S6K1 phosphorylation, respectively, in a mTORC1-dependent manner (Krause et al. 2002; Kimura et al. 2003). Interestingly, it has been reported that AMPK activators trigger mTOR phosphorylation on T2446 (Cheng et al. 2004); however, whether this influences mTOR activity requires further investigation.

LKB1 is a tumor suppressor gene, the mutation of which is responsible for Peutz–Jeghers syndrome; characterized by colorectal hamartomas (Table 7.1). LKB1 is a major upstream activating kinase for AMPK (Hawley et al. 2003; Woods et al. 2003), and has a permissive role on AMPK-dependent energy level sensing (Corradetti et al. 2004, Shaw et al. 2004). Importantly, hamartomatous gastrointestinal polyps in LKB1 mutant mice exhibit mTORC1 effector hyperactivation (Shaw et al. 2004), providing in vivo evidence of a molecular link between LKB1 and mTOR.

An alternative mechanism whereby energy levels impinge on mTORC1 involves REDD1 (for Regulated in Development and DNA-damage response), a protein with no obvious functional domain. REDD1 is induced by an array of cellular stresses, while its contribution seems dispensable under normal conditions (Reiling and Hafen 2004; Sofer et al. 2005). REDD1 is involved in glucose and oxygen deprivation-induced inhibition of mTORC1 effectors, acting independently of AMPK (Reiling and Hafen 2004; Brugarolas et al. 2004; Sofer et al. 2005), suggesting that REDD1 and AMPK act in parallel pathways in response to energy stresses. Additionally, REDD orthologs in Drosophila have also been shown to regulate mTORC1 in response to starvation (Reiling and Hafen 2004). However, REDD1 does not appear to modulate amino acid regulation of mTORC1 signaling (Sofer et al. 2005). Interestingly, REDD1 mRNA expression is induced in hypoxic conditions in a PI3K- and mTORC1-dependent manner, possibly through upregulation of hypoxia-inducible factor HIF1 (Schwarzer et al. 2005), suggesting a complex negative feedback loop involving PI3K/Akt, mTOR, HIF, and REDD1.

It is also documented that the PI3K/Akt pathway impinges on glucose metabolism via upregulation of glucose transporter and glycolytic enzyme expression (Majumder et al. 2004). Regulation of ATP levels by Akt was suggested as an essential mechanism whereby Akt signals to mTOR, as impaired mTORC1 signaling in Akt1/Akt2-deficient MEFs is rescued by a dominant-negative allele of AMPK (Hahn-Windgassen et al. 2005). Similarly, overexpression of REDD1 impairs Akt-induced regulation of S6K1, suggesting that REDD1 functions downstream of PI3K/Akt to inhibit mTORC1 signaling (Reiling and Hafen 2004; Corradetti et al. 2005, Schwarzer et al. 2005). Therefore, an array of pathways participate in the translation of energy levels to mTORC1. There appear to be two independent arms, LKB1/AMPK and REDD1, that receive inputs from energy cues, both arms cross talking with PI3K/Akt signaling. Although it was initially accepted that PI3K/Akt is specific for growth factor signaling, a deeper understanding of the upstream regulators of mTOR places the PI3K/Akt module as a mediator of additional inputs signaling to mTORC1.

Amino Acids Impinge on mTORC1, Possibly via TSC/Rheb

Tuberous sclerosis complex (TSC) is an autosomal dominant disorder characterized by hamartomas in a variety of organs (Table 7.1). TSC is caused by mutations in TSC1 (coding for hamartin) and TSC2 (coding for tuberin) tumor suppressor genes. TSC1 and TSC2 function as a heterodimer, the formation and stability of which is dependent on TSC2 phosphorylation. A role for TSC in mTORC1 signaling was suspected following the observation that TSC functions to decrease cell growth (Fig. 7.1; Reviewed in Shamji et al. 2003). In TSC1- or TSC2-null cells, both S6K1 and 4E-BP1 are constitutively phosphorylated, and tumor growth in the Ecker rat model of TSC is exquisitely sensitive to rapamycin (Kenerson et al. 2002).

Finally, cells derived from patients affected by TSC exhibit overactivation of S6K1 (Kenerson et al. 2002), further supporting the molecular link between TSC and mTOR.

The mTORC1 pathway is particularly sensitive to amino acid levels, in particular branched-chain amino acids like leucine, but the mechanism is debated. Sabatini and colleagues have reported conformational changes in the mTORC1 complex on amino acid starvation, suggesting that the configuration of the complex is dependent on nutrient sufficiency (Kim et al. 2002, 2003). Whether TSC is involved in the nutrient-sensing mechanism is controversial (Inoki et al. 2002; Gao et al. 2002; Smith et al. 2005; Roccio et al. 2005; Nobukuni et al. 2005). Numerous TSC2 point mutations identified in patients are localized in the GAP domain, indicating that TSC most probably acts as a small GTPase-activating protein for the small GTPase Rheb (Ras homolog enriched in brain), promoting the conversion of GTP- to GDP-bound Rheb (Fig. 7.1; reviewed in Manning and Cantley 2003). Although Rheb is the only small GTPase (among 17 potential candidates) that mediates TSC effects on S6K1 activity (Zhang et al. 2003b), it has been postulated that TSC has additional (mTOR-dependent?) small GTPase target(s) involved in the regulation of growth and proliferation (Stocker et al. 2003). Rheb is conserved in all eukaryotes. In mammalian cells and Drosophila models, Rheb signals positively to mTORC1 in the absence of nutrient support (Garami et al. 2003, Tee et al. 2003b), in a rapamycin-sensitive manner (reviewed in Manning and Cantley 2003). In fission yeast, Rheb is required for cells to grow normally under limited amounts of nitrogen (Mach et al. 2000), raising the possibility that Rheb might stimulate mTORC1 indirectly by promoting nutrient import. This would be consistent with the subcellular localization of Rheb, located at the membrane through a farnesyl moiety in the carboxy-terminal region. Furthermore, farnesylation of Rheb was suggested to be essential for optimal mTORC1 activation (Castro et al. 2003; Tee et al. 2003b), although others contradict this (Li et al. 2004). Alternatively, Avruch and colleagues demonstrated that Rheb binds directly to the catalytic domain of mTOR (as well as to GβL), independently of TSC (Long et al. 2005a). Rheb binding to the mTORC1 complex does not require GTP loading. Activation of the complex is, however, strictly dependent on the presence of GTP-loaded Rheb (Long et al. 2005a). Importantly, Rheb binding to mTOR is reversibly inhibited by amino acid withdrawal (Long et al. 2005b). Deletion studies indicated that amino acid depletion acts upon the carboxy-terminal lobe of the mTOR catalytic domain to interfere with Rheb binding to the adjacent amino-terminal lobe. As amino acid withdrawal does not modulate mTOR kinase activity in vitro (Hara et al. 1998; Long et al. 2005b), it has been speculated that nutrient deprivation generates an inhibitor of Rheb/mTOR interaction that interferes with the ability of mTOR to phosphorylate raptor-recruited substrates.

TSC/Rheb/mTORC1 Functions as a Broad Integrator for Cell Growth

TSC/Rheb integrates signals not only from nutrients but also from growth factors and energy cues, conveying them to mTORC1 to drive cell growth. Under energy-starved conditions, AMPK phosphorylates and activates TSC2 to inhibit mTORC1 effector phosphorylation (Inoki et al. 2003). Furthermore, cell size reduction triggered by energy starvation appears dependent on TSC2 (Inoki et al. 2003; Shaw et al. 2004), although this has been queried (Hay and Sonenberg 2004). The former would be consistent with a linear model in which AMP-to-ATP ratio is sensed by AMPK in a LKB1-dependent manner and then translated to mTORC1 via TSC/Rheb (Corradetti et al. 2004; Shaw et al. 2004). Alternatively, AMPK activation has been reported to phosphorylate mTOR on T2446 (Cheng et al. 2004), and this might account for the TSC-independent inhibitory mechanism discussed by Hay and Sonenberg (Hay and Sonenberg 2004). TSC/Rheb also mediate REDD-induced effects of oxygen and energy deprivation on mTORC1 (Reiling and Hafen 2004; Brugarolas et al. 2004). REDD1 overexpression is sufficient to downregulate S6K1 phosphorylation in a TSC-dependent manner, while its disruption abrogates the hypoxia-induced inhibition of mTORC1 (Brugarolas et al. 2004).

A number of concomitant studies in Drosophila and mammalian models pointed to TSC2 as a direct substrate of Akt (reviewed in Shamji et al. 2003). Several residues located outside the GAP domain are phosphorylated by Akt in vitro (S939 and T1462 in humans; conserved in Drosophila) and in vivo. However, although overexpression studies in Drosophila indicated that TSC functions to inhibit the insulin-signaling pathway downstream of Akt, gene-replacement studies demonstrated that a nonphosphorylatable TSC2 mutant has little effect on Drosophila development (Dong and Pan et al. 2004), indicating the need to further investigate the relationship between growth factor-stimulated Akt and TSC/Rheb/mTORC1 in in vivo models.

Growth factor-induced regulation of mTORC1 signaling has long been thought to be mediated exclusively by PI3K/Akt. However, Pandolfi and colleagues described another mitogenic pathway possibly regulating TSC/Rheb/mTORC1 (Ma et al. 2005a). They reported that Erk might play a critical role in a parallel pathway to PI3K/Akt converging on TSC, consistent with the activation of Erk kinases in a subset of TSC lesions. They showed that Ras-induced, Erk-dependent phosphorylation of TSC2 on S540 and S664 (residues located outside the catalytic domain and conserved in higher eukaryotes) impairs TSC2's ability to inhibit mTORC1 and oncogenic transformation. Both these effects were prevented by a nonphosphorylatable allele. Similarly, the Ras/Erk signaling pathway has been suggested to impinge on mTOR (Tee et al. 2003a; Roux et al. 2004) by RSK1-mediated phosphorylation of TSC2 on S1798, leading to inactivation of TSC and increased S6K1 phosphorylation (Roux et al. 2004). However, Erk/RSK1 effects on translation and cell growth have not yet been directly addressed.

7.1.3.2 Survival Function

Mediator of Akt Survival Activity

Akt is a key regulator of cell survival, thought to mediate its effects through multiple down-stream effectors, like forkhead proteins, mdm2, Bad, or ASK1. PI3K/Akt activation of mTORC1 regulates cell growth. However, in vivo work suggests that mTOR might also mediate some aspects of PI3K/Akt-driven survival. Therefore, although inhibition of mTORC1 in the presence of basal PI3K/Akt activation has strictly cytostatic effects, PI3K/Akt dependence or overactivation might result in some levels of dependence on mTORC1 for survival. For instance, it was shown that rapamycin derivatives restrain the growth of PTEN-deficient xenograft tumors by increasing apoptosis (Neshat et al. 2001). Importantly, they can restore chemosensitivity and endocrine therapy responsiveness in Akt-driven cancer models (Wendel et al. 2004; deGraffenried et al. 2004). Moreover, treatment with the rapamycin derivative RAD001 induced massive apoptosis and complete reversal of the neoplastic phenotype in an Akt-dependent murine prostate intraepithelial neoplasia intraepithelial neoplasia model (Majumder et al. 2004).

Mediator of Autophagy

Cell homeostasis requires maintenance of a constant supply for intracellular precursors of macromolecular biosynthesis. Besides importing nutrients and energy sources from their extracellular environment, higher eukaryotes retain intracellular catabolic processes like autophagy, also referred to as programmed cell death type II (reviewed in Kondo 2005; Lum 2005). Autophagy is characterized by sequestration of cytoplasmic components into autophagosome vacuoles for bulk degradation; breakdown products provide metabolites to support biosynthesis. It was initially characterized as a response to nutrient deprivation but has been more recently implicated in cell survival, development, and tumor suppression (Kondo et al. 2005; Lum et al. 2005). Interestingly, although cancer cells generally exhibit reduced autophagy, it can be induced in response to some therapies. However, the role of autophagy in cancer therapy (defensive or destructive) is still controversial (Ng and Huang 2005).

In yeast, TOR lies upstream of autophagy-associated genes and acts as a gatekeeper for initiating the autophagic pathway. In mammalian cells, rapamycin stimulates autophagy, implicating mTORC1 as an important regulator (Kanazawa et al. 2004). A number of pathways feeding into mTORC1 have been implicated; however, mTORC1-independent effects also exist (Mordier et al. 2000; Kanazawa et al. 2004). Consistent with the positive role of growth factors on nutrient uptake (Edinger et al. 2002) and its role in the regulation of glucose metabolism, the PI3K/Akt pathway impairs autophagy (Lum et al. 2005), and rapamycin reverses some aspects of this. Interestingly, a synergistic increase of rapamycin-induced autophagy by PI3K or Akt inhibitors was recently demonstrated in malignant glioma cells (Takeuchi et al. 2005).

7.1.3.3 Angiogenic Function

It is well documented that rapamycin and rapamycin derivatives are potent inhibitors of tumor cell proliferation, exhibiting activity in a broad range of tumor cells (Lane et al. 2003a; Dutcher 2004; Beuvink et al. 2005; Boulay et al. 2005). Xenografts derived from indifferent tumor lines display relative sensitivity in vivo, despite tumor drug levels never reaching the IC50 for inhibition of cell proliferation (Lane et al. 2002; O'Reilly et al. 2005). Moreover, human vascular endothelial and smooth muscle cell (SMC) proliferation is exquisitely sensitive to mTORC1 inhibition (Lane et al. 2002; Guba et al. 2002; O'Reilly et al. 2005; Marx et al. 1995). Consistently, rapamycin and its derivatives inhibit tumor growth by reducing VEGF production (Guba et al. 2002; Brugarolas et al. 2003), dramatically decreasing tumor neovascularization (Guba et al. 2002; Shinohara et al. 2005) and the density of perfused vessels in primary tumors and metastases (Lane et al. 2002, O'Reilly et al. 2005), strongly supporting a direct antiangiogenic activity. In the case of RAD001, a reduction in SMC coverage of tumor-associated vessels has also been observed (O'Reilly et al. 2005). Additionally, mTORC1 regulates HIF1α and its target genes in an array of in vitro and animal models (Brugarolas et al. 2003; Majumder et al. 2004), suggesting that mTOR inhibitors have potential for the treatment of highly vascularized tumors, as for instance those occurring in patients affected by TSC (reviewed in Inoki et al. 2005) or von Hippel–Lindau (VHL) syndrome (Thomas et al. 2006).

7.1.3.4 Feedback Regulatory Mechanisms

mTORC1 Signals Negatively to PI3K/Akt via IRS

Insulin is a critical factor for PI3K/Akt/mTORC1-mediated cell growth. Insulin responsiveness is regulated at the level of the adaptor protein insulin receptor substrates (IRS1 and IRS2) that are recruited by engaged receptors to activate PI3K/Akt among other pathways. On activation, IRS proteins are phosphorylated and downregulated, restraining insulin signaling, a phenomenon known as insulin resistance (reviewed in Manning 2004). S6K1 was reported to mediate insulin resistance in a rapamycin-sensitive manner (Harrington et al. 2004; Shah 2004). Moreover, S6K1-deficient mice are hypersensitive to insulin and are protected against age- and diet-induced obesity (Um et al. 2004), supporting the idea that S6K1 signals back to restrain insulin-induced PI3K/Akt activation.

Strikingly, this feedback mechanism raises concerns regarding the use of rapamycin derivatives in the clinic for patients harboring tumors with overactivated mTORC1 pathway, as it might lead to enhancement of Akt-dependent survival pathways. Indeed, there are reports that the negative feedback loop is active in tumor models (Manning et al. 2005; Ma et al. 2005b; O'Reilly et al. 2006) and in solid tumors in patients (Tabernero et al. 2005; O'Reilly et al. 2006). Specifically, on-treatment pharmacodynamic evaluation of the effects of RAD001 on the tumors of advanced cancer patients suggests that in some patients phosphorylated Akt (S473) levels increase with dose (Tabernero et al. 2005). As yet, it is too early for any correlations with response to be made.

mTORC2 Signals Positively to Akt

The functions of mTORC2 are still poorly understood. Sabatini and collaborators have recently suggested that mTORC2 acts as an Akt kinase (Sarbassov et al. 2005). Akt requires phosphorylation of T308 in the activation loop (mediated by PDK1) and S473 in the hydrophobic motif, a site homologous to the mTORC1-dependent site T389 in S6K1. The identity of the S473 kinase has been controversial, although mTOR may fulfill a number of criteria for being the elusive S473 kinase. RNAi-mediated down-regulation of mTOR and rictor, but not raptor, resulted in a reduction in Akt phosphorylation on both S473 and T308 in a number of mammalian cell lines, indicating that mTOR and rictor share a positive role in Akt activation. Furthermore, immunopurified mTORC2 phosphorylated Akt in vitro. The biological relevance of mTORC2-dependent Akt phosphorylation is unclear (reviewed in Guertin and Sabatini 2005; Hay 2005). Although it is unknown what inputs regulate mTORC2, there may be some level of dependence on growth factors (Jacinto et al. 2004; Sarbassov et al. 2004, 2005), possibly through PI3K. This feedback mechanism would place mTORC2 upstream of Akt, as a potential activator of rapamycin-sensitive mTORC1 in response to growth factor stimulation. Conversely, Akt-induced mTORC1 activation might ultimately restrain Akt activation by eventually impinging on the levels or activity of mTORC2, and might therefore represent an alternative negative feedback mechanism. Indeed, prolonged treatment with rapamycin might decrease mTORC2 levels below those needed to maintain Akt signaling in certain cell types (Sarbassov et al. 2006), a mechanism that would strengthen the therapeutic potential of mTORC1 inhibition.

7.2 mTOR Pathway Activation in Cancer

Mutation or overexpression of mTOR has not been described in human cancers. However, its essential checkpoint activity, its regulation by signaling pathways often deregulated in tumors, and its role in the translation of well-characterized oncogenes, strongly support the potential of mTOR as well as components of the mTORC1 pathway as valuable therapeutic targets in oncology. Optimization of the use of rapamycin derivatives in the clinic necessitates a better understanding of the molecular events that drive mTOR dependence in human tumors, as well as the identification of biomarkers that may predispose to increased sensitivity or are associated with resistance mechanisms.

7.2.1 Deregulation of RTK/PI3K/Akt Signaling in Cancer

The PI3K/Akt pathway is heavily deregulated in numerous tumors by various mechanisms, indicating a fundamental role in the development and progression of many tumor types (Table 7.1; reviewed in Vivanco and Sawyers 2002; Hennessy et al. 2006). Activated Akt triggers a number of responses including increased proliferation, survival, and motility, altogether driving malignant progression. A large body of evidence supports an essential contribution of the mTORC1 pathway in PI3K/Akt-dependent effects on cancer progression, suggesting that activation of the PI3K/Akt pathway may induce some level of dependence on mTORC1 signaling and, ultimately, sensitize these tumors to inhibition of mTORC1. Loss of function of the tumor suppressor PTEN is a common alteration in both familial and sporadic cancers. PTEN deficiency has been postulated as a major sensitivity determinant for mTORC1 inhibitors (Neshat et al. 2001; Podsypanina et al. 2001; Yu et al., 2001; Shi et al. 2002), although this correlation may be dependent on tumor type (Lane et al 2003a). Interestingly, in a phase II safety trial in women with heavily treated, advanced breast cancer, three of the four PTEN-negative patients showed objective response to mTORC1 inhibition, whereas only 37% of the overall patient population exhibited evidence of clinical benefit (Chan 2004). Hence, further analysis of patient tumors under treatment with rapamycin derivatives is warranted. PTEN deficiency is correlated with increased Akt activation (Choe et al. 2003); however, additional genetic alterations can result in Akt deregulation, including mutations of PI3K subunits and Akt amplification (Table 7.1; reviewed in Vivanco and Sawyers 2002, Samuels and Ericson 2006). In this respect, Akt activation might be a broader predisposition marker for mTOR inhibitor sensitivity (Boulay et al. 2003; Noh et al. 2004). Indeed, we have demonstrated that levels of Akt phosphorylation on serine 473 correlate highly with the in vitro antiproliferative response of tumor cell lines to RAD001 (Fig. 7.2). In agreement with this finding, mTORC1 inhibition has also been demonstrated to have activity or revert therapeutic resistance in Akt-driven cancer models (Wendel et al. 2004; Majumder et al. 2004; deGraffenried et al. 2004). Evaluation of the relevance of measuring Akt phosphorylation levels as a potential stratification marker in cancer patients is awaited.

7.2.2 Hamartoma Syndromes

Hamartomas are benign hyperproliferative disorders, which are hallmarks of a number of inherited syndromes. Several regulators of mTORC1 (i.e., TSC1 and TSC2, LKB1, PTEN, and NF1; see Fig. 7.1) have tumor suppressor function, inactivation of which drives the development of histologically-related hamartomas in various organs (Table 7.1; reviewed in Inoki et al. 2005). Importantly, mTORC1 signaling is upregulated in lesions from tuberous sclerosis (TSC1 or TSC2 mutations) and neurofibromatosis type 1 (NF1) patients (Kenerson et al. 2002; Johannessen et al. 2005; Dasgupta et al. 2005) and in animal models of Peutz–Jeghers syndrome (PJS, mutations in LKB1; Coradetti et al. 2004; Shaw et al. 2004), supporting a functional relationship between these diseases and mTORC1 activation. Hamartomas in TSC and PJS rarely become malignant, in contrast to tumors resulting from PTEN inactivation (e.g., Cowden disease). Negative feedback mechanisms impairing PI3K/Akt activation have been proposed to prevent the progression to malignancy. For example, TSC inactivation was shown to disrupt PI3K/Akt signaling through downregulation of PDGFR expression (Zhang et al. 2003a). Additionally, S6K1 overactivation was demonstrated to inactivate IRS/PI3K/Akt signaling, a mechanism recently supported in PTEN/TSC2 compound heterozygous mice,

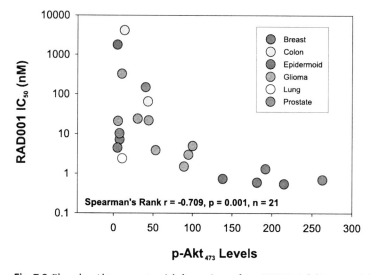

Fig. 7.2 Phospho-Akt as a potential determinant for mTORC1 inhibitor sensitivity. Analysis of a panel of 21 tumor cell lines derived from various tumor types demonstrated a strong association between higher phospho-Akt (serine 473) levels (as measured by ELISA) and increased in vitro sensitivity to the antiproliferative activity of the mTORC1 inhibitor RAD001 (IC50). The y-axis represents RAD001 IC50 for antiproliferative response. The x-axis represents phospho-AKT levels (arbitrary units normalized against an internal control). The correlation coefficient (r) and significance level (p) were calculated with the Spearman rank order coefficient

where PTEN haploinsufficiency overcomes the effect of TSC2 haploinsufficiency, consistent with a dominant effect on the PI3K/Akt pathway downstream of TSC2 (Manning et al. 2005; Ma et al. 2005b). These feedback mechanisms raise a number of concerns regarding the potential benefit of mTORC1 inhibitors in the treatment of TSC, and other hamartoma syndromes, as treatment could lead to reactivation of Akt survival pathways. However, in this regard, a recent report showed that oral rapamycin therapy did indeed induce regression of astrocytomas associated with TSC in all five patients treated, a very promising observation (Franz et al. 2006). More extensive trials in TSC patients will help to clarify this issue.

7.3 mTOR Inhibitors in Cancer

All mTOR inhibitors that have entered clinical development so far, including RAD001 (everolimus), CCI-779 (temsirolimus) and AP23573, are rapamycin derivatives and, therefore, target mTORC1 only (Table 7.2). Here we will concentrate on preclinical and clinical aspects of the development of RAD001 in oncology.

7.3.1 Preclinical Development

Rapamycin derivatives have antiproliferative activity against a variety of tumor cell lines

in vitro (Neshat et al. 2001; Shi et al. 2002; Lane et al. 2003a; Noh et al. 2004; reviewed in Hidalgo and Rowinsky 2000; Huang and Houghton 2003; Dutcher 2004, Beuvink et al. 2005, Boulay et al. 2005), triggering prolonged G1 accumulation in sensitive cells (Fingar et al. 2004; Ohanna et al. 2005, Boulay et al. 2005). Significant growth inhibition was also observed in a number of mouse and human cancer models (Podsypanina et al. 2001; Yu et al. 2001; O'Reilly et al. 2002; Guba et al. 2002; Majumder et al. 2004; Wendel et al. 2004; Wu et al. 2005, Boulay et al. 2004). Furthermore, combined antiproliferative and antiangiogenic activities in animal models clearly support the potential of these agents in cancer patients. Although the primary effect of mTORC1 inhibition is cytostatic, a number of genetically defined tumor models indicate that these agents can exert cytotoxic activities in particular settings (Majumder et al. 2004; Wendel et al. 2004). Finally, given the increased sensitivity of tumor cells to nutrient and energy supply, the checkpoint function of mTORC1 for cellular stresses (reviewed in Proud 2004) suggests that inhibition can sensitize cells to a number of other cytotoxics or targeted agents.

7.3.1.1 Potentiation of Chemotherapy and Radiotherapy

In preclinical models, there are a number of reports that the combination of mTORC1 inhibitors with standard chemotherapeutic agents, targeting DNA and microtubules, provides

Table 7.2 mTOR inhibitors in the clinic

Drug	Type	Administration	Company	Status/indication
RAD001 (everolimus)	Rapamycin derivative	Oral	Novartis	Phase II, broad focus development including NSCLC, breast, renal cell carcinoma (RCC), neuroendocrine tumors
CCI-779 (temsirolimus)	Prodrug of rapamycin	Intravenous	Wyeth Ayerst	Phase III: mantle cell lymphoma and RCC
		Oral		Phase II: metastatic endometrial cancer
AP23573	Rapamycin derivative	Intravenous	ARIAD	Phase II: bone and soft tissue sarcoma

a greater antitumor effect than either agent alone (Shi et al. 1995; Grunwald et al. 2002; O'Reilly et al. 2003; Mondesire et al. 2004; Wu et al. 2005). In this context, mTORC1 signaling is impaired by various genotoxic stresses in both normal and tumor cells (reviewed in Proud 2004), an event preceding the onset of cell death. Additionally, it has been reported that p53 regulates mTORC1 by means of the AMPK/TSC energy sensor pathway (Feng et al. 2005), supporting coordinated regulation of cellular checkpoints to ensure normal growth and proliferation. Taking this to the therapeutic setting, and consistent with previous work (Shi et al. 1995), we have observed more profound effects on tumor cell proliferation and survival after concomitant exposure to the DNA-damaging anticancer agent cisplatin and RAD001 (Beuvink et al. 2005). Indeed, RAD001 sensitized tumor cell lines with wild-type p53 status to enter the apoptotic program in the presence of suboptimal concentrations of cisplatin. Detailed molecular analysis demonstrated that mTORC1 inhibition potentiated p53-dependent, DNA damage-induced cytotoxicity, by impairing p53-dependent upregulation of the cyclin-dependent kinase inhibitor p21 (Fig. 7.3). This was attributed to effects of mTORC1 inhibition on global translation, resulting in the reduced expression of proteins, like p21, that have a high turnover (Beuvink et al. 2005). It has recently become evident that p21 not only prevents cells from proceeding through replication but also has a profound antiapoptotic function by inhibiting several proapoptotic components (reviewed in Weiss 2003). Hence, attenuation of p21 induction caused by suboptimal DNA damage, which would normally cause cells to enter the DNA repair program, could explain the entry into apoptosis caused by RAD001, a conclusion supported by siRNA approaches (Beuvink et al. 2005). From these data, it is tempting to speculate that combination with mTORC1 inhibitors could expand the narrow therapeutic window associated with platins and other DNA-damaging agents. In this respect, although we have seen positive interactions between RAD001 and DNA-damaging agents with other mechanisms of action (such as topoisomerase inhibitors; O'Reilly et al. 2003 and unpublished results), it remains to be seen whether this can be ex-

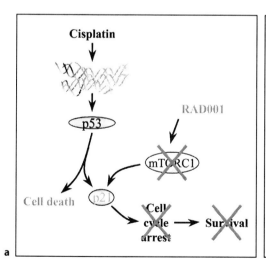
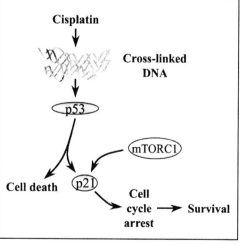

Fig. 7.3a,b. mTORC1 enhances DNA damage-induced cell death by reducing the expression of the antiapoptotic protein p21. DNA-damaging agents like cisplatin induce the activation of the p53 checkpoint pathway, resulting in either cell death through activation of proapoptotic genes or cell cycle arrest and DNA repair through activation of antiapoptotic genes like the cyclin-dependent kinase inhibitor p21 (**a**). The rapamycin derivative RAD001 sensitizes tumor cells to the cytotoxic effect of DNA-damaging agents by preventing the upregulation of p21, and therefore shifting the equilibrium toward cell death (**b**).

plained by similar effects on p53/p21 response. Considering that >50% tumors harbor mutations in the p53 checkpoint, it also remains to be clarified whether other mechanisms may enhance chemotherapeutic-induced cell death independently of p53 function (Grunwald et al. 2002; Mondesire et al. 2004; Wendel et al. 2004; Wu et al. 2005).

Radiotherapy is widely used to treat certain types of tumors, in particular glioblastomas (GBM). Considering the fatal outcome for these patients, there is a need to define novel therapeutic approaches combining radiotherapy with novel therapeutics targeting mediators of known resistance mechanisms. In these highly vascularized tumors, radiation activates the PI3K/Akt pathway, one of the mechanisms suggested to lead to resistance and tumor recurrence. It has recently been shown that mTORC1 signaling is also induced in tumor and vascular endothelial cells after radiation therapy in a PI3K-dependent manner (Shinohara et al. 2005; Albert et al. 2006), indicating that radioresistance might be associated with mTORC1 pathway activation. Inhibition of mTORC1 enhances the radiosensitivity of breast cancer cells in vitro (Albert et al. 2006) and GBM xenografts by acting on tumor cells (Eshleman 2002) or dramatically reducing vascular density and endothelial cell survival (Shinohara et al. 2005). On the basis of these promising results, combined mTORC1 inhibition and radiotherapy is worthy of clinical evaluation.

7.3.1.2 Combination with Targeted Therapies

A rational approach to test the impact of impaired mTORC1 signaling is to evaluate rapamycin derivatives in patients bearing tumors that exhibit overactivation of PI3K/Akt signaling. For instance, it has become evident that there is potential for combination with therapeutics targeting tyrosine kinases that are at least partly dependent on Akt for their oncogenic activity, such as Bcr-Abl in chronic myelogenous leukemia (Mohi et al. 2004; Dengler et al. 2005) and ErbB and IGF-1 receptors in solid tumors (reviewed in Hynes and Lane 2005; O'Reilly et al. 2006). Interestingly, combinations of RAD001 with AEE788 (a multifunction inhibitor of EGFR, ErbB2, and the VEGFR) in animal models of GBM caused inhibition of xenograft growth and increased survival in mice with intracranial tumors to an extent greater than either agent as monotherapy (Goudar et al. 2005). Consistent with IGF-1 receptor inhibition reducing the increased Akt phosphorylation associated with mTORC1 inhibition in vitro, combination with rapamycin also exhibited more profound effects on tumor cell proliferation (O'Reilly et al. 2006).

Recently, we have also evaluated the effect of combining RAD001 with the aromatase inhibitor letrozole in estrogen-sensitive breast cancer models. The role of estrogen in breast cancer progression is well established. Consequently, its treatment and prevention with hormonal (endocrine) antiestrogenic therapies, such as tamoxifen and more recently aromatase inhibitors, has proven quite successful (Goss 2003a; Cuzick et al. 2003; Veronesi et al. 2005; Early Breast Cancer Trialists' Collaborative Group 2005). Letrozole is a potent, third-generation aromatase inhibitor successfully applied in the adjuvant and advanced breast cancer settings (Goss et al. 2003b; Rose et al. 2003; Smith 2004; Janicke et al. 2004; Thurlimann et al. 2005), which inhibits the aromatase enzyme required for the production of estrogen from androgens. We therefore carried out our studies in human breast cancer cells expressing endogenous aromatase enzyme (known as MCF7/Aro and T47D/Aro) (Boulay et al. 2005). Although estradiol-stimulated proliferation of MCF7/Aro cells was associated with modulation of the mTOR pathway and suppressed by RAD001 treatment, in agreement with previous work with rapamycin (Pang et al. 2001; Castoria et al 2001), a striking combinatorial effect between RAD001 and letrozole was demonstrated. In both cell lines, each single agent dose-dependently inhibited aromatase-mediated, estrogen-induced proliferation. However, in combination, a synergistic effect on proliferation was observed, which correlated with more profound effects on cell cycle progression and significant decreases in cell viability. Increased cell death was particularly evident with optimal drug combinations and was defined as apoptosis by TUNEL analysis.

These results demonstrate that combination of letrozole and RAD001 holds promise for the rational treatment of estrogen-dependent breast cancers in a scenario where the tumor cells are sensitive to both agents alone. However, the Akt/mTOR pathway may also be involved in the development of resistance to endocrine therapies (reviewed in Johnston 2005). Indeed, Akt activation is associated with a more aggressive clinical phenotype and a worse clinical outcome for endocrine-treated patients with breast cancers (Perez-Tenorio and Stal 2002). Moreover, long-term estrogen deprivation, mimicking to some extent the effect of aromatase inhibitors, can result in estrogen hypersensitivity associated with increased Akt activation and mTOR effector phosphorylation (Yue et al. 2003). It is therefore tempting to propose that this drug combination may also have potential as an approach to circumvent or combat resistance. This hypothesis is supported by recent work showing that mTOR inhibition can restore tamoxifen response in a breast cancer xenograft model expressing a constitutively active allele of Akt (deGraffenried et al 2004).

7.3.2 Clinical Development

7.3.2.1 Evaluation of Biologically Effective Doses

Rapamycin or rapamycin derivatives, such as RAD001, were initially developed as immunosuppressants for prevention of allograft rejection. As immune suppression is an undesired side effect in cancer patients, it might be advisable to define a therapeutic window to differentiate both activities. In this regard, prolonged ($\geq$3-day) effects on downstream mTOR effector molecules (e.g., p70S6K1 and 4E-BP1) in tumor cells is seen after a single pulse treatment with RAD001 in vitro (Beuvink et al. 2001) and in a rat pancreatic tumor model, an observation correlating with the antitumor efficacy of intermittent (weekly) dosing strategies in the latter (Boulay et al 2004). Using a rat model that recapitulates T cell-dependent responses, we demonstrated that the same weekly dosing regimen allows for recovery of the immune system as compared to daily dosing, allowing clear differentiation between antitumor and unwanted immunosuppressive effects (Boulay et al. 2004). These data show that it is possible to evaluate therapeutic windows preclinically.

Such work leads the way to improving on empirical drug development, where drug level is chosen based on the maximally tolerated dose. In contrast to classic cytotoxic agents, for targeted therapeutics the relationship between dose and response is suggested to plateau above a threshold dose, whereas the relationship between dose and toxicity is still linear (O'Donnell et al. 2003; Chan 2004). Hence, it would seem logical in this case to instead define the optimal biologically effective dose. Such an approach might reduce side effects and facilitate the design of combination trials. Hence, to most efficiently exploit the pharmacological profile of rapamycin derivatives, it is important to carefully monitor the dose given to a cancer patient, especially considering the observation that treatment can be less effective if overdosed (Guba et al. 2002). Evaluation of the optimal effective dose requires a reliable biomarker whose modulation closely correlates with pathway inactivation. mTORC1 has two highly specific effectors, 4E-BP1 and S6K1; the activity of the latter can be accurately measured ex vivo from specimens derived from tumors and surrogate tissues such as skin or peripheral blood mononucleocytes (PBMCs; Boulay et al. 2004; O'Donnell et al. 2003; Lane et al. 2003b). Strikingly, with a syngeneic rat pancreatic tumor model, significant antitumor efficacy of weekly RAD001 treatment regimens was correlated with inactivation of S6K1 in PBMCs for 1 week (Boulay et al. 2004). Importantly, pharmacodynamic analysis of PBMC-derived S6K1 activity in a phase IA clinical study, including 18 patients with advanced solid tumors receiving RAD001 in weekly doses (5, 10, 20, and 30 mg/week orally), demonstrated S6K1 inactivation for 1 week in seven of eight patients treated with the two highest doses (O'Donnell et al. 2003; Lane et al. 2003b). Subsequent pharmacokinetic and pharmacodynamic modeling, based on the rat tumor model data and patient pharmacokinetics, helped to define both weekly (50–70 mg) and daily (10 mg) optimal biological doses of RAD001 (O'Donnell et al. 2003; Lane et al. 2003b). These were confirmed to provide continuous suppression of tumor mTORC1 activity through direct immunohistochemical analysis of patient tumors (Tabernero et al. 2005), and are currently being further evaluated in the clinical setting.

7.3.2.2 Safety and Response in Advanced Solid Tumors; Evaluation of Combination with Letrozole in Advanced Breast Cancer Patients

In phase I trials, as a single agent RAD001 has shown clinical activity in breast cancer, non-small cell lung cancer (NSCLC) and colorectal cancer. A mild myelosuppression was observed, and the most commonly observed, mild (grade 1/2) nonhematologic adverse events were fatigue, rash, and stomatitis. Cardiotoxicity, alopecia, and peripheral edema were not observed. Severe adverse events occurred in fewer than 5% of patients. (Tabernero et al. 2005; O'Donnell et al. 2003). Hence, the side effect profile is in accordance with that seen in the organ transplantation setting and is similar to that observed with CCI-779 in single-agent safety trials (reviewed in Chan 2004; Vignot et al. 2005).

On the basis of the promising preclinical data, RAD001 in combination with the aromatase inhibitor letrozole (Femara®) is being evaluated in the advanced breast cancer setting. An open-label, phase IB, escalating-dose design study of the safety and pharmacokinetics of the combination in patients with advanced breast cancer has been performed (Awada et al. 2004, Awada et al. manuscript in preparation). Treatment with letrozole 2.5 mg/day and RAD001 at 5 mg/day or 10 mg/day was examined in 18 breast cancer patients who had not experienced an objective response to letrozole alone after at least 4 months treatment. No dose-limiting toxicities were observed in the patients receiving RAD001 at 5 mg/day; hence, the dose was increased to 10 mg/day with acceptable tolerability. The most frequently reported adverse events were stomatitis, anorexia/decreased appetite, fatigue, diarrhea, headache, and rash. One case of dose-limiting toxicity (grade 3 thrombocytopenia) was observed in a patient treated with 10 mg RAD001. No significant alteration in plasma and whole blood levels of letrozole or RAD001 were observed when coadministered. From a total of 16 patients, there was one complete response in the 10-mg RAD001 cohort, with no partial responses. Stable disease (8–20 months) occurred in two and four patients receiving 5 and 10 mg/day RAD001, respectively (Awada et al. 2004, Awada et al. manuscript in preparation). Hence, there was evidence of a more profound antitumor effect as a result of adding RAD001 to the letrozole treatment regimen, reflecting the preclinical observations.

The results of the preclinical and early phase IB studies demonstrate the feasibility and tolerability of combination therapy with RAD001 and letrozole. On the basis of these results, a dose of 10 mg/day RAD001 has been recommended for further trials (Awada et al. 2004, Awada et al. manuscript in preparation). Additionally, further drug combination partners are also being assessed in the clinical setting.

7.3.2.3 Patient Stratification

Identification of molecularly defined patient populations more likely to respond to treatment is of great value for the development of targeted therapeutics. Recent progresses in the basic knowledge of mTOR signaling provided some clues for patient stratification. First, mTORC1 activation is a common feature in a number of hyperproliferative diseases and hamartoma syndromes (such as tuberous sclerosis), indicating potential dependence on the mTORC1 pathway (Kenerson et al. 2002; Johannessen et al. 2005; Dasgupta et al. 2005). Although it appears probable that mTORC1 inhibitors will essentially be developed in oncology as combination therapeutics, hamartoma diseases might represent potential indications for a monotherapy approach (Table 7.1). Consequently, RAD001 is currently being assessed in tuberous sclerosis patients.

Expression and activation of PI3K/Akt/mTOR pathway components have been profiled in human tumor biopsies. For example, PTEN deficiency was highly correlated with increased Akt activation in a set of glioblastomas (Choe et al. 2003). Similarly, phospho-Akt (S473) and phospho-S6K1 (T421/S424) levels were significantly correlated in a mixed panel of solid tumors (Xu et al. 2004). Modeling of in vitro sensitivity studies suggested that, overall, one-fourth of the tumors in the latter study exhibited low PTEN, higher phospho-Akt (S473), and higher phospho-S6K1 (T421/S424), and might thus be predicted to be sensitive to mTORC1 inhibitors. In a larger study, there was a significant correlation between the levels of phospho-Akt, phospho-4E-BP1, and phospho-S6K1 (Rojo et al. 2004), further supporting that pharmacodynamic analysis of these markers could help define patient populations. Preliminary results in a phase II trial in patients with recurrent GBM indicated that higher baseline tumor phospho-S6K1 (T421/S424) levels, rather than PTEN status or phospho-Akt (S473) levels, were associated with neuroimaging response to mTORC1 inhibition (Galanis et al. 2005). However, in a limited study of heavily pretreated patients with advanced breast tumors, both PTEN loss and ErbB2 overexpression were suggested to be associated with response to mTORC1 inhibition (Chan 2004). These studies are by no means conclusive, but they highlight the need for large prospective pharmacodynamic analyses of multiple markers of PI3K/Akt/mTOR pathway activation in various tumor types to establish a broader view of their use as potential predisposition biomarkers. Taking this further, the clinical consequences of rapamycin-induced Akt activation are also a major concern. Further clinical studies combining pharmacodynamic evaluation of Akt activation and efficacy are warranted to clarify this issue.

In conclusion, increased activation of the PI3K/PTEN/mTOR pathway might be associated with a higher dependence on mTORC1 signaling for proliferation and/or survival of tumor cells. Clearly, as discussed above, preclinical profiling studies support this hypothesis. The need is there to thoroughly evaluate clinically whether molecular profiling can indeed aid patient stratification efforts in the arena of mTORC1 inhibitors. This is a major emphasis in the case of the RAD001 clinical development program, which is currently ongoing.

Acknowledgements. We would like to acknowledge all those researchers whose work we were unable to cite because of space restrictions. We would also like to thank Dr. Thomas Radimerski, Dr. David Lebwohl and Dr. Philippe Thevenaz (Novartis Pharma AG) for their critical reading of the manuscript and Dr. Sauveur-Michel Maira, Dr. Terence O'Reilly, Marc Hattenberger and Sabine Zumstein-Mecker (Novartis Pharma AG) for kindly performing the ELISA assay and correlations presented in Fig. 7.2.

References

Abraham RT (2004) PI 3-kinase related kinases:'big' players in stress-induced signaling pathways. DNA Repair (Amst) 3:883–887

Albert JM, Kim KW, Cao C, Lu B (2006) Targeting the Akt/mammalian target of rapamycin pathway for radiosensitization of breast cancer. Mol Cancer Ther 5:1183–1189

Ali SM, Sabatini DM (2005) Structure of S6 kinase 1 determines whether raptor-mTOR or rictor-mTOR phosphorylates its hydrophobic motif site. J Biol Chem 280:19445–19448

Aoki M, Blazek E, Vogt PK (2001) A role of the kinase mTOR in cellular transformation induced by the oncoproteins P3K and Akt. Proc Natl Acad Sci USA 98:136–141

Avdulov S, Li S, Michalek V, Burrichter D, Peterson M, Perlman DM, Manivel JC, Sonenberg N, Yee D, Bitterman PB, Polunovsky VA (2004) Activation of translation complex eIF4F is essential for the genesis and maintenance of the malignant phenotype in human mammary epithelial cells. Cancer Cell 5:553–563

Awada A, Cardoso F, Fontaine C, Dirix L, De Grve J, Sotiriou C, Steinseifer J, Wouters C, Tanaka C, Ressayre-Djaffer C, Piccart M (2004) A phase Ib study of the mTOR inhibitor RAD001(everolimus) in combination with letrozole (Femara), investigating safety and pharmacokinetics in patients with advanced breast cancer stable or progressing on letrozole. Breast Cancer Res Treat 88(suppl 1):S234

Awada A, Cardoso F, Fontaine C, Dirix L, De Grève J, Sotiriou C, Steinseifer J, Wouters C, Tanaka C, Zoellner U, Tang P, Piccart M (Manuscript in preparation) The mTOR inhibitor RAD001 (everolimus) in combination with letrozole in patients with advanced breast cancer. Results of a phase 1 study with pharmacokinetics.

Beuvink I, O'Reilly T, Zumstein-Mecker S, Zilbermann F, Sedrani R, Kozma SC, Thomas G, Lane HA (2001) Antitumor activity of RAD001, an orally active rapamycin derivative. Proc Am Assoc Cancer Res 42:366

Beuvink I, Boulay A, Fumagalli S, Zilbermann F, Ruetz S, O'Reilly T, Natt F, Hall J, Lane HA, Thomas G (2005) The mTOR inhibitor RAD001 sensitizes tumor cells to DNA-damaged induced apoptosis through inhibition of p21 translation. Cell 120:747–759

Boulay A, Hattenberger M, Maira SM, Thomas G, Merlo A, O'Reilly T, Lane HA (2003) Phospho-Akt levels as potential biomarker of in vitro sensitivity of tumor cell lines to the mTOR pathway inhibitor RAD001. Proc AACR-NCI-EORTC Abstract 1096

Boulay A, Zumstein-Mecker S, Stephan C, Beuvink I, Zilbermann F, Haller R, Tobler S, Heusser C, O'Reilly T, Stolz B, Marti A, Thomas G, Lane HA (2004) Antitumor efficacy of intermittent treatment schedules with the rapamycin derivative RAD001 correlates with prolonged inactivation of ribosomal protein S6 kinase 1 in peripheral blood mononuclear cells. Cancer Res 64:252–261

Boulay A, Rudloff J, Ye J, Zumstein-Mecker S, O'Reilly T, Evans DB, Chen S, Lane HA (2005) Dual inhibition of mTOR and estrogen receptor signaling in vitro induces cell death in models of breast cancer. Clin Cancer Res 11:5319–5328

Brugarolas J, Vazquez F, Reddy A, Sellers WR, Kaelin WG (2003) TCS2 regulates VEGF through mTOR-dependent and -independent pathways. Cancer Cell 4:147–158

Brugarolas J, Lei K, Hurley RL, Manning BD, Reiling JH, Hafen E, Witters LA, Ellisen LW, Kaelin WG Jr. (2004) Regulation of mTOR function in response to hypoxia by REDD1 and the TSC1/TSC2 tumor suppressor complex. Genes Dev 18:2893–2904

Burnett PE, Barrow RK, Cohen NA, Snyder SH, Sabatini DM (1998) RAFT1 phosphorylation of the translational regulators p70 S6 kinase and 4E-BP1. Proc Natl Acad Sci USA 95:1432–1437

Carling D (2004) The AMP-activated protein kinase cascade-a unifying system for energy control. Trends Biochem Sci 29:18–24

Castoria G, Migliaccio A, Bilancio A, Di Domenico M, de Falco A, Lombardi M, Fiorentino R, Varricchio L, Barone MV, Auricchio F (2001) PI3-kinase in concert with Src promotes the S-phase entry of oestradiol-stimulated MCF-7 cells. EMBO J 20:6050–6059

Castro AF, Rebhun JF, Clark GJ, Quilliam LA (2003) Rheb binds tuberous sclerosis complex 2 (TSC2) and promotes S6 kinase activation in a rapamycin- and farnesylation-dependent manner. J Biol Chem 278:32493–32496

Chan S (2004) Targeting the mammalian target of rapamycin (mTOR):a new approach to treating cancer. Br J Cancer 91:1420–1424

Cheng SW, Fryer LG, Carling D, Shepherd PR (2004) Thr2446 is a novel mammalian target of rapamycin (mTOR) phosphorylation site regulated by nutrient status. J Biol Chem 279:15719–15722

Chiang GG, Abraham RT (2005) Phosphorylation of mammalian target of rapamycin (mTOR) at Ser-2448 is mediated by p70S6 kinase. J Biol Chem 280:25485–25490

Choe G, Horvath S, Cloughesy TF, Crosby K, Seligson D, Palotie A, Inge L, Smith BL, Sawyers CL, Mischel PS (2003) Analysis of the phosphatidylinositol 3'-kinase signaling pathway in glioblastoma patients in vivo. Cancer Res 63:2742–2746

Conde E, Angulo B, Tang M, Morente M, Torres-Lanzas J, Lopez-Encuentra A, Lopez-Rios F, Sanchez-Cespedes M (2006) Molecular context of the EGFR mutations: evidence for the activation of mTOR/S6K signaling. Clin Cancer Res 12:710–717

Corradetti MN, Inoki K, Bardeesy N, DePinho RA, Guan KL (2004) Regulation of the TSC pathway by LKB1: evidence of a molecular link between tuberous sclerosis complex and Peutz-Jeghers syndrome. Genes Dev 18:1533–1538

Corradetti MN, Inoki K, Guan KL (2005) The stress-inducted proteins RTP801 and RTP801L are negative regulators of the mammalian target of rapamycin pathway. J Biol Chem 280:9769–9772

Cuzick J, Powles T, Veronesi U, Forbes J, Edwards R, Ashley S, Boyle P (2003) Overview of the main outcome in breast-cancer prevention trials. Lancet 361:296–300

Dasgupta B, Yi Y, Chen DY, Weber JD, Gutmann DH (2005) Proteomic analysis reveals hyperactivation of the mammalian target of rapamycin pathway in neurofibromatosis 1-associated human and mouse brain tumors. Cancer Res 65:2755–2760

De Benedetti A, Graff JR (2004) eIF-4E expression and its role in malignancies and metastases. Oncogene 23:3189–3199

deGraffenried LA, Friedrichs WE, Russell DH, Donzis EJ, Middleton AK, Silva JM, Roth RA, Hidalgo M (2004) Inhibition of mTOR activity restores tamoxifen response in breast cancer cells with aberrant Akt activity. Clin Cancer Res 10:8059–8067

Dengler J, von Bubnoff N, Decker T, Peschel C, Duyster J (2005) Combination of imatinib with rapamycin or RAD001 acts synergistically only in Bcr-Abl-positive cells with moderate resistance to imatinib. Leukemia 19:1835–1838

Dennis PB, Jaeschke A, Saitoh M, Fowler B, Kozma SC, Thomas G (2001) Mammalian TOR:a homeostatic ATP sensor. Science 294:1102–1105

Dong J, Pan D (2004) Tsc2 is not a critical target of Akt during normal Drosophila development. Genes Dev 18:2479–2484

Dutcher JP (2004) Mammalian target of rapamycin (mTOR) Inhibitors. Curr Oncol Rep 6:111–115

Early Breast Cancer Trialists' Collaborative Group (EBCTCG) (2005) Effects of chemotherapy and hormonal therapy for early breast cancer on recurrence and 15-year survival:an overview of the randomized trials. Lancet 365:1687–1717

Edinger AL, Thompson CB (2002) Akt maintains cell size and survival by increasing mTOR-dependent nutrient uptake. Mol Biol Cell 13:2276–2288

Edinger AL, Linardic CM, Chiang GG, Thompson CB,Abraham RT (2003) Differential effects of rapamycin on mammalian target of rapamycin signaling functions in mammalian cells. Cancer Res 63:8451–8460,

Eshleman JS, Carlson BL, Mladek AC, Kastner BD, Shide KL, Sarkaria JN (2002) Inhibition of the mammalian target of rapamycin sensitizes U87 xenografts to fractionated radiation therapy. Cancer Res 62:7291–7297

Feng Z, Zhang H, Levine AJ, Jin S (2005) The coordinate regulation of the p53 and mTOR pathways in cells. Proc Natl Acad Sci USA 102:8204–8209

Fingar DC, Salama S, Tsou C, Harlow E, Blenis J (2002) Mammalian cell size is controlled by mTOR and its downstream targets S6K1 and 4EBP1/eIF4E. Genes Dev 16:1472–1487

Fingar DC, Richardson CJ, Tee AR, Cheatham L, Tsou C, Blenis J (2004) mTOR controls cell cycle progression through its cell growth effectors S6K1 and 4E-BP1/eukaryotic translation initiation factor 4E. Mol Cell Biol 24:200–216

Franz DN, Leonard J, Tudor C, Chuck G, Care M, Sethuraman G, Dinopoulos A, Thomas G, Crone KR (2006) Rapamycin causes regression of astrocytomas in tuberous sclerosis complex Ann Neurol 59:490–498

Galanis E, Buckner JC, Maurer MJ, Kreisberg JI, Ballman K, Boni J, Peralba JM, Jenkins RB, Dakhil SR, Morton RF, Jaeckle KA, Scheithauer BW, Dancey J, Hidalgo M, Walsh DJ (2005) Phase II trial of temsirolimus (CCI-779) in recurrent glioblastoma multiforme:a North Central Cancer Treatment Group Study. J Clin Oncol 23:5294–5304

Gangloff YG, Mueller M, Dann SG, Svoboda P, Sticker M, Spetz JF, Um SH, Brown EJ, Cereghini S, Thomas G, Kozma SC (2004) Disruption of the mouse mTOR gene leads to early postimplantation lethality and prohibits embryonic stem cell development. Mol Cell Biol 24:9508–9516

Gao X, Zhang Y, Arrazola P, Hino O, Kobayashi T, Yeung RS, Ru B, Pan D (2002) Tsc tumour suppressor proteins antagonize amino-acid-TOR signalling. Nat Cell Biol 4:699–704

Garami A, Zwartkruis FJ, Nobukuni T, Joaquin M, Roccio M, Stocker H, Kozma SC, Hafen E, Bos JL, Thomas G (2003) Insulin activation of Rheb, a mediator of mTOR/S6K/4E-BP signaling, is inhibited by TSC1 and 2. Mol Cell 11:1457–1466

Gera JF, Mellinghoff IK, Shi Y, Rettig MB, Tran C, Hsu JH, Sawyers CL, Lichtenstein AK (2004) AKT activity determines sensitivity to mammalian target of rapamycin (mTOR) inhibitors by regulating cyclin D1 and c-myc expression. J Biol Chem 279:2737–2746

Gingras AC, Gygi SP, Raught B, Polakiewicz RD, Abraham RT, Hoekstra MF, Aebersold R, Sonenberg N (1999) Regulation of 4E-BP1 phosphorylation:a novel two-step mechanism. Genes Dev 13:1422–1437,

Gingras AC, Raught B, Sonenberg N (2001) Regulation of translation initiation by FRAP/mTOR. Genes Dev 15:807–826

Goss PE (2003a) Emerging role of aromatase inhibitors in the adjuvant setting. Am J Clin Oncol 26:S27–33

Goss PE, Ingle JN, Martino S, Robert NJ, Muss HB, Piccart MJ, Castiglione M, Tu D, Shepherd LE, Pritchard KI, Livingston RB, Davidson NE, Norton L, Perez EA, Abrams JS, Therasse P, Palmer MJ, Pater JL (2003b) A randomized trial of letrozole in postmenopausal women after five years of tamoxifen therapy for early-stage breast cancer. N Engl J Med 349:1793–1802

Goudar RK, Shi Q, Hjelmeland MD, Keir ST, McLendon RE, Wikstrand CJ, Reese ED, Conrad CA, Traxler P, Lane HA, Reardon DA, Cavenee WK, Wang XF, Bigner DD, Friedman HS, Rich JN (2005) Combination therapy of inhibitors of epidermal growth factor receptor/vascular endothelial growth factor receptor 2 (AEE788) and the mammalian target of rapamycin (RAD001) offers improved glioblastoma tumor growth inhibition. Mol Cancer Ther 4:101–112

Grunwald V, DeGraffenried L, Russel D, Friedrichs WE, Ray RB, Hidalgo M (2002) Inhibitors of mTOR reverse doxorubicin resistance conferred by PTEN status in prostate cancer cells. Cancer Res 62:6141–6145,

Guarneri V, Conte PF (2004) The curability of breast cancer and the treatment of advanced disease. Eur J Nucl Med Mol Imaging 31 Suppl 1:S149–S161

Guba M, von Breitenbuch P, Steinbauer M, Koehl G, Flegel S, Hornung M, Bruns CJ, Zuelke C, Farkas S, Anthuber M, Jauch KW, Geissler EK (2002) Rapamycin inhibits primary and metastatic tumor growth by antiangiogenesis:involvement of vascular endothelial growth factor. Nat Med 8:128–135

Guertin DA, Sabatini DM (2005) An expanding role for mTOR in cancer. Trends Mol Med 11:353–361

Hahn-Windgassen A, Nogueira V, Chen CC, Skeen JE, Sonenberg N, Hay N (2005) Akt Activates the mammalian target of rapamycin by regulating cellular ATP level and AMPK Activity. J Biol Chem 280:32081–32089

Hara K, Yonezawa K, Weng QP, Kozlowski MT, Belham C, Avruch J (1998) Amino acid sufficiency and mTOR regulate p70 S6 kinase and eIF-4E BP1 through a common effector mechanism. J Biol Chem 273:14484–14494

Hara K, Maruki Y, Long X, Yoshino K, Oshiro N, Hidayat S, Tokunaga C, Avruch J, Yonezawa K (2002) Raptor, a binding partner of target of rapamycin (TOR), mediates TOR action. Cell 110:177–189

Harrington LS, Findlay GM, Gray A, Tolkacheva T, Wigfield S, Rebholz H, Barnett J, Leslie NR, Cheng S, Shepherd PR, Gout I, Downes CP, Lamb RF (2004) The TSC1–2 tumor suppressor controls insulin-PI3K signaling via regulation of IRS proteins. J Cell Biol 166:213–223

Hawley SA, Boudeau J, Reid JL, Mustard KJ, Udd L, Makela TP, Alessi DR, Hardie DG (2003) Complexes between the LKB1 tumor suppressor, STRAD alpha/beta and MO25 alpha/beta are upstream kinases in the AMP-activated protein kinase cascade. J Biol 2:28

Hay N, Sonenberg N (2004) Upstream and downstream of mTOR. Genes Dev 18:1926–1945

Hay N (2005) The Akt-mTOR tango and its relevance to cancer. Cancer Cell 8:179–183

Hennessy BT, Smith DL, Ram PT, Lu Y, Mills GB (2006) Exploiting the PI3K/Akt pathway for cancer drug discovery. Nat Rev Drug Discovery 4:988–1004

Hidalgo M, Rowinsky EK (2000) The rapamycin-sensitive signal transduction pathway as a target for cancer therapy. Oncogene 19:6680–6686

Holz MK, Blenis J (2005) Identification of S6 kinase 1 as a novel mammalian target of rapamycin (mTOR)-phosphorylating kinase. J Biol Chem 280:26089–26093

Horman S, Browne G, Krause U, Patel J, Vertommen D, Bertrand L, Lavoinne A, Hue L, Proud C, Rider M (2002) Activation of AMP-activated protein kinase leads to the phosphorylation of elongation factor 2 and an inhibition of protein synthesis. Curr Biol 12:1419–1423

Huang S, Houghton PJ (2003) Targeting mTOR signaling for cancer therapy. Curr Opin Pharmacol 3:371–377

Hynes NE, Lane HA (2005) ERBB receptors and cancer: the complexity of targeted inhibitors. Nat Rev Cancer 5:341–354

Inoki K, Li Y, Zhu T, Wu J, Guan KL (2002) TSC2 is phosphorylated and inhibited by Akt and suppresses mTOR signalling. Nat Cell Biol 4:648–657

Inoki K, Zhu T, Guan KL (2003) TSC2 mediates cellular energy response to control cell growth and survival. Cell 115:577–590

Inoki K, Corradetti MN, Guan KL (2005) Dysregulation of the TSC-mTOR pathway in human disease. Nat Genet 37:19–24

Jacinto E, Loewith R, Schmidt A, Lin S, Ruegg MA, Hall A, Hall MN (2004) Mammalian TOR complex 2 controls the actin cytoskeleton and is rapamycin insensitive. Nat Cell Biol 6:1122–1128

Janicke F (2004) Are all aromatase inhibitors the same? A review of the current evidence. Breast 13 Suppl 1: S10–S18

Jefferies HB, Fumagalli S, Dennis PB, Reinhard C, Pearson RB, Thomas G (1997) Rapamycin suppresses 5'TOP mRNA translation through inhibition in p70s6k. EMBO J 16:3693–3704

Johannessen CM, Reczek EE, James MF, Brems H, Legius E, Cichowski K (2005) The NF1 tumor suppressor critically regulates TSC2 and mTOR. Proc Natl Acad Sci USA 102:8573–8578

Johnston SR (2005) Combinations of endocrine and biological agents:present status of therapeutic and presurgical investigations. Clin Cancer Res 11:889s–899s

Kanazawa T, Taneike I, Akaishi R, Yoshizawa F, Furuya N, Fujimura S, Kadowaki M (2004) Amino acids and insulin control autophagic proteolysis through different signaling pathways in relation to mTOR in isolated rat hepatocytes. J Biol Chem 279:8452–8459

Kenerson HL, Aicher LD, True LD, Yeung RS (2002) Activated mammalian target of rapamycin pathway in the pathogenesis of tuberous sclerosis complex renal tumors. Cancer Res 62:5645–5650

Kim DH, Sarbassov DD, Ali SM, King JE, Latek RR, Erdjument-Bromage H, Tempst P, Sabatini DM (2002) mTOR interacts with raptor to form a nutrient-sensitive complex that signals to the cell growth machinery. Cell 110:163–175

Kim DH, Sarbassov DD, Ali SM, Latek RR, Guntur KV, Erdjument-Bromage H, Tempst P, Sabatini DM (2003) GbetaL, a positive regulator of the rapamycin-sensitive pathway required for the nutrient-sensitive interaction between raptor and mTOR. Mol Cell 11:895–904

Kimura N, Tokunaga C, Dalal S, Richardson C, Yoshino K, Hara K, Kemp BE, Witters LA, Mimura O, Yonezawa K (2003) A possible linkage between AMP-activated protein kinase (AMPK) and mammalian target of rapamycin (mTOR) signalling pathway. Genes Cells 8:65–79

Kondo Y, Kanzawa T, Sawaya R, Kondo S (2005) The role of autophagy in cancer development and response to therapy. Nat Rev Cancer 5:726–734

Krause U, Bertrand L, Hue L (2002) Control of p70 ribosomal protein S6 kinase and acetyl-CoA carboxylase by AMP-activated protein kinase and protein phosphatases in isolated hepatocytes. Eur J Biochem 269:3751–3759

Lane HA, Schnell A, Theuer T, O'Reilly T, Wood J (2002) Antiangiogenic activity of RAD001, an orally active anticancer agent. Proc Am Assoc Cancer Res 43:922

Lane HA, Boulay A, Hattenberger M, Maira SM, Thomas G, Merlo A, O'Reilly T (2003a) The orally active rapamycin derivative RAD001 has potential as an antitumor agent with a broad antiproliferative activity: PTEN as a molecular determinant of response. Proc Am Assoc Cancer Res 44:314

Lane HA, Tanaka C, Kovarik J, O'Reilly T, Zumstein-Mecker S, McMahon LM, Cohen P, O'Donnell A, Judson I, Raymond E (2003b) Preclinical and clinical pharmacokinetic/pharmacodynamic (PK/PD) modeling to help define an optimal biological dose for the oral mTOR inhibitor, RAD001, in oncology. Proc Am Soc Clin Oncol 22:237

Li Y, Inoki K, Guan KL (2004) Biochemical and functional characterizations of small GTPase Rheb and TSC2 GAP activity. Mol Cell Biol 24:7965–7975

Liu L, Cash TP, Jones RG, Keith B, Thompson CB, Simon MC (2006) Hypoxia-induced energy stress regulates mRNA translation and cell growth. Mol Cell 21:521–531

Loewith R, Jacinto E, Wullschleger S, Lorberg A, Crespo JL, Bonenfant D, Oppliger W, Jenoe P, Hall MN (2002) Two TOR complexes, only one of which is rapamycin sensitive, have distinct roles in cell growth control. Mol Cell 10:457–468

Long X, Lin Y, Ortiz-Vega S, Yonezawa K, Avruch J (2005a) Rheb binds and regulates the mTOR kinase. Curr Biol 15:702–713

Long X, Ortiz-Vega S, Lin Y, Avruch J (2005b) Rheb binding to mammalian target of rapamycin (mTOR) is regulated by amino acid sufficiency. J Biol Chem 280:23433–23436

Lum JJ, DeBerardinis RJ, Thompson CB (2005) Autophagy in metazoans:cell survival in the land of plenty. Nat Rev Mol Cell Biol 6:439–448

Ma L, Chen Z, Erdjument-Bromage H, Tempst P, Pandolfi PP (2005a) Phosphorylation and functional inactivation of TSC2 by Erk implications for tuberous sclerosis and cancer pathogenesis. Cell 121:179–193,

Ma L, Teruya-Feldstein J, Behrendt N, Chen Z, Noda T, Hino O, Cordon-Cardo C, Pandolfi PP (2005b) Genetic analysis of Pten and Tsc2 functional interactions in the mouse reveals asymmetrical haploinsufficiency in tumor suppression. Genes Dev 19:1779–1786

Mach KE, Furge KA, Albright CF (2000) Loss of Rhb1, a Rheb-related GTPase in fission yeast, causes growth arrest with a terminal phenotype similar to that caused by nitrogen starvation. Genetics 155:611–622,

Majumder PK, Febbo PG, Bikoff R, Berger R, Xue Q, McMahon LM, Manola J, Brugarolas J, McDonnell TJ, Golub TR, Loda M, Lane HA, Sellers WR (2004) mTOR inhibition reverses Akt-dependent prostate intraepithelial neoplasia through regulation of apoptotic and HIF-1-dependent pathways. Nat Med 10:594–601

Manning BD, Cantley LC (2003) Rheb fills a GAP between TSC and TOR. Trends Biochem Sci 28:573–576

Manning BD (2004) Balancing Akt with S6K:implications for both metabolic diseases and tumorigenesis. J Cell Biol 167:399–403

Manning BD, Logsdon MN, Lipovsky AI, Abbott D, Kwiatkowski DJ, Cantley LC (2005) Feedback inhibition of Akt signaling limits the growth of tumors lacking Tsc2. Genes Dev 19:1773–1778

Marx SO, Jayaraman T, Go LO, Marks AR (1995) Rapamycin-FKBP inhibits cell cycle regulators of proliferation in vascular smooth muscle cells. Circ Res 76:412–417

Mohi MG, Boulton C, Gu TL, Sternberg DW, Neuberg D, Griffin JD, Gilliland DG, Neel BG (2004) Combination of rapamycin and protein tyrosine kinase (PTK) inhibitors for the treatment of leukemias caused by oncogenic PTKs. Proc Natl Acad Sci USA 101:3130–3135

Mondesire WH, Jian W, Zhang H, Ensor J, Hung MC, Mills GB, Meric-Bernstam F (2004) Targeting mammalian target of rapamycin synergistically enhances chemotherapy-induced cytotoxicity in breast cancer cells. Clin Cancer Res 10:7031–7042

Mordier S, Deval C, Bechet D, Tassa A, Ferrara M (2000) Leucine limitation induces autophagy and activation of lysosome-dependent proteolysis in C2C12 myotubes through a mammalian target of rapamycin-independent signaling pathway. J Biol Chem 275:29900–29906

Mothe-Satney I, Brunn GJ, McMahon LP, Capaldo CT, Abraham RT, Lawrence JC Jr (2000) Mammalian target of rapamycin-dependent phosphorylation of PHAS-I in four (S/T)P sites detected by phospho-specific antibodies. J Biol Chem 275:33836–33843

Murakami M, Ichisaka T, Maeda M, Oshiro N, Hara K, Edenhofer F, Kiyama H, Yonezawa K, Yamanaka S (2004) mTOR is essential for growth and proliferation in early mouse embryos and embryonic stem cells. Mol Cell Biol 24:6710–6718

Nave BT, Ouwens M, Withers DJ, Alessi DR, Shepherd PR (1999) Mammalian target of rapamycin is a direct target for protein kinase B:identification of a convergence point for opposing effects of insulin and amino-acid deficiency on protein translation. Biochem J 344 Pt 2:427–431

Neshat MS, Mellinghoff IK, Tran C, Stiles B, Thomas G, Petersen R, Frost P, Gibbons JJ, Wu H, Sawyers CL (2001) Enhanced sensitivity of PTEN-deficient tumors to inhibition of FRAP/mTOR. Proc Natl Acad Sci USA 98:10314–10319

Ng Grace, Huang J (2005) The significance of autophagy in cancer. Mol Carcinogenesis 43:183–187

Nobukuni T, Joaquin M, Roccio M, Dann SG, Kim SY, Gulati P, Byfield MP, Backer JM, Natt F, Bos JL, Zwartkruis FJ, Thomas G (2005) Amino acids mediate mTOR/raptor signaling through activation of class 3 phosphatidylinositol 3OH-kinase. Proc Natl Acad Sci USA

Noh WC, Mondesire WH, Peng J, Jian W, Zhang H, Dong J, Mills GB, Hung MC, Meric-Bernstam F (2004) Determinants of rapamycin sensitivity in breast cancer cells. Clin Cancer Res 10:1013–1023

O'Donnell A, Faivre S, Judson I, Delbado C, Brock C, Lane HA, Shand N, Hazell K, Armand JP, Raymond E (2003) A phase I study of the oral mTOR inhibitor RAD001 as monotherapy to identify the optimal biologically effective dose using toxicity, pharmacokinetic (PK) and pharmacodynamic (PD) endpoints in patients with solid tumors. Proc Am Soc Clin Oncol 22:200

Ohanna M, Sobering AK, Lapointe T, Lorenzo L, Praud C, Petroulakis E, Sonenberg N, Kelly PA, Sotiropoulos A, Pende M (2005) Atrophy of S6K1(-/-) skeletal muscle cells reveals distinct mTOR effectors for cell cycle and size control. Nat Cell Biol 7:286–294

O'Reilly T, Vaxelaire J, Muller M (2002) In vivo activity of RAD001, an orally active rapamycin derivative, in experimental tumor models. Proc Am Asso Cancer Res 43:71

O'Reilly T, Muller M, Hattenberger M, Vaxelaire J, Lane HA (2003) Antitumor activity of RAD001 in combination with cytotoxic agents. Proc Am Assoc Cancer Res 44:136

O'Reilly T, Wood J, Littlewood-Ewans A, Boulay A, Schnell C, Sini P, Maira MS, Martiny-Baron G, Lane HA (2005) Differential anti-vascular effects of mTOR or VEGFR pathway inhibition: A rational basis for combining RAD001 and PTK787/ZK222584. Proc Am Assoc Cancer Res 46:715

O'Reilly KE, Rojo F, She QB, Solit D, Mills GB, Smith D, Lane HA, Hofmann F, Hicklin DJ, Ludwig DL, Baselga J, Rosen N (2006) mTOR inhibition induces upstream receptor tyrosine kinase signaling and activates Akt. Cancer Res 66:1500–1508

Pang H, Faber LE (2001) Estrogen and rapamycin effects on cell cycle progression in T47D breast cancer cells. Breast Cancer Res Treat 70:21–26

Pende M, Um SH, Mieulet V, Sticker M, Goss VL, Mestan J, Mueller M, Fumagalli S, Kozma SC, Thomas G (2004) S6K1(-/-)/S6K2(-/-) mice exhibit perinatal lethality and rapamycin-sensitive 5'-terminal oligopyrimidine mRNA translation and reveal a mitogen-activated protein kinase-dependent S6 kinase pathway. Mol Cell Biol 24:3112–3124

Peng T, Golub TR, Sabatini DM (2002) The immunosuppressant rapamycin mimics a starvation-like signal distinct from amino acid and glucose deprivation. Mol Cell Biol 22:5575–5584

Peng XD, Xu PZ, Chen ML, Hahn-Windgassen A, Skeen J, Jacobs J, Sundararajan D, Chen WS, Crawford SE, Coleman KG, Hay N (2003) Dwarfism, impaired skin development, skeletal muscle atrophy, delayed bone development, and impeded adipogenesis in mice lacking Akt1 and Akt2. Genes Dev 17:1352–1365

Perez-Tenorio G, Stal O (2002) Activation of AKT/PKB in breast cancer predicts a worse outcome among endocrine treated patients. Br J Cancer 86:540–545

Podsypanina K, Lee RT, Politis C, Hennessy I, Crane A, Puc J, Neshat M, Wang H, Yang L, Gibbons J, Frost P, Dreisbach V, Blenis J, Gaciong Z, Fisher P, Sawyers C, Hedrick-Ellenson L, Parsons R (2001) An inhibitor of mTOR reduces neoplasia and normalizes p70/S6 kinase activity in Pten+/- mice. Proc Natl Acad Sci USA 98:10320–10325

Proud CG (2004) The multifaceted role of mTOR in cellular stress responses. DNA Repair (Amst) 3:927–934

Reiling JH, Hafen E (2004) The hypoxia-induced paralogs Scylla and Charybdis inhibit growth by down-regulating S6K activity upstream of TSC in Drosophila. Genes Dev 18:2879–2892

Roccio M, Bos JL, Zwartkruis FJ (2005) Regulation of the small GTPase Rheb by amino acids. Oncogene 25:657–664

Rojo F, Iglesias C, Tabernerro J, Jimenez J, Rodriguez S, Bellmunt J, Ramon S, Baselga J (2004) Molecular markers of the mTOR pathway activation in human tumors:a baseline analysis. Proc Am Soc Clin Oncol 22:14S

Rose C, Vtoraya O, Pluzanska A, Davidson N, Gershanovich M, Thomas R, Johnson S, Caicedo JJ, Gervasio H, Manikhas G, Ben Ayed F, Burdette-Radoux S, Chaudri-Ross HA, Lang R (2003) An open randomised trial of second-line endocrine therapy in advanced breast cancer. comparison of the aromatase inhibitors letrozole and anastrozole. Eur J Cancer 39:2318–2327

Rousseau D, Gingras AC, Pause A, Sonenberg N (1996) The eIF4E-binding proteins 1 and 2 are negative regulators of cell growth. Oncogene 13:2415–2420

Roux PP, Ballif BA, Anjum R, Gygi SP, Blenis J (2004) Tumor-promoting phorbol esters and activated Ras inactivate the tuberous sclerosis tumor suppressor complex via p90 ribosomal S6 kinase. Proc Natl Acad Sci USA 101:13489–13494

Ruvinsky I, Sharon N, Lerer T, Cohen H, Stolovich-Rain M, Nir T, Dor Y, Zisman P, Meyuhas O (2005) Ribosomal protein S6 phosphorylation is a determinant of cell size and glucose homeostasis. Genes Dev 19:2199–2211

Samuels Y, Ericson K (2006) Oncogenic PI3K and its role in cancer. Curr Opin Onc 18:77–82

Sarbassov DD, Ali SM, Kim DH, Guertin DA, Latek RR, Erdjument-Bromage H, Tempst P, Sabatini DM (2004) Rictor, a novel binding partner of mTOR, defines a rapamycin-insensitive and raptor-independent pathway that regulates the cytoskeleton. Curr Biol 14:1296–1302

Sarbassov DD, Guertin DA, Ali SM, Sabatini DM (2005) Phosphorylation and regulation of Akt/PKB by the rictor-mTOR complex. Science 307:1098–1101

Sarbassov DD, Ali SM, Sengupta S, Sheen JH, Hsu PP, Bagley AF, Markhard AL, Sabatini DM (2006) Prolonged rapamycin treatment inhibits mTORC2 assembly and Akt/PKB. Mol Cell 22:159–168

Schalm SS, Blenis J (2002) Identification of a conserved motif required for mTOR signaling. Curr Biol 12:632–639

Schalm SS, Fingar DC, Sabatini DM, Blenis J (2003) TOS motif-mediated raptor binding regulates 4E-BP1 multisite phosphorylation and function. Curr Biol 13:797–806

Scheper GC, Proud CG (2002) Does phosphorylation of the cap-dependent protein eIF4E play a role in translation initiation. Eur J Biochem 269:5350–5359

Schmelzle T, Hall MN (2000) TOR, a central controller of cell growth. Cell 103:253–262

Schwarzer R, Tondera D, Arnold W, Giese K, Klippel A, Kaufmann J (2005) REDD1 integrates hypoxia-mediated survival signaling downstream of phosphatidylinositol 3-kinase. Oncogene 24:1138–1149

Scott PH, Brunn GJ, Kohn AD, Roth RA, Lawrence JC, Jr. (1998) Evidence of insulin-stimulated phosphorylation and activation of the mammalian target of rapamycin mediated by a protein kinase B signaling pathway. Proc Natl Acad Sci USA 95:7772–7777

Sekulic A, Hudson CC, Homme JL, Yin P, Otterness DM, Karnitz LM, Abraham RT (2000) A direct linkage between the phosphoinositide 3-kinase-AKT signaling pathway and the mammalian target of rapamycin in mitogen-stimulated and transformed cells. Cancer Res 60:3504–3513

Shah OJ, Wang Z, Hunter T (2004) Inappropriate activation of the TSC/Rheb/mTOR/S6K cassette induces IRS1/2 depletion, insulin resistance, and cell survival deficiencies. Curr Biol 14:1650–1656

Shamji AF, Nghiem P, Schreiber SL (2003) Integration of growth factor and nutrient signaling:implications for cancer biology. Mol Cell 12:271–280

Shaw RJ, Bardeesy N, Manning BD, Lopez L, Kosmatka M, DePinho RA, Cantley LC (2004) The LKB1 tumor suppressor negatively regulates mTOR signaling. Cancer Cell 6:91–99

Shi Y, Frankel A, Radvanyi LG, Penn LZ, Miller RG, Mills GB (1995) Rapamycin enhances apoptosis and increases sensitivity to cisplatin in vitro. Cancer Res 55:1982–1988

Shi Y, Gera J, Hu L, Hsu JH, Bookstein R, Li W, Lichtenstein A (2002) Enhanced sensitivity of multiple myeloma cells containing PTEN mutations to CCI-779. Cancer Res 62:5027–5034

Shima H, Pende M, Chen Y, Fumagalli S, Thomas G, Kozma SC (1998) Disruption of the p70(s6k)/p85(s6k) gene reveals a small mouse phenotype and a new functional S6 kinase. EMBO J 17:6649–6659

Shinohara ET, Cao C, Niermann K, Mu Y, Zeng F, Hallahan DE, Lu B (2005) Enhanced radiation damage of tumor vasculature by mTOR inhibitors. Oncogene 24:5414–5422

Smith EM, Finn SG, Tee AR, Browne GJ, Proud CG (2005) The tuberous sclerosis protein TSC2 is not required for the regulation of the mammalian target of rapamycin by amino acids and certain cellular stresses. J Biol Chem 280:18717–18727

Smith IE (2004) Aromatase inhibitors in early breast cancer therapy. Semin Oncol 31:9–14

Sofer A, Lei K, Johannessen CM, Ellisen LW (2005) Regulation of mTOR and cell growth in response to energy stress by REDD1. Mol Cell Biol 25:5834–5845

Stocker H, Radimerski T, Schindelholz B, Wittwer F, Belawat P, Daram P, Breuer S, Thomas G, Hafen E (2003) Rheb is an essential regulator of S6K in controlling cell growth in Drosophila. Nat Cell Biol 5:559–565

Sun SY, Rosenberg LM, Wang X, Zhou Z, Yue P, Fu H, Khuri FR (2005) Activation of Akt and eIF4E survival pathways by rapamycin-mediated mammalian target of rapamycin inhibition. Cancer Res 65:7052–7058

Tabernero J, Rojo F, Burris E, Casado E, Macarulla T, Jones S, Dimitrijevic S, Hazell K, Shand N, Baselga J (2005) A phase I study with tumor molecular pharmacodynamic (MPD) evaluation of dose and schedule of the oral mTOR-inhibitor Everolimus (RAD001) in patients (pts) with advanced solid tumors. Proc Am Soc Clin Oncol Abstract 3007

Takeuchi H, Kondo Y, Fujiwara K, Kanzawa T, Aoki H, Mills GB, Kondo S (2005) Synergistic augmentation of rapamycin-induced autophagy in malignant glioma cells by phosphatidylinositol 3-kinase/protein kinase B inhibitors. Cancer Res 65:3336–3346

Tang H, Hornstein E, Stolovich M, Levy G, Livingstone M, Templeton D, Avruch J, Meyuhas O (2001) Amino acid-induced translation of TOP mRNAs is fully dependent on phosphatidylinositol 3-kinase-mediated signaling, is partially inhibited by rapamycin, and is independent of S6K1 and rpS6 phosphorylation. Mol Cell Biol 21:8671–8683

Tee AR, Anjum R, Blenis J (2003a) Inactivation of the tuberous sclerosis complex-1 and –2 gene products

occurs by phosphoinositide 3-kinase/Akt-dependent and -independent phosphorylation of tuberin. J Biol Chem 278:37288–37296

Tee AR, Manning BD, Roux PP, Cantley LC, Blenis J (2003b) Tuberous sclerosis complex gene products, Tuberin and Hamartin, control mTOR signaling by acting as a GTPase-activating protein complex toward Rheb. Curr Biol 13:1259–1268

Thomas GV, Tran C, Mellinghoff IK, Welsbie DS, Chan E, Fueger B, Czernin J, Sawyers CL (2006) Hypoxia-inducible factor determines sensitivity to inhibitors of mTOR in kidney cancer. Nat Med 12:122–127

Thurlimann B, Keshaviah A, Coates AS, Mouridsen H, Mauriac L, Forbes JF, Paridaens R, Castiglione-Gertsch M, Gelber RD, Rabaglio M, Smith I, Wardley A, Price KN, Goldhirsch A, Breast International Group (BIG) 1–98 Collaborative Group (2005) A comparison of letrozole and tamoxifen in postmenopausal women with early breast cancer. N Engl J Med 353:2747–2757

Um SH, Frigerio F, Watanabe M, Picard F, Joaquin M, Sticker M, Fumagalli S, Allegrini PR, Kozma SC, Auwerx J, Thomas G (2004) Absence of S6K1 protects against age- and diet-induced obesity while enhancing insulin sensitivity. Nature 431:200–205

Veronesi U, Boyle P, Goldhirsch A, Orecchia R, Viale G (2005) Breast cancer. Lancet 365:1727–41

Vignot S, Faivre S, Aguirre D, Raymond E (2005) mTOR-targeted therapy of cancer with rapamycin derivatives. Ann Oncol 16:525–537

Vivanco I, Sawyers CL (2002) The phosphatidylinositol 3-Kinase AKT pathway in human cancer. Nat Rev Cancer 2:489–501

Weiss RH (2003) p21Waf1/Cip1 as a therapeutic target in breast and other cancers. Cancer Cell 4:425–429

Wendel HG, De Stanchina E, Fridman JS, Malina A, Ray S, Kogan S, Cordon-Cardo C, Pelletier J, Lowe SW (2004) Survival signalling by Akt and eIF4E in oncogenesis and cancer therapy. Nature 428:332–337

Woods A, Johnstone SR, Dickerson K, Leiper FC, Fryer LG, Neumann D, Schlattner U, Wallimann T, Carlson M, Carling D (2003) LKB1 is the upstream kinase in the AMP-activated protein kinase cascade. Curr Biol 13:2004–2008

Wu L, Birle DC, Tannock IF (2005) Effects of the mammalian target of rapamycin inhibitor CCI-779 used alone or with chemotherapy on human prostate cancer cells and xenografts. Cancer Res 65:2825–2831

Wullschleger S, Loewith R, Oppliger W, Hall MN (2005) Molecular organization of target of rapamycin complex 2. J Biol Chem 280:30697–30704

Xu G, Zhang W, Bertram P, Zheng XF, McLeod H (2004) Pharmacogenomic profiling of the PI3K/PTEN-AKT-mTOR pathway in common human tumors. Int J Oncol 24:893–900

Yu K, Toral-Barza L, Discafani C, Zhang WG, Skotnicki J, Frost P, Gibbons JJ (2001) mTOR, a novel target in breast cancer:the effect of CCI-779, an mTOR inhibitor, in preclinical models of breast cancer. Endocr Relat Cancer 8:249–258

Yue W, Wang JP, Conaway MR, Li Y, Santen RJ (2003) Adaptive hypersensitivity following long-term estrogen deprivation:involvement of multiple signal pathways. J Steroid Biochem Mol Biol 86:265–274

Zhang H, Cicchetti G, Onda H, Koon HB, Asrican K, Bajraszewski N, Vazquez F, Carpenter CL, Kwiatkowski DJ (2003a) Loss of Tsc1/Tsc2 activates mTOR and disrupts PI3K-Akt signaling through downregulation of PDGFR. J Clin Invest 112:1223–1233

Zhang Y, Gao X, Saucedo LJ, Ru B, Edgar BA, Pan D (2003b) Rheb is a direct target of the tuberous sclerosis tumour suppressor proteins. Nat Cell Biol 5:578–581

The Ras Signalling Pathway as a Target in Cancer Therapy

Kathryn Graham and Michael F. Olson

Recent Results in Cancer Research, Vol. 172
© Springer-Verlag Berlin Heidelberg 2007

8.1 Introduction

The Ras GTPase proteins and their downstream effectors regulate specific intracellular signalling pathways involved in numerous biological processes. Their actions directly influence progression through the cell cycle and the delicate balance of pro- and anti-apoptotic factors. The variety of functions controlled by Ras, and the emerging evidence indicating that aberrations in Ras as well as at multiple points in downstream signalling pathways contribute to tumourigenesis, suggest that Ras signal transduction mechanisms have significant potential as anti-cancer therapeutic targets.

A number of novel therapies based on the concept of targeting Ras signalling pathways are in various stages of pre-clinical and clinical development. The introduction of the first 'anti-Ras' agents, the farnesyl transferase inhibitors (FTIs), which were proposed to interrupt the crucial post-translational modification of Ras, led to much anticipation of their potential therapeutic benefits, but their overall performance in clinical trials has failed to live up to these high expectations. This has prompted a re-evaluation of their utility in cancer management, and where they have had some efficacy their mode of action as Ras inhibitors remains hotly debated.

The advent of antisense oligonucleotide therapies and small-molecule inhibitors has resulted in the production of several agents directed against Ras or specific pathway components. The efficacy of these agents in model systems, as well as the increasing knowledge of the contribution made by various Ras effectors to the incidence and progression of cancer, has encouraged the development of further novel therapies.

Here we will discuss the significance of Ras signal transduction in the neoplastic process, highlighting the proteins which have been targeted for drug development and the effectiveness of these novel targeted therapies in clinical trials. The potential of inhibiting post-translational modification by alternative means will also be explored. Finally we will suggest future aims and directions for cancer therapies that target Ras function.

8.2 Structure and Function of Ras GTPases

8.2.1 Ras Biology

The Ras genes encode four highly homologous 21-kDa proteins: H-Ras, N-Ras, K-Ras4A and K-Ras4B (mRNA splice variants from a single K-Ras gene with K-Ras4B being the ubiquitously expressed form). These proteins alternate between an active GTP-bound state and an inactive GDP-bound state (Fig. 8.1). This cycling process permits Ras proteins to act as molecular switches. The activation/deactiva-

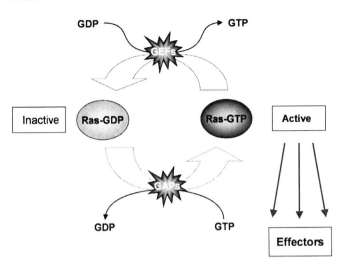

Fig. 8.1 Activation/inactivation of Ras GTPases. Ras GTPases are small-molecular-weight guanine nucleotide binding proteins which are inactive when associated with GDP and active when bound to GTP. This molecular switch mechanism is regulated by the opposing forces of guanine nucleotide exchange factors (GEFs), which catalyse the exchange of GDP for GTP, and GTPase activating proteins (GAPs), which promote hydrolysis of GTP to GDP. Active GTP-loaded Ras interacts with and/or activates numerous downstream signalling effectors

tion mechanism is regulated by two classes of proteins: guanine nucleotide exchange factors (GEFs) and GTPase activating proteins (GAPs). A trigger from an upstream signal (e.g. ligand stimulation of a receptor tyrosine kinase) promotes GEFs to catalyse the exchange of GDP for GTP, thereby activating Ras. To extinguish the resultant activated state, GAPs drive the hydrolysis of GTP to GDP and the Ras protein returns to its quiescent state. Mutations to specific codons (12, 13 or 61) result in decreased GTP hydrolysis (Sprang 1997). As a consequence, mutated Ras proteins remain constitutively in the active GTP-bound state, resulting in sustained signalling via downstream effector pathways, which ultimately is the key contributory factor in Ras-related oncogenesis.

8.2.2 Post-translational Modification

Newly synthesized Ras protein is a cytosolic precursor which must undergo a series of enzymatic reactions in order to fulfil its biological functions (Fig. 8.2). This process of post-translational modification consists of prenylation, proteolysis and carboxymethylation, the end result of which is the localisation of Ras to appropriate lipid membranes. Proper and complete post-translational modification is important not only for normal signal transduction but also for malignant transformation (Jackson et al. 1990; Kato et al. 1992). Prenylation of Ras proteins (more specifically farnesylation or geranylgeranylation) is a primary and essential component of post-translational modification. This involves the covalent attachment of a 15-carbon farnesyl, or a 20-carbon geranylgeranyl isoprenoid, catalysed by the protein farnesyl transferase (FTase) or geranylgeranyl transferase I (GGTase I) enzymes, respectively. The lipid molecules are incorporated into Ras proteins at a specific sequence motif situated at the C-terminus, typically referred to as the CAAX box, where C represents cysteine, A are aliphatic amino acids and X is usually methionine, serine, glutamine or leucine. Prenylation is thought to increase the hydrophobicity of the target protein, thereby anchoring it in the appropriate subcellular position. However, it is also likely that the prenylation reactions have a wider range of functions, in addition to the modification of Ras proteins, which are not yet fully characterised.

The geranylgeranylation reaction can be catalysed by an additional enzyme, geranylgeranyl transferase type II (GGTase II). GGTase II is not linked specifically to Ras, but instead has a role in the modification of Rab GTPases, a group of Ras-related proteins involved in the regulation of vesicular transport (Farnsworth et al. 1994). Only a small percentage of cellular proteins are isoprenylated, the majority of which undergo geranylgeranylation. However,

H-, N- and K-Ras proteins are preferred substrates for FTase rather than GGTase I, although K-Ras and N-Ras may also be modified by GGTase I in the context of FTase inhibition (Whyte et al. 1997).

After prenylation, the three terminal amino acids are removed by the Rce1 (ras converting enzyme) endopeptidase, an integral membrane protein resident in the endoplasmic reticulum. The final modification common to all forms of Ras is carboxymethylation (Clark et al. 1997), in which the remaining isoprenylated cysteine residue is methylated by the enzyme isoprenylcysteine carboxyl methyltransferase (ICMT). H-Ras, N-Ras and K-Ras4A are subject to a further palmitoylation modification in the carboxyl-terminal region of the protein (Hancock et al. 1989). K-Ras4B is thought not to require this additional lipid modification for proper membrane association because of the presence of a stretch of six basic lysine amino acids proximal to the CAAX box (McCoy et al. 1984).

8.2.3 Ras Signal Transduction Pathways

The Ras GTPases are centrally situated in an extensive and complex signalling network, which is further complicated by multiple mechanisms of cross talk and feedback regulation. The pathways downstream of Ras which

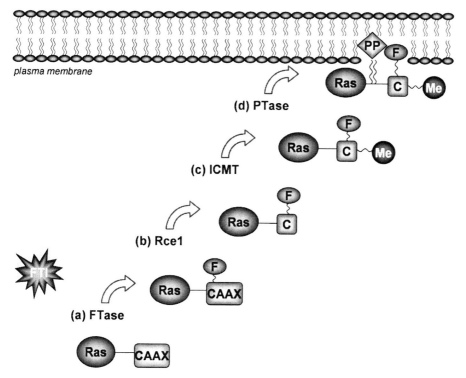

Fig. 8.2 Post-translational modifications of Ras proteins. (*a*) A 15-carbon farnesyl group is incorporated into the CAAX box at the cysteine residue by the enzyme farnesyl transferase (FTase). (*b*) The three terminal amino acids are removed by endoproteolytic digestion catalysed by ras converting enzyme 1 (Rce1). (*c*) The cysteine residue is methylated by isoprenylcysteine carboxyl methyltransferase (ICMT). (*d*) H-Ras, N-Ras and K-Ras 4A undergo a further modification, catalysed by palmitoyltransferase (PTase), which facilitates localisation to the inner surface of the plasma membrane. K-Ras 4B is anchored to the membrane by a different mechanism. The only agents in clinical development designed to interrupt Ras post-translational modification are the farnesyl transferase inhibitors (FTIs); however, their anti-cancer effects may be achieved through the inhibition of non-Ras protein farnesylation

have been subject to most research, and which therefore represent the most well-developed pharmaceutical targets, are Raf, PI3K and, to a lesser extent, RalGDS. However, this list is not comprehensive, and it may be the case that additional Ras effectors will eventually prove also to be effective targets for anti-cancer therapies. A simplified outline of the main Ras-regulated signal transduction pathways is illustrated in Fig. 8.3.

8.2.3.1 Raf/MAP Kinase Pathway

The A-Raf, B-Raf and C-Raf (also known as Raf-1) serine/threonine kinases are the most extensively studied Ras effector molecules. Although they display extensive sequence homology, especially within their kinase domains, each has a distinct pattern of tissue distribution and has been found to play subtly different roles in intracellular signalling and

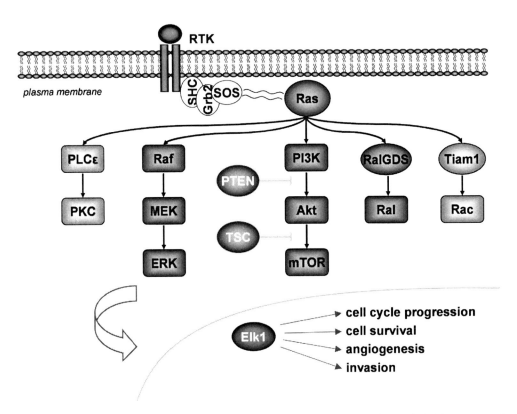

Fig. 8.3 Ras signal transduction pathway. The stimulation of a receptor tyrosine kinase (RTK) by an extracellular ligand results in the assembly of multi-molecular complexes (e.g., SHC, Grb2, SOS) that interact with Ras at the plasma membrane, thereby promoting the exchange of GDP for GTP. Activated Ras then participates in a cascade of signalling events, the most notable pathway being Raf/MEK/ERK. The end product of ERK activation is the phosphorylation of cytoplasmic and nuclear targets, such as the Elk1 transcription factor, which regulates transcription of genes involved in crucial cellular processes including cell cycle progression, survival, angiogenesis and invasion. Activation of PI3K leads to activation of Akt and mTOR, which play critical roles in the control of apoptosis and protein synthesis. Downstream of PI3K, the tumour suppressor genes PTEN and TSC also contribute to the regulation of Akt and mTOR. RalGDS is a guanine nucleotide exchange factor (GEF) for Ral, which has roles in regulating gene transcription and vesicle transport. Similarly, Tiam1 is a GEF that activates Rac, leading to changes in the architecture of the actin cytoskeleton, which is critically important in the processes of tumour cell invasion and metastasis. Phospholipase C (PLC) mediates cross talk between small GTPase signalling pathways and activates protein kinase C (PKC), which has numerous effects on tumour cells including stimulation of proliferation

embryonic development. Raf is activated by association of GTP-loaded Ras to the Ras-binding domain (RBD), accompanied by a series of phosphorylations; the sum total of these events is a conformational change permissive for catalytic activity. B-Raf has a higher relative level of constitutive kinase activity due to the presence of negatively charged glutamic acid residues, which are tyrosines at homologous positions in A-Raf and C-Raf that require phosphorylation for full activation (Mason et al. 1999). As a result, B-Raf is a more potent activator of downstream effectors and is more readily activated by single hit mutations than are A-Raf or C-Raf. Although initial research efforts focussed largely on C-Raf, because of the biological properties of B-Raf and the dramatically higher incidence of tumour-associated B-Raf mutations than either A-Raf or C-Raf, B-Raf has recently become the centre of attention.

The principal function of activated Raf is phosphorylation of the mitogen-activated protein (MAP) kinase kinases MEK1 and MEK2, which are dual-specificity kinases which phosphorylate the MAP kinases ERK1 and ERK2 on threonine and tyrosine residues within their activation loops, resulting in profound stimulation of catalytic activity. On activation, the ERK MAP kinases phosphorylate both cytoplasmic and nuclear substrates, including a number of transcription factors such as Elk-1, and promote a transcriptional program which collectively influences diverse biological processes including cell cycle progression and proliferation, cell survival, angiogenesis and invasion, which contribute to the oncogenic process.

8.2.3.2 PI3K/Akt/mTOR pathway

Phosphoinositide 3-kinases (PI3Ks) are lipid kinases, comprised of catalytic and regulatory subunits, which mediate the phosphorylation of phosphatidylinositol (Ptdlns) on the third carbon of the inositol ring. PI3K actually consists of three different types: Class IA enzymes consist of any p110α, p110β, or p110δ catalytic subunits associated with one p85α, p85β or p55γ regulatory subunits. There is a

single Class IB PI3K that is comprised of p110γ catalytic and p101 regulatory subunits. There are also three Class II PI3Ks (CIIα, CIIβ, and CIIγ) and one Class III PI3K. Each of these three classes of PI3K enzymes is normally activated by distinct upstream mechanisms. One way that activation may be achieved is through the association of Ras-GTP with the catalytic subunit, which stimulates the generation of 3-phosphorylated Ptdlns second messengers. Elevated levels of 3-phosphorylated Ptdlns have been associated with a number of biological phenomena which contribute to the malignant phenotype, such as suppression of apoptosis, increased angiogenesis and cell motility (Vivanco and Sawyers 2002). The actions of PI3K are normally countered by the tumour suppressor PTEN (phosphatase and tensin homologue), a lipid phosphatase which de-phosphorylates phosphorylated Ptdlns second messengers. Acting downstream of PI3K is the protein kinase Akt (also known as protein kinase B or PKB), which is an important regulator of apoptosis and cell growth (Altomare and Testa 2005). One of the critical targets of Akt is mTOR (mammalian target of rapamycin), which plays a significant role in regulation of protein synthesis by influencing the activity of the p70 and p85 S6 ribosomal protein kinases (p70S6K and p85S6K). Activity of these two kinases are also influenced by the tuberous sclerosis complex (TSC), which is comprised of TSC1 (also known as hamartin) and TSC2 (tuberin), and which acts as a GAP for the GTP-binding protein Rheb. The activity of S6K is regulated by Rheb through its binding to mTor, which facilitates activation of the mTOR kinase function. In the absence of TSC function, Rheb-GTP levels rise, leading to increased mTOR and consequently S6K activity.

8.2.3.3 RalGDS

Ral proteins comprise a distinct family of Ras-related GTPases (Chardin and Tavitian 1986). They are controlled by a specific set of guanine nucleotide exchange factors (RalGEFs) that promote GDP/GTP exchange, including the Ral-GDP dissociation stimulator (RalGDS).

Ral GTPases have been implicated in the regulation of vesicle trafficking, cell morphology and transcription, processes which may directly or indirectly contribute to the development and progression of cancer (Feig 2003).

8.3 Oncogenic Associations of the Aberrant Ras Signal Tranduction Pathway

8.3.1 Ras

Since the identification of Ras as a proto-oncogene over 20 years ago, Ras mutations have been implicated in a wide spectrum of human malignancies. A recent COSMIC (Catalogue of Somatic Mutations in Cancer) update indicates that approximately 1/3 of all human cancers are associated with Ras mutations (K-Ras=22.1%, N-Ras=7.6%, H-Ras=3.8%; www.sanger.ac.uk/genetics/CGP/cosmic/). K-Ras mutations are most frequently observed and typically encountered in adenocarcinomas, particularly of the pancreas (90%), lower gastrointestinal tract (50%) and lung (30%) (Bos 1989). N-Ras mutations are commonly associated with thyroid malignancy of follicular derivation. In addition, they are also the most common Ras mutation in haematological malignancies, with a frequency of up to 70% in certain types of leukaemia (Reuter et al. 2000). H-Ras mutations occur least frequently, and are most often linked to tumours of the urothelial tract. It is currently debated whether specific Ras mutations influence prognostic outcome. The results from retrospective studies have largely proved inconclusive. Despite a recent meta-analysis performed on lung cancer which suggests a connection between K-Ras mutation and unfavourable outcome (Mascaux et al. 2005), a similar review of colorectal malignancy was more equivocal (Anwar et al. 2004).

The most commonly observed mutations are located at codons 12, 13 and 61 (Bos 1989), which appear to be critical sites for GTP hydrolysis-mediated Ras regulation (Sprang 1997), and when mutated lead to uncontrolled activity. However, GTPase function may also be compromised by the loss of a Ras GAP, such as the tumour suppressor NF1 (neurofibrin) (Martin et al. 1990; Xu et al. 1990a, 1990b), although this is relatively uncommon. The hereditary clinical syndrome associated with NF1, neurofibromatosis, is characterised by multiple benign peripheral nerve sheath tumours. There is, however, a risk of malignant transformation and predisposition for myeloid leukaemias. The underlying abnormality in Ras regulation is postulated to contribute to tumour development and the possibility of employing an anti-Ras strategy in this condition has been suggested.

8.3.2 Raf/MAP Kinase Pathway

Although it came to be generally accepted that Ras-mediated oncogenesis required the simultaneous input of several downstream signalling pathways, it was only recently discovered that activating B-Raf mutations are associated with human cancer, with an overall incidence of approximately 7% (Davies et al. 2002). B-Raf and Ras mutations tend to occur in a similar range of tumour types, although concomitant mutations are rare (Davies et al. 2002; Rajagopalan et al. 2002; Singer et al. 2003). These findings suggested that the Raf/MEK/ERK pathway is the principal mechanism mediating Ras-induced oncogenesis in particular cancers. The highest frequency of B-Raf mutation was noted in malignant melanoma (60%–70%), followed by papillary thyroid cancer (35%–50%), serous epithelial ovarian cancer (30%) and colorectal cancer (5%–20%). A lower mutation frequency has been reported in a variety of other tumour types including breast, renal, sarcoma, hepatobiliary tract and haematological malignancies.

Over 40 B-Raf mutations have been identified; most are rare, with the exception of the V600E mutant (a single T to A substitution at nucleotide position 1799 in exon 15 resulting in the conversion of valine 600 to glutamate) which accounts for 80% of the total (Davies et al. 2002). B-Raf mutations are predominantly localised within the kinase domain and generally result in the generation of constitutively active mutant proteins. The evidence supporting oncogenic activity of B-Raf include its ability to transform cultured murine fibroblasts and constitutively stimulate ERK activity independent of Ras (Davies et al. 2002; Wan et al. 2004). The exact timing of B-Raf alterations in the oncogenic process is unclear. Some evidence exists indicating that gain-of-function mutations may be an early occurrence, for example, the observation that B-Raf aberrations can be detected in a large proportion of benign naevi (up to 80%) (Pollock et al. 2003). Yet, these lesions rarely progress to invasive melanoma (Zaal et al. 2004). From this information, it can be inferred that B-Raf activation may be an early promotional event that is insufficient to induce tumours alone, consistent with a multi-step model of carcinogenesis. Recent data show that B-Raf V600E can induce a senescence-like cell cycle arrest of human naevi, suggesting that additional steps are required to overcome this limit and allow for progression to unrestricted neoplastic growth (Michaloglou et al. 2005).

C-Raf mutations have been documented (Emuss et al. 2005) but appear to be very rare and subsequently information is limited. One current model suggests that B-Raf is rate-limiting and that the function of C-Raf is to amplify B-Raf signalling from the context of B-Raf/C-Raf heterodimers, which may account for the lack of activating C-Raf mutations in association with human cancer. To date, no A-Raf mutations have been reported in the context of malignancy.

8.3.3 PI3K/Akt/mTOR Pathway

Accumulating evidence exists which supports the role of the PI3K/Akt/mTOR pathway in oncogenesis. A recent screening survey demonstrated mutations in the PI3K catalytic subunit in breast, lung, colorectal and brain tumours (Samuels et al. 2004), with more than three-quarters of the mutations located within two cluster regions, the helical and kinase domains. Functional assays of one of the predominant kinase mutations (H1047R) revealed elevated lipid kinase activity (Samuels et al. 2004). In addition, expression of H1047R in mammary

epithelial cells induced phenotypic manifestations characteristic of malignancy (Isakoff et al. 2005). Amplification and/or overexpression of PI3K and Akt have also been documented in a range of tumours, particularly breast, ovarian and endometrial cancers (Bellacosa et al. 1995; Micci et al. 2004; Shayesteh et al. 1999). The presence of elevated Akt protein levels in breast cancer is intriguing given that gene amplification is unusual. This phenomenon may instead result from the amplification, overexpression and increased signalling activity of growth factor receptors such as HER2/neu. The possible contribution of Akt overexpression to malignancy has been addressed in studies which demonstrated transforming ability in murine fibroblasts (Cheng et al. 1997; Sun et al. 2001) and tumour-inducing capabilities in nude mice (Sun et al. 2001). In addition, the Akt2 isoform has been linked to increased invasive and metastatic properties of human breast and ovarian cancer cells in vitro (Arboleda et al. 2003).

The most compelling evidence for the involvement of the PI3K pathway in cancer, however, has arisen from work based on the tumour suppressor PTEN. Knockout mouse models have demonstrated a strong cancer phenotype in heterozygous animals (Podsypanina et al. 1999; Stambolic et al. 2000). In the human setting, germline mutations in PTEN produce familial syndromes such as Cowden's disease, which is associated with a heightened risk of breast, thyroid and endometrial cancers (Eng 2003). More importantly, inactivation of this gene, acquired through a variety of genetic and epigenetic mechanisms, has been associated with up to 40% of sporadic human tumours, making PTEN the second most commonly affected tumour suppressor after p53. Its function is most frequently altered in endometrial cancer and glioblastoma multiforme, and to a lesser degree in a range of solid tumours including pancreatic, prostatic and renal carcinomas (Sansal and Sellars 2004). Germline mutations in the TSC genes have also been identified and are responsible for the clinical syndrome of tuberous sclerosis, characterised by multiple organ hamartomas. Although this results in a less aggressive cancer phenotype than PTEN loss, there is evidence that these patients are at a slightly increased risk of malignancy, including renal cell carcinoma (Mak and Yeung 2004). The resultant constitutive activation of Akt and/or mTOR resulting from disruption of these important tumour suppressors and their influence over critical cellular functions highlights the significance of this signal transduction pathway in oncogenesis. The frequency of mutations in this pathway, especially PTEN inactivation, has led to speculation about potential prognostic implications. The data are conflicting and do not reach any significant conclusions, possibly because patient numbers tend to be small in individual studies, and because the results are in direct opposition in the two most common PTEN-related malignancies, endometrial cancer and glioblastoma multiforme (Risinger et al. 1998; Smith et al. 2001).

8.4 Therapies

A wide variety of agents directed against Ras and its downstream signalling components have reached clinical development, as shown in Table 8.1. The first group of compounds to enter the clinic were the farnesyl transferase inhibitors, which target the enzymatic post-translational modification of Ras. Although they appeared to be safe and well-tolerated for the most part, their efficacy in solid tumours was insufficient to merit monotherapy. In addition, where therapeutic benefit has been noted, the precise mode of action remains unclear. A more specific means of inactivating Ras proteins may be achieved by downregulating protein expression. This can be accomplished with specific antisense oligonucleotides, but again efficacy appears to be suboptimal, particularly as a single agent. Raf has also been targeted by antisense oligonucleotides, but the principal method for inhibition of the Raf/MAPK pathway has been achieved by the development of protein kinase inhibitors against Raf or MEK.

Table 8.1 Anti-Ras signalling agents in clinical development

Farnesyl transferase inhibitors	R115777 (tipafarnib)	Phase III
	SCH66336 (lonafarnib)	Phase III
	BMS-214662	Phase II
	L778123[a]	Phase I
Ras antisense inhibitors	ISIS 2503	Phase I
Raf antisense inhibitors	ISIS 5132	Phase II
	LErafAON	Phase I
Raf kinase inhibitors	BAY-439006 (sorafenib)	Phase III
MEK kinase inhibitors	CI-1040	Phase II
	PD-325901	Phase II
	ARRY-142886	Phase I
Alkylphospho-cholines	Miltefosine[a]	Phase I
	Perifosine	Phase II
mTOR inhibitors	CCI-779	Phase III
	RAD001	Phase II
	AP23573	Phase II
Hsp90 inhibitors	17-AAG	Phase I
	17-DMAG	Phase I

[a] Denotes agents which have been withdrawn because of concerns over demonstrated or potential toxicity

In order to target the PI3K signalling cascade, natural and synthetic fungal derivative inhibitors have been developed, but have yet to reach clinical testing, compromised by problems with chemical stability and toxicity. As a result, efforts have concentrated primarily on derivatives of the antibiotic rapamycin, which inhibit mTOR and to a lesser extent on a novel class of alkylphosphocholines that inhibit Akt. One type of inhibitor known to have multiple targets within the Raf and PI3K pathways, in addition to upstream growth factor receptors, are Hsp90 inhibitors. In the sections below, we will discuss the progress in the development of these inhibitors towards clinical deployment.

8.4.1 Inhibition of Post-translational Prenylation

As post-translational modifications of Ras proteins are necessary for biological activity, each individual enzyme in the process is a potential target for the development of anti-cancer drugs. Only agents targeting the first reaction in the process, prenylation, have reached clinical phases of testing. The fact that Ras proteins are typically modified by farnesylation, rather than geranylgeranylation, concentrated early efforts on the farnesyl transferase enzyme, leading to identification and development of farnesyl transferase inhibitors (FTIs), which could be termed the first 'anti-Ras' agents. Several FTIs demonstrated notable in vitro and in vivo efficacy, and progressed to phase I–III clinical trials in solid and haematological malignancies. However, the results from these trials were disappointing for the most part. The realisation that K-Ras and N-Ras, the most commonly occurring Ras mutants, could be geranylgeranylated in the context of farnesyl transferase inhibition (Whyte et al. 1997) made blocking geranylgeranyl transferase type I, either alone or in combination with the farnesyl transferase inhibition, an additional goal for drug development.

8.4.1.1 Farnesyl Transferase Inhibitors

This class of enzyme inhibitor can be categorized as:

- CAAX-peptidomimetics which compete with the protein CAAX motif for binding to farnesyl transferase
- Analogues of farnesyl pyrophosphate which compete with the prenyl substrate for binding to farnesyl transferase
- Bi-substrate inhibitors which combine the properties of the above

A number of specific inhibitors have been developed in each of these categories, and subjected to rigorous testing in pre-clinical studies. In the laboratory setting, FTIs revealed the ability to inhibit growth of a wide range of human tumour cell lines, as well as in xenograft and transgenic models (Appels et al. 2005). The anti-tumour outcome has been linked with pleiotropic effects on apoptosis, angiogenesis and the cell cycle.

Following the encouraging results with FTIs in laboratory experimentation, there were high expectations for their potential efficacy in combating human cancer. Several agents advanced to clinical trials, including; R115777 (Tipafarnib), SCH66336 (Lonafarnib), BMS-214662 and L778123. Phase I dose escalation studies revealed that these agents were generally well tolerated with a toxicity profile consisting of gastrointestinal upset, mild to moderate myelosuppression, fatigue and peripheral sensory neuropathy. The major exception to this occurred during infusional therapy with L778123, which can result in a prolonged QT interval, thereby inducing a potential risk of life-threatening ventricular dysrhythmia. As a result, this agent has been withdrawn from further studies. Of the two most studied inhibitors, notable side effects were myelosuppression for R115777 and gastrointestinal upset for SCH66336. Major toxicity was also absent in murine models. This is perhaps surprising, given that farnesylation is not restricted to Ras proteins. A wide variety of proteins with CAAX sequences which can potentially be farnesylated have been identified. Some studies applied this knowledge to identify pharmacodynamic markers, such as the chaperone protein HDJ-2, in order to assess FTI-related biological activity.

The results from early phase studies were somewhat unexpected in that FTIs failed to demonstrate significant efficacy in a range of solid tumours (Sebti and Adjei 2004) but did evoke response rates of 10%–30% in a mixture of rather unexpected malignancies, including breast cancer (Johnston et al. 2003), glioblastoma multiforme (Cloughesy et al. 2005) and haematological malignancies (Cortes 2003; Karp et al. 2001; Kurzrock et al. 2003). The most striking aspect of these results is that breast and brain tumours infrequently possess mutant Ras, thereby calling to question the underlying mechanism of action leading to disease response. Recent evidence implies that farnesylated proteins other than Ras may be responsible for the therapeutic effects of FTIs. Genetic deletion of the FT catalytic β-subunit in mice did not effect tumour initiation in two Ras-dependent models but did have a limited but significant effect on restricting tumour progression (Mijimolle et al. 2005). However, the ability of active H-Ras to associate with cellular membranes was not affected by the absence of FT activity, possibly because palmitoyl residues attached to cysteines in positions 181 and 184 were sufficient for this subcellular localisation. These data are consistent with the proposal that alternative targets are responsible for the anti-tumour effects of FTIs; possible candidates include Rheb (Clark et al. 1997), RhoB (Du et al. 1999; Lebowitz et al. 1997; Liu et al. 2000), PTP-CAAX (Zeng et al. 2000, 2003) and CENP-E and F (Ashar et al. 2000; Hussein and Taylor 2002). However, direct experimental evidence of the role of each of these proteins in FTI action is not fully conclusive.

Two phase III studies have been published employing R115777 in advanced colorectal (Rao et al. 2004) and pancreatic (Van Cutsem et al. 2004) malignancies, the latter in combination with the cytotoxic pyrimidine analogue gemcitabine. Both trials reported an acceptable toxicity profile, even in combination with cytotoxic chemotherapy (Van Cutsem et al. 2004) but there was no statistically significant increase in progression-free or overall survival.

Combination of Farnesyl Transferase Inhibitors with Conventional Therapies

Chemotherapy. Although the results from initial phase III studies were disappointing, a number of questions were raised regarding the optimal use of FTIs. Firstly, the study by Van Cutsem et al. illustrated that FTIs can be safely combined with other forms of conventional therapy (Van Cutsem et al. 2004). Secondly, tumour grade and stage may be significant factors as FTIs are predominantly cytostatic rather than cytotoxic. A major criticism of studies to date is that they have been performed in patients with advanced refractory disease and were assessed using standard criteria that may not have been applicable. Combination therapy may still prove to be an efficacious application of FTIs in the correct clinical context. FTIs have displayed synergistic effects in vitro with a variety of cytotoxic agents (Sun et al. 1999) and have been safely administered with a variety of chemotherapeutic agents in early phase trials including anthracyclines, topoisomerase inhibitors, antimetabolites, platinum derivatives and taxanes. The combination of FTIs and taxanes is of particular interest as the mitotic block caused by taxane-induced microtubule disruption may be enhanced by FTIs (Moasser et al. 1998). The molecular mechanism of the synergistic action is unknown but recent work has shown the ability of SCH66336 to increase microtubule stabilization and acetylation and suppress microtubule dynamics, proposing a link between farnesyl transferase and tubulin acetylation (Marcus et al. 2005).

Radiotherapy. It is well documented that the efficacy of radiotherapy can be increased by the co-administration of cytotoxic chemotherapeutic agents, and the same relationship may also apply to more selective targeted agents. As a result, potential synergy between ionizing radiation and FTIs has been investigated. This possibility is supported by work indicating that activating Ras mutations induce relative radioresistance (Bernhard et al. 2000; Ling and Endlich 1989; McKenna et al. 1990a, 1990b; Samid et al. 1991) (although this does not seem to be a feature which can be generalized to all cell lines and tumour types) and the reversal of this phenomenon by FTIs in vitro (Bernhard et al. 1996, 1998) and in vivo (Cohen-Jonathan et al. 2000). Just as FTIs have demonstrated anti-tumour activity in cancer cell lines without Ras mutations (End et al. 2001), wild-type Ras cell lines may exhibit increased radiosensitivity when treated with FTIs (Cohen-Jonathan et al. 1999; Delmas et al. 2002). However, these findings have not been completely replicated (Bernhard et al. 1998). Mechanisms other than Ras inhibition may explain the apparent radiosensitising properties of FTIs, for instance cell cycle redistribution (Morgan et al. 2001). These results could, therefore, have important clinical implications regarding the potential treatment of many tumour types, and suggest that therapy need not be restricted to tumours with activated Ras mutations.

Two dose escalation studies combining external beam radiotherapy with infusional FTI administration have been reported; one study included head and neck cancer and advanced inoperable non-small-cell lung cancer (Hahn et al. 2002), while the other study was restricted to pancreatic carcinoma (Martin et al. 2004). There were several partial and complete responses reported, and the dual modality approach was reasonably well tolerated with no significant increase in radiation-related toxicity. However, the FTI utilised in each case was L778123 and these studies were terminated early when this drug was withdrawn. Therefore, a number of questions remain unanswered, including; the most appropriate agent to combine with radiation, the optimal dose to achieve maximum potency and the tumour types most likely to respond.

Current Studies. Monotherapy with FTI is unlikely to be an efficacious treatment option, with the exception of certain groups of haematological malignancy. Their value in cancer treatment is therefore contentious, and the future of these agents relies on their performance in combination with either conventional forms of cancer management or newer molecular therapies. A number of studies are currently under way employing FTIs and various cytotoxic compounds in locally advanced and metastatic breast cancer, glioma and acute myeloid leukaemia. In addition, the effectiveness of FTIs in conjunction with external beam radiotherapy continues to be examined; there are several phase I and II studies recruiting patients with glioblastoma, pancreatic carcinoma and non-small-cell lung cancer. There are also ongoing trials combining FTIs with first- or second-line hormonal therapy in locally advanced and metastatic breast cancer, due to evidence of an additive effect with tamoxifen in vitro (Ellis et al. 2003). Similarly, a synergistic effect of FTIs with the c-kit tyrosine kinase inhibitor Imatinib has been reported (Brodsky et al. 2003; Nakajima et al. 2003). As a result, combination therapy of R115777 with Imatinib in chronic myeloid leukaemia is being explored. An overview of current combination studies is provided in Table 8.2.

Table 8.2 Current combination studies employing farnesyl transferase inhibitors (R115777 or SCH66336)

Cytotoxic chemotherapy		
Alkylating agents	I/II	Glioblastoma
Antimetabolites	I/II	Breast
Taxanes	I/II	Breast
Topoisomerase inhibitors	I	AML advanced solid tumours
Endocrine therapy		
Aromatase inhibitors	II	Breast
Anti-oestrogen	II	Breast
Targeted therapy		
Trastuzumab	I	Breast
Sorafenib	I	Advanced solid tumours
Bortezomib	I/II	Myeloma
Imatinib	I	CML
Ionising radiation		
External beam radiotherapy	I	Pancreas/lung/ glioblastoma

8.4.1.2 Geranylgeranyl Transferase Type I Inhibitors

The dramatic effects of FTIs observed in early experimental systems were predominantly based on H-Ras-induced cancer model systems (Kohl et al. 1993), which may explain the relative lack of efficacy in human studies where K-Ras or N-Ras is more commonly mutated. The realisation that N-Ras and K-Ras are modified by geranylgeranylation in the presence of FTIs (Whyte et al. 1997) generated interest in developing GGTase I inhibitors to overcome the apparent FTI resistance of the two most common Ras mutations. Several compounds have been developed with evident effects in in vitro and in vivo model systems (Sebti and Hamilton 2000). However, none has yet advanced to clinical trials because of adverse factors including dose-limiting toxicity in pre-clinical animal models (Lobell et al. 2001). Given that N-Ras and K-Ras may be either farnesylated or geranylgeranylated, an alternative approach has been to develop compounds that target both

FTase and GGTase I enzymes. Combination FTase and GGTase I inhibitors effectively block K-Ras isoprenylation and have synergistic actions in vitro, principally increased induction of apoptosis (Lobell et al. 2001). However, dual prenyltransferase inhibition was poorly tolerated and resulted in lethality in mice. Of note, L778123 exhibits dual FTase and GGTase I inhibitory activity, and was withdrawn because of toxicity as previously discussed. Therefore, it may prove to be impossible that agents with the required level of potency for inhibiting both enzymes could be developed without producing unacceptable levels of toxicity.

8.4.2 Inhibition of Ras Protein Expression

An alternative approach to inhibiting Ras signalling has been to design antisense oligonucleotides to reduce the protein levels of Ras or the downstream effector Raf. This form of targeted approach makes use of short synthetic nucleotide strands which act by hybridizing with mRNA transcripts corresponding to the gene of interest, leading to reduced protein levels through inhibition of translation and/or mRNA destabilisation. The concept of antisense interference as a therapeutic strategy has been forwarded for a considerable period, but the development of effective antisense therapeutic agents has been fraught with difficulties, specific problems being inefficient delivery and rapid degradation. One way that these complications have at least been partially surmounted is through the use of stable phosphorothioate bases. As a result, there are now a large number of antisense oligonucleotides directed against genes involved in tumour cell survival and proliferation, including Ras and Raf.

ISIS 2503 is a 20-mer phosphorothioate antisense oligonucleotide which targets the translation initiation site of H-Ras mRNA. It was shown to specifically reduce the expression of H-Ras mRNA and protein in vitro (Chen et al. 1996; Monia et al. 1992) and inhibited the growth of human tumour xenografts (Holmlund et al. 1999). Despite concerns that

the inhibition of H-Ras might lead to detrimental effects on normal tissue, overt toxicity was minimal, and therefore this did not present a barrier for progression into clinical studies.

Phase I trials in solid tumours using prolonged infusional administration regimens revealed that ISIS 2503 was relatively non-toxic in humans, with typical adverse effects consisting of nausea, fatigue and myelosuppression which were not dose limiting (Adjei et al. 2003; Cunningham et al. 2001). Fever was also frequently observed, which appears to be a common class effect from oligonucleotide therapy. ISIS 2503 has been evaluated as a monotherapy in a phase II setting in advanced non-small-cell lung cancer, breast cancer, colorectal cancer and pancreatic carcinoma (Cox and Der 2002), with combination studies under way with taxanes. While there were some cases of disease regression noted in phase I studies, there were no objective responses in the single-agent groups in the phase II studies. The efficacy of ISIS 2503 has also been examined in a combination approach with gemcitabine in pancreatic cancer. A response rate of 10.4% was elicited (Alberts et al. 2004), although the contribution of the oligonucleotide component is difficult to assess. Similar to the shortcomings of FTIs, much of the research with antisense oligonucleotides, including ISIS 2503, has focussed on H-Ras, which is the least frequently mutated isoform. There are K-Ras specific oligonucleotides which have been tested in the laboratory setting, resulting in the inhibition of K-Ras expression and reduced ERK phosphorylation in colon cancer cell lines (Ross et al. 2001), but have yet to progress to clinical development. Therefore, the full potential of the antisense approach to inhibit Ras has yet to be clarified.

8.4.3 Inhibition of Downstream Effectors

8.4.3.1 Raf/MAP Kinase Pathway

In view of the strong evidence indicating a role for the Raf/MAP kinase pathway in tumourigenesis, several different strategies have been advanced to target Raf or its downstream effectors. Pre-clinical efforts are underway with

MCP1, a small-molecule Ras–Raf interaction inhibitor which blocks Raf activation by Ras. In addition, antisense oligonucleotides targeting C-Raf have advanced to phase I testing. However, most efforts to date have focussed on protein kinase inhibitors that target Raf or MEK kinases.

Raf Antisense Inhibitors

ISIS 5132 is a 20-nucleotide phosphorothioate antisense oligonucleotide which targets the 3'-untranslated region of C-Raf mRNA. Clear inhibitory effects consisting of a reduction in synthesis of C-Raf protein in vitro and corresponding diminished tumour growth in lung and breast cancer xenograft models have been reported (Monia et al. 1996a, 1996b). Feasibility studies using continuous or intermittent dosing regimens in humans have been undertaken. Generally, ISIS 5132 was well tolerated and displayed toxicities similar to those previously detected with other unrelated antisense oligonucleotides, although haemolytic anaemia and renal impairment were observed at higher doses (Rudin et al. 2001). Stable disease was reported as the best outcome in phase II studies of patients with breast, ovarian and hormone refractory prostate cancer (Coudert et al. 2001; Cripps et al. 2002; Oza et al. 2003; Tolcher et al. 2002).

To overcome degradation and improve intracellular delivery, a liposomal formulation of a C-Raf antisense oligonucleotide, LErafAON, has been developed. Encapsulation with liposomes is an attractive option as this method has been used successfully to facilitate drug delivery of other anti-cancer agents. The main advantage for antisense oligonucleotides is that this type of formulation can eliminate the requirement for extensive phosphorothioate modification (LErafAON contains only modifications to the 5' and 3' termini), thereby removing a potential source of toxicity. LErafAON has now entered phase I dose finding studies in advanced solid malignancies alone, or in combination with external beam radiotherapy following on from the finding that Raf antisense oligonucleotides can radiosensitise cells in vitro (Gokhale et al. 1999).

The lack of clinically significant responses with ISIS 5132 may result from a fundamental cytostatic effect or insufficient delivery, or it may indicate that targeting C-Raf alone is insufficient. Consistent with this latter possibility, RNAi-mediated knockdown of C-Raf in a melanoma cell line failed to appreciably alter the phosphorylation of the downstream target MEK, although B-Raf RNAi produced significant inhibition (Hingorani et al. 2003). The results of trials involving alternative delivery modes, such as liposomal formulation, are eagerly awaited.

Raf Kinase Inhibitors

The leading Raf kinase inhibitor in clinical development is BAY 43-9006 (Sorafenib), an orally administered bi-aryl urea compound, which was originally identified in high-throughput screening against C-Raf (Lyons et al. 2001). This agent is currently subject to extensive phase II and III clinical testing. It is a competitive inhibitor of ATP binding in the catalytic domains of C-Raf, wild-type B-Raf and the V600E B-Raf mutant. Further biochemical studies revealed that BAY 43-9006 also inhibited a number of receptor tyrosine kinases known to be instrumental in tumourigenesis and angiogenesis, including; VEGFR, PDGFR-β and c-Kit (Wilhelm et al. 2004). This feature may reflect a degree of structural homology between the domains of these kinases in which BAY 43-9006 binds.

In vitro, BAY 43-9006 demonstrated the ability to reduce downstream ERK phosphorylation in a variety of tumour cell lines. Potent anti-tumour activity was observed with in vivo tumour models containing wild-type or mutant B-Raf and/or K-Ras (Wilhelm et al. 2004). Initial studies employing oral administration schedules revealed dose-related toxicities of gastrointestinal upset, hypertension and dermatological manifestations, including palmar-plantar syndrome, which were generally mild to moderate in nature (Hotte and Hirte 2002). Perhaps the most interesting data from the phase II setting have arisen from a large randomised discontinuation study. Five hundred patients with a range of tumour types including melanoma and renal cell carcinoma were entered into this trial and assigned to either BAY 43-9006 or placebo after evidence of disease stability or response following a 12-week introductory period with the drug. The most notable effect was seen in renal cell carcinoma, where 70% of study participants had evidence of disease response or stability at the end of a second 12-week assessment period (Ratain et al. 2005). A subsequent randomised phase III study in renal cancer demonstrated a doubling of progression-free survival from 3 months to 6 months at interim analysis with a trend towards increased survival (Escudier et al. 2005a, 2005b), prompting the Food and Drug Administration to approve sorafenib for use in advanced renal cell carcinoma in the US.

The prevalence of Raf mutations in malignant melanoma (Davies et al. 2002) sparked much hope for Raf kinase inhibitors in combating this particular disease, which is typically resistant to conventional forms of therapy. A limited number of cases of stable disease and partial response were reported in the melanoma cohort, but the striking results seen in renal cell carcinoma were not replicated (Ahmad et al. 2004). One possible explanation for the suboptimal effect of sorafenib as monotherapy in a tumour type with a high frequency of B-Raf mutations is that BAY 43-9006 alone does not sufficiently inhibit B-Raf in vivo. Consistent with this possibility, BAY 43-9006 has been shown to inhibit the activity of B-Raf V600E in vitro, but considerably less effectively than the inhibition of activated C-Raf (Karasarides et al. 2004). In addition, the range of kinases inhibited by BAY 43-9006 suggests that where anti-tumour results have been observed, inhibition of alternative or additional targets may be involved. The fact that the most significant results to date were seen in renal cell carcinoma may result from anti-angiogenic effects of BAY 43-9006. Renal cell carcinomas typically express elevated levels of VEGF (Nicol et al. 1997), commonly due to mutations in the Von-Hippel Lindau (VHL) gene. As a result, novel agents designed to target angiogenesis can exert inhibitory effects on renal cell carcinoma, such as the VEGF monoclonal antibody Bevacizumab, which delayed time to disease progression in a phase III study (Yang et al. 2003). Sorafenib may therefore prove to be useful against tumours which depend on VEGF receptor function for the establishment and maintenance of the tumour vasculature.

BAY 43-9006 continues to be evaluated in malignant melanoma in combination regimens. Phase I/II studies combining sorafenib with cytotoxic chemotherapy, notably carboplatin and paclitaxel (Flaherty et al. 2004), have shown promise, which has paved the way for phase III trials in advanced/metastatic disease. A pivotal phase III trial is also under way in hepatocellular carcinoma, prompted by modest activity in phase I/II studies, with plans for a further single-agent phase III trial in non-small-cell lung cancer. A variety of other solid malignancies are currently undergoing phase I/II studies with sorafenib in combination with cytotoxic agents following encouraging toxicity and pharmacokinetic profiles in pre-clinical models (Wilhelm et al. 2004). An expanded programme of development has also been extended to combination studies with other novel therapeutic agents such as FTIs, interferon-α, VEGF receptor inhibitors or EGF receptor inhibitory monoclonal antibodies.

MEK Kinase Inhibitors

Small-molecule inhibitors of MEK1 and MEK2 (collectively called MEK) have been identified and the first candidate drug to enter clinical trials, CI-1040 (PD184352), is an orally active non-ATP-competitive MEK inhibitor. Anti-tumour effects in preclinical models correlated with reduced ERK phosphorylation in a fashion similar to Raf kinase inhibition (Sebolt-Leopold et al. 1999). The anti-tumour effects of MEK inhibition also appeared to extend to proliferation, differentiation and apoptosis (Ahn et al. 2001). An additional role for the MAPK pathway in angiogenesis has been proposed and recent data indicate that expression of dominant-negative MEK in the tumour vasculature can suppress angiogenesis and tumour growth, suggesting that inhibitors of MEK may act at the level of tumour cells and endothelial cells (Mavria et al. 2006). Phase I studies confirmed the safety of CI-1040, with toxicity generally grade 2 (NCI-CTC). Phase II trials generally resulted in stable disease at best (Rinehart et al. 2004). The lack of robust objective responses by traditional means of assessment, coupled with suboptimal pharmacokinetics (Wallace et al. 2005) has resulted in diminished interest in this particular compound. PD0325901, a second-generation MEK inhibitor with improved pharmacological properties resulting in a longer duration of action and increased potency, has recently entered the clinical arena. ARRY-142886 also demonstrates high MEK selectivity and promising pharmacokinetics and has just commenced phase I testing.

There are currently no specific agents reported which directly inhibit ERK, but since this effector molecule is a critical factor in cell proliferation and survival, it may be a potentially valid target for drug development.

8.4.3.2 PI3K/Akt/mTOR Pathway

Increasing knowledge of aberrant Ras signalling mechanisms, in addition to Raf/MAP kinase, has heightened interest in targeting elements of the PI3K/Akt/mTOR pathway. A number of natural and synthetic compounds capable of inhibiting PI3K and Akt are under investigation, but have largely met with setbacks due to problems with stability, specificity and toxicity. Most success to date has been attained by rapamycin derivatives which inhibit mTOR and which are currently recruiting into phase I–III trials.

PI3K Inhibitors

The most well-known and commonly used PI3K inhibitors in the laboratory setting are wortmannin, a fungal metabolite, and the flavanoid derivative LY294002. Both compounds inhibit PI3K activity by targeting the ATP binding domain of the p110 catalytic subunit, resulting in reduced proliferation of tumour cell lines and growth inhibition in xenograft models (Hu et al. 2000; Schultz et al. 1995). A synergistic effect on the induction of apoptosis was observed in response to the combination of classical PI3K inhibitors with cytotoxic agents

in vitro (West et al. 2002) or with paclitaxel in murine models (Hu et al. 2002). Both wortmannin and LY294002 also potentiate the effect of radiotherapy (Brognard et al. 2001; Sarkaria et al. 1998), raising the possibility of their use in combination with radiation. However, pharmaceutical development has been thwarted by difficulties pertaining to the stability, solubility and toxicity of these compounds. Newer second-generation compounds with more favourable physicochemical properties are being developed, but as yet none of the classical or second-generation inhibitors has progressed beyond preclinical testing. The first-generation compounds are relatively non-specific, which may explain their toxicity profile. Although a clearer view of the significance of the various PI3K isoforms in human disease is emerging, particularly regarding inflammation and the immune response from work using knock-out mouse models, there is currently no evidence that targeted selection is merited in cancer therapy.

Akt Inhibitors

Kinase inhibitors typically act as ATP analogues that block catalytic activity. However, one way that Akt activity has been targeted is with alkylphosphocholines, which are analogues of ether lipids which interact with the cell membrane. Their exact mode of action is unclear, but they do appear to interfere with phosphoinositide metabolism and consequently with the phosphorylation and activation of Akt (Kondapaka et al. 2003). Growth inhibitory activity was observed in an array of human tumour cell lines, including melanoma, lung, prostate, breast and central nervous system tumours and mouse mammary tumours in vivo (Hilgard et al. 1997). One of the earliest compounds, miltefosine, was originally developed as a topical anti-cancer agent. Administration of an orally available form resulted in severe gastrointestinal toxicity (Hilgard et al. 1997), prompting the search for a less toxic analogue which led to the development of perifosine. Parenteral administration with perifosine is contraindicated because of the propensity of these agents to cause haemaolysis via the intravenous route. Similarly, phase I studies revealed a degree of gastrointestinal upset following oral administration (Crul et al. 2002; Van Ummersen et al. 2004), with a suggestion of anti-tumour activity in sarcoma. Various dosing schedules are under review to limit adverse effects, and there are plans for further phase I and phase II studies either alone or in combination with standard cancer therapeutics.

A number of other phosphatidylinositol lipid analogues are in development, but there have been concerns regarding specificity of lipid analogue compounds. Another approach is to design specific small-molecule inhibitors targeted at Akt, a number of which are currently undergoing pre-clinical evaluation, with indications that they can delay the progression of tumours in vivo (Luo et al. 2005). However, Akt is involved in crucial metabolic pathways including transduction of the insulin response. Preliminary studies have illustrated that Akt inhibitors appear to induce a pattern of insulin resistance (Luo et al. 2005), which is in keeping with the hyperinsulinaemic state observed in knockout mouse models (Cho et al. 2001). The potential metabolic upset generated by such agents may prove to be dose limiting and prevent full-scale development.

mTOR Inhibitors

Rapamycin, the prototypical mTOR inhibitor, is a macrocyclic lactone derived from Streptomyces hygroscopicus. Its antiproliferative effect is mediated through the association of rapamycin with the cytoplasmic receptor FK506 binding protein-12 (FKBP12). The resultant inhibition of mTOR prevents phosphorylation of p70S6K and other proteins involved in cell cycle regulation, which leads to arrest in the G1 phase of the cell cycle. Rapamycin's anti-cancer properties were discovered two decades ago during a National Cancer Institute screening programme, but it failed to undergo further evaluation at that time. However, it is approved for use as an immunosuppressant, and because of its proven safety record in animal models and in human organ transplantation, interest in its anti-cancer actions

resurfaced. Subsequent studies revealed the ability to induce apoptosis in certain human cancer cell lines including melanoma (Busca et al. 1996) and tumour growth inhibition and anti-angiogenic effects in in vivo mouse models (Humar et al. 2002).

Rapamycin is poorly soluble in water and is relatively unstable in solution; therefore, it is a poor candidate for parenteral administration. These unfavourable properties led to the synthesis of several ester analogues with improved pharmacological characteristics which demonstrated similar efficacy in vitro. Of these analogues, CCI-779 (temsirolimus) has undergone extensive phase II testing, RAD001 (everolimus) has also reached phase I/II trials and more recently studies of AP23573 have started recruiting in the clinical setting.

CCI-779 results in significant growth inhibition in vitro and delayed tumour growth in vivo (Dudkin et al. 2001; Frost et al. 2004; Geoerger et al. 2001). Anti-tumour activity was observed in renal, breast and to a lesser extent in lung, neuroendocrine, sarcoma and gynaecological cancers in phase I monotherapy trials. Pre-treated renal and breast cancer patients were then selected for phase II studies. Typical toxicity consisted of myelosuppression (predominantly thrombocytopenia at higher doses), mucositis, asthenia and dermatological reactions. Metabolic upset has been reported, notably hyperglycaemia and hypertriglyceridaemia. Interestingly, psychological disturbance including bipolar disorder has also been documented as has pneumonitis, which was a feature in original organ transplantation studies. An overall response rate of 9.2% was reported for breast cancer (Chan et al. 2005) and 7% for renal carcinoma (Atkins et al. 2004). The potential of CCI-779 to synergise with interferon-α has been clinically investigated in advanced renal cancer and was reasonably well tolerated (Smith et al. 2004), prompting the initiation of phase III investigation. Combination treatment is also under way in other solid and haematological malignancies with a variety of small-molecule inhibitors. The prospect of combination with chemotherapy is appealing, particularly as the PI3K/Akt/mTOR pathway is critical in cell survival, but attempts so far combining with anti-metabolites have met with considerable toxicity (Punt et al. 2003).

RAD001 is an orally bioavailable derivative of rapamycin currently under investigation in phase I/II trials. Originally an immuno-suppressant approved for use in solid organ transplantations, extensive safety data exist indicating that it can induce hypercholester-olemia, hypertriglyceridemia and reduced tes-tosterone following prolonged treatment. Early toxicity reported for RAD001 from cancer tri-als includes mucositis, elevated serum lipid levels and mild myelosuppression. It is cur-rently being evaluated in refractory haemato-logical malignancies, as well as a range of solid tumours including breast, prostate and endo-metrial cancers, of which the latter display a high frequency of PTEN mutations. AP23573 is the latest rapamycin analogue to undergo ex-panded clinical development and patients are currently being enrolled into urological and gynaecological cancer studies with early indi-cations that oral mucositis is the dose-limiting toxicity.

8.4.4 Multi-targeted Ras Inhibitors

The complicated nature of Ras signal transduc-tion pathways may be favourable in presenting numerous options for developing novel thera-peutics, but the potential input from cross talk and alternate signalling mechanisms, many of which are not yet fully recognised or under-stood, may lead to substantially reduced ef-ficacy. One way of combating this particular problem might be to employ therapeutic agents with a broad range of targets. The multi-tar-geted nature of sorafenib has sparked much interest in its true mechanism of action in pa-tients. In fact, many of the more efficacious molecular therapies exhibit multiple targets of potential action. It may be possible, and in-deed desirable, to exploit other agents which have multiple targets to simultaneously inhibit several components of the Ras signal transduc-tion pathway, or other pathways in addition to Ras, in order to maximise clinical benefit. Heat shock proteins, which act as molecular chaperones for a variety of essential proteins,

can be inhibited by derivatives of the antibi-otic geldanamycin. The resultant inhibition of both Raf/MAPK pathway and PI3K/Akt/mTOR pathway components may prove to be more effective for cancer treatment.

8.4.4.1 Hsp90 Inhibitors

Heat shock protein 90 (Hsp90) is a member of the ubiquitous molecular chaperone super-family which promote proper protein folding, function and stability. Unlike many other Hsp family members, which are involved in general maintenance, Hsp90 interacts with a specific set of gene products, including several known to be mutated or overexpressed in cancer, such as Her2, Raf and Akt (Whitesell and Lindquist 2005). These client proteins form stable com-plexes with Hsp90, which supports their struc-tural integrity. Inhibition of Hsp90 leads to the degradation of the client protein in a protea-some-dependent fashion. Overexpression of heat shock proteins is a common feature of human malignancy (Whitesell and Lindquist 2005) and the clinical significance of this has been demonstrated in breast cancer, where overexpression of Hsp90 correlated with ad-verse outcome (Yano et al. 1996).

The anti-tumour effect of geldanamycin and related benzoquinone antibiotics was found to act through inhibition of Hsp90 by attaching to the N-terminal ATP-binding site (Whitesell et al. 1994). Exposure to Hsp90 inhibitors such as the ansamycin derivative 17-AAG (17-allyl-amino,17-demethoxygeldanamycin) results in depletion of Akt (Basso et al. 2002), B-Raf (da Rocha Dias et al. 2005), including the V600E B-Raf mutant (Grbovic et al. 2006), and C-Raf (Basso et al. 2002; Beliakoff et al. 2003; Schulte et al. 1996; Solit et al. 2002), highlighting its potential use as a multi-targeted anti-Ras sig-nalling agent. 17-AAG has been studied in sev-eral phase I trials with a cytostatic effect noted (Neckers and Ivy 2003). Phase II studies are un-der way in a variety of solid tumours, includ-ing; breast, thyroid and melanoma, in addition to renal cancers associated with von Hippel-Lindau disease. The molecular hallmark of this rare inherited disorder is inactivation of VHL leading to the accumulation of hypoxia-inducible factors (HIF) which promote increased expression of several genes, including VEGF and PDGF. The subunit of HIF-1 is known to interact with Hsp90 and is therefore the main target of 17-AAG in this particular scenario. Because of poor solubility and extensive hepatic metabolism via the cytochrome P450 enzyme complex, work is ongoing to identify and develop novel Hsp90 inhibitors with more favourable pharmacological properties. In fact, the water-soluble, orally bioavailable 17-DMAG (17-dimethylamino,17-demethoxygeldanamycin) is now available for phase I testing.

Despite the ubiquitous role of Hsp90, significant toxicity has not been observed clinically. It has been speculated that cancer cells may be more sensitive to Hsp inhibition than normal cells because of increased levels of abnormal, misfolded proteins (Ferrarini et al. 1992). The favourable toxicity profile suggests that combination with conventional therapy may be appropriate. 17-AAG can sensitize cells to the induction of apoptosis by ionizing radiation (Bisht et al. 2003; Enmon et al. 2003) and chemotherapy (Munster et al. 2001). An alternative means of combination therapy is being investigated in which Hsp90 inhibitors are conjugated to other targeted agents such as trastuzumab, an antibody directed against erbB2 (Mandler et al. 2004).

The clinical evaluation of anti-Ras agents has generated interesting and thought-provoking results, but much is still to be learned about how best to predict which patients are likely to benefit from their use. An intriguing outcome in myeloma models where PTEN-deficient cell lines exhibited heightened sensitivity to CCI-779 resulting in G1 arrest (Shi et al 2002) led to speculation that it might be possible to predict sensitivity to mTOR inhibitors on the basis of PTEN mutations. If this were indeed the case, there would be important implications for cancer therapy as PTEN loss/inactivation is a relatively frequent event. Biomarker studies with the MEK inhibitor CI-1040, using ERK phosphorylation as the read-out, have shown target inhibition in patients, but it is unclear how this might be associated with tumour response. There is recent evidence from pre-clinical models indicating that B-Raf mutational sta-

tus may predict response to MEK inhibition. Pharmacological inhibition of MEK reduced growth of B-Raf-mutant cell lines and xenograft tumours, mediated by cyclin D1 downregulation (Solit et al. 2006). The results from this work are likely to promote the development of further disease-directed phase II studies. Overall, there are currently no definitive biomarkers or mutational phenotypes capable of predicting response in human tumours. The identification of relevant biomarkers or even pertinent mutational status from well-designed clinical trials is imperative in order to tailor therapy regimens to the appropriate patient population.

8.5 Future Directions

Increased understanding of the complexities of Ras activation, localisation and downstream signal transduction pathways opens up the possibility of a future generation of novel cancer therapeutics. This may encompass improving the efficacy and safety profiles of existing agents, or alternatively the development of entirely new compounds. Possible avenues include interrupting the constitutively activated state of mutated Ras, exploring alternate means of disrupting membrane localisation, and designing specific inhibitors against other Ras-related GTPases and downstream effectors. The role of oncolytic reovirus therapy is under investigation in early-phase studies, as is immunotherapy, incorporating peptide vaccination schemes, most notably directed against mutant K-Ras in pancreatic cancer. Further techniques that have not progressed beyond the relatively preliminary experimental stage consist of gene-silencing mechanisms, such as RNAi and epigenetic modification.

8.5.1 Inhibition of Ras Activation

The Ras mutations associated with human cancer result in defective intrinsic GTPase activity leading to the oncogenic constitutively activated state. In theory, by designing inhibitors against the GTP-binding site of Ras, it might be possible to inhibit the activity of oncogenic Ras. However, the strong affinity of Ras for GTP and its high intracellular concentration make this approach unlikely to be successfully realised. Restoration of its self-regulatory GTPase activity could theoretically be achieved by substrate-assisted catalysis employing a synthetic GTP mimetic. The GTP analogue DABP-GTP (3,4-diaminobenzo-phenone-phosphoamidate-GTP) has shown some promise and can rescue the GTP-hydrolysing property of Ras in vitro. Interestingly, this analogue is hydrolysed more efficiently by mutant than wild-type Ras (Ahmadian et al. 1999). Ideally, this concept will lead to specific compounds which selectively target defective Ras without affecting the wild-type protein.

8.5.2 Inhibition of Ras Post-translational Modification

Most efforts to disrupt post-translational modification of Ras, and consequently its association with plasma membranes, have concentrated on inhibition of the prenyl transferase enzymes, especially farnesyl transferase, fuelled by early indications that farnesylation was essential for transformation (Jackson et al. 1990; Kato et al. 1992). Despite the lack of overtly positive results, the knowledge from the clinical use of FTIs brings to light future lines of study. If inhibiting the farnesylation of critical proteins is truly the mechanism of FTI action, then it may be useful to block prenylation by alternative methods, such as limiting the production of enzyme substrates (i.e. farnesyl pyrophosphate). Alternatively, it may prove advantageous to target the post-prenylation enzymes Rce1 endopeptidase and ICMT, which catalyse proteolysis and carboxymethylation respectively and which are required for correct membrane localisation.

8.5.2.1 Rce1 Endoprotease Inhibitors

The Rce1 endoprotease is essential for cleavage of the C-terminal AAX tripeptide following farnesylation of the Cysteine residue. The importance of this enzyme has been demonstrated in mouse models, where Rce1 deletion results in defective proteolysis that is embryonic lethal (Kim et al. 1999). Studies of Rce1 disruption in vitro produced modest effects in transformed cells, but notably less than those effects observed in similar studies employing FTIs (Bergo et al. 2002). Loss of Rce1-induced proteolysis does appear to sensitise cells to FTIs, however, again highlighting the role of combination therapies with targeted treatments, and suggesting that this would be the most effective means of employing anti-Rce1 compounds. A number of peptide and nonpeptide inhibitors of Rce1 have been developed as potential therapeutic agents (Dolence et al. 2000; Schlitzer et al. 2001) but there is a potential for adverse toxicity which might limit the development of such agents given the dilated cardiomyopathy observed in Rce1-null mice (Bergo et al. 2004b). Therefore, two issues threaten the further development of this class of inhibitor: suboptimal performance as a monotherapy, combined with potential toxicity.

8.5.2.2 Isoprenylcysteine Carboxyl Methyltransferase Inhibitors

The final step in Ras post-translational modification is methylation of the isoprenylated carboxyl-terminal cysteine residue by ICMT. Gene deletion studies indicate that interfering with methylation, which resulted in altered localisation of K-Ras (Bergo et al. 2000) and reduced transformation by oncogenic K-Ras and B-Raf in murine fibroblasts (Bergo et al. 2004a), had more pronounced effects than deletion of Rce1, suggesting a more requisite biological function. In order to inhibit Ras carboxyl methylation, it would be possible to develop prenylcysteine analogue compounds to compete with the substrate, S-adenosylhomocysteine (AdoHcy) mimetics, or AdoHcy hydrolase inhibitors to elevate intracellular AdoHcy levels given that ICMT is competitively inhibited by this product of the methyl transfer reaction. Interestingly, methotrexate, which is a widely used chemotherapeutic agent, inhibits ICMT by increasing AdoHcy levels, resulting in decreased Ras methylation and reduced cell proliferation. The main drawback for ICMT inhibition by manipulating AdoHcy levels is that other cellular methyl transferases would also be inhibited, thereby potentially increasing the risk of toxicity. One factor which may drive further development of this strategy as a possible anti-cancer treatment is that inhibition of ICMT activity has been reported to induce endothelial cell apoptosis (Kramer et al. 2003). These results suggest that ICMT inhibition may prove to be a useful anti-cancer therapy because of its effects on angiogenesis as well as tumour cells.

8.5.2.3 Isoprenyl Synthesis Pathway Inhibitors

One advantage for the strategy of inhibiting farnesyl pyrophosphate and geranylgeranyl pyrophosphate production is that well-tolerated bioactive compounds called statins, which were created for other indications, are already either in trials or even approved for routine clinical use. Statins were designed to inhibit 3-hydroxy-3-methylglutaryl coenzyme A (HMG CoA) reductase, a crucial enzyme in the biosynthesis of mevalonate, which is required for production of cholesterol as well as substrates required by the isoprenylation enzymes. Their major clinical application is the prevention of cardiovascular disease by lowering low-density lipoprotein cholesterol levels, but their effects are much more complex and they exhibit anti-inflammatory, anti-angiogenic and immunomodulatory properties. The potential role of statins as cancer chemo-prevention agents based on the interpretation of secondary endpoint data from cardiovascular trials is controversial, with conflicting results regarding the incidence of specific types of malignancy. However, there is emerging evidence on the basis of prospective evaluation to suggest significant statin-associated reductions in overall cancer incidence (Demierre et al. 2005). In addition, experimental work has illustrated that this class of drugs demonstrate an anti-cancer effect. Data from in vitro and in vivo model systems (Graaf et al. 2004) indicate that statins inhibit primary tumour growth by induction of growth arrest and apoptosis, possibly mediated through inhibition of geranylgeranylated Rho proteins. Work is currently ongoing to further assess the potential anticancer effect of statins, particularly as combination therapy with conventional forms of cancer management.

Another class of therapeutic compounds which may work by inhibiting FTase and GGTase I precursors are nitrogen-containing bisphosphonates, which inhibit farnesyl synthase and possibly geranylgeranyl synthase. Nitrogen-containing bisphosphonates affect the modification, localisation, protein levels and/or activation of Ras and Rho proteins, and it has been proposed that the anti-proliferative and pro-apoptotic effects of these compounds result from the inhibition of modifications to Ras, Rho or both. It remains to be seen whether the anti-tumour effects observed in vitro (Diel et al. 2000; Senaratne et al. 2000; Tassone et al. 2000) will translate to useful cancer therapies for soft-tissue tumours. It has also been proposed that a combination therapy of statins plus bisphosphonates may be an effective strategy (Vincenzi et al. 2003) because of the greater inhibition of isoprenyl biosynthesis induced by blocking the biosynthetic pathway at two points.

8.5.3 Novel Inhibitors of Downstream Targets

Although the Raf/MAP kinase and PI3K/AKt/mTOR/S6K pathways regulated by Ras signalling have been the subject of intense scrutiny, results from genetic deletion studies in mice have revealed that additional Ras effectors likely contribute to the development of malignancy. Deletion of the Rac GEF Tiam1 reduced the formation of skin tumours caused by a two-stage chemical carcinogenesis protocol which acts by inducing oncogenic activation of H-Ras (Malliri et al. 2002). In addition, deletion of RalGDS, a guanine nucleotide exchange factor for Ral GTPases, similarly reduced tumour incidence, size and progression in the skin cancer model (Gonzalez-Garcia et al. 2005). These results highlight that multiple Ras-regulated signal transduction pathways contribute to oncogenesis, suggesting that these pathways may also be effective anti-cancer targets. One reason that the Raf and PI3K pathways have been favoured for drug development is that the key targets are kinases, which are readily druggable proteins. To inhibit Tiam1 or RalGDS function might require the development of protein-protein interaction inhibitors, an approach which has been relatively neglected. However, increasingly sophisticated structural information is available for the interactions between Rac and its activator Tiam1 and for Ral interaction with RalGDS. Resultant small-molecule screens are being performed in the hope of identifying effective inhibitors. Indeed, a small-molecule antagonist has been described which selectively inhibits Rac-Tiam1 (Gao et al. 2004). The progress made with inhibitors against Raf, MEK and mTOR may extend to the development of agents against less central effectors in the Ras pathway such as Tiam1, RalGDS or PLC.

8.6   Conclusions

Given the compelling clinical evidence, as well as substantial experimental data, relating elevated Ras signalling to tumour growth and progression, targeting Ras signalling pathways has become a major undertaking in the development of novel cancer therapeutics. To achieve this goal, there have largely been two types of therapeutic strategies adopted: either inhibition of Ras post-translational modifications or inhibition of downstream effectors. While FTIs have produced encouraging outcomes in the treatment of a limited specific set of cancers, as single agents they have proven to be ineffective for the majority of cancer types. Further complicating the issue is the strong possibility that the major FTI targets in responsive tumours are proteins other than Ras. However, these findings do not eliminate the drug discovery strategy of targeting Ras post-translational modifications as an approach which might eventually lead to the development of effective therapeu-

tics. For example, it may be more efficacious to generate therapeutic agents which target multiple Ras proteins by inhibiting upstream biosynthetic steps required for the production of isoprenoid lipids. Clinical trials examining the anti-cancer efficacy of HMG-CoA reductase inhibitors (statins) and bisphosphonates are currently under way. An additional tactic would be to target the enzymes which function after the prenylation step, namely, Rce1 or ICMT. Ultimately, the greatest value for Ras post-translational modification inhibitors may lie in their use in combination modalities, with conventional therapies such as cytotoxic agents, endocrine inhibitors, targeted therapeutics or ionising radiation. Progress in this approach is not necessarily limited by the production of novel agents, but is dependent on the intelligent design and implementation of informative clinical studies.

Although inhibition of Ras modifications are well advanced experimentally and clinically, more recent efforts have focussed principally on the inhibition of downstream effector proteins, including Raf and MEK. A prime reason for this is that kinases are very druggable, most kinase inhibitors being ATP analogues. Despite early fears that ATP analogues would be difficult to engineer with sufficient selectivity, combinatorial chemistry and high-throughput screening methods have produced highly selective and potent kinase inhibitors. Kinases were initially concentrated upon for practical reasons, but recent developments in basic research have shown that alterations in signalling downstream of Ras (e.g. B-Raf, PTEN, TSC1/2) also contribute substantially to cancer. As a result, the most progress in targeting Ras signalling may well result from these efforts to block effector function. Although combination therapies with Ras effector inhibitors have not been extensively studied to date, multi-agent therapeutic regimens may well prove to be the most efficacious.

In summary, the success of novel therapeutics which target signal transduction proteins has provided further impetus to drug development efforts aimed at Ras signalling pathways. It is anticipated that significant advancements will be made, both in the development of novel agents and in the refinement of combination regimens with existing and future compounds. These efforts will hopefully make significant contributions to cancer therapy.

Acknowledgements. Many thanks to Professor TRJ Evans and Dr LM Tho for reviewing the manuscript. Research in the Olson laboratory is supported by Cancer Research UK and a grant from the NIH (CA-030721).

References

Adjei AA, Dy GK, Erlichman C, Reid JM, Sloan JA, Pitot HC, Alberts SR, Goldberg RM, Hanson LJ, Atherton PJ, Watanabe T, Geary RS, Holmlund J, Dorr FA (2003) A phase I trial of ISIS 2503, an antisense inhibitor of H-ras, in combination with gemcitabine in patients with advanced cancer. Clin Cancer Res 9:115-123

Ahmad T, Marais R, Pyle L, James M, Schwartz B, Gore M, Eisen T (2004) BAY 43-9006 in patients with advanced melanoma: The Royal Marsden experience. J Clin Oncol (Meeting Abstracts) 22:7506

Ahmadian MR, Zor T, Vogt D, Kabsch W, Selinger Z, Wittinghofer A, Scheffzek K (1999) Guanosine triphosphatase stimulation of oncogenic Ras mutants. Proc Natl Acad Sci USA 96:7065-7070

Ahn NG, Nahreini TS, Tolwinski NS, Resing KA (2001) Pharmacologic inhibitors of MKK1 and MKK2. Methods Enzymol 332:417-431

Alberts SR, Schroeder M, Erlichman C, Steen PD, Foster NR, Moore DF, Jr, Rowland KM, Jr, Nair S, Tschetter LK, Fitch TR (2004) Gemcitabine and ISIS-2503 for patients with locally advanced or metastatic pancreatic adenocarcinoma: A North Central Cancer Treatment Group Phase II Trial. J Clin Oncol 22:4944-4950

Altomare DA, Testa JR (2005) Perturbations of the AKT signaling pathway in human cancer. Oncogene 24:7455-7464

Anwar S, Frayling IM, Scott NA, Carlson GL (2004) Systematic review of genetic influences on the prognosis of colorectal cancer. Br J Surg 91:1275-1291

Appels NMGM, Beijnen JH, Schellens JHM (2005) Development of farnesyl transferase inhibitors: A review. Oncologist 10:565-578

Arboleda MJ, Lyons JF, Kabbinavar FF, Bray MR, Snow BE, Ayala R, Danino M, Karlan BY, Slamon DJ (2003) Overexpression of AKT2/protein kinase Bbeta leads to up-regulation of beta1 integrins, increased invasion, and metastasis of human breast and ovarian cancer cells. Cancer Res 63:196-206

Ashar HR, James L, Gray K, Carr D, Black S, Armstrong L, Bishop WR, Kirschmeier P (2000) Farnesyl transfer-

ase inhibitors block the farnesylation of CENP-E and CENP-F and alter the association of CENP-E with the microtubules. J Biol Chem 275:30451-30457

Atkins MB, Hidalgo M, Stadler WM, Logan TF, Dutcher JP, Hudes GR, Park Y, Liou S-H, Marshall B, Boni JP, Dukart G, Sherman ML (2004) Randomized Phase II study of multiple dose levels of CCI-779, a novel mammalian target of rapamycin kinase inhibitor, in patients with advanced refractory renal cell carcinoma. J Clin Oncol 22:909-918

Basso AD, Solit DB, Chiosis G, Giri B, Tsichlis P, Rosen N (2002) Akt forms an intracellular complex with heat shock protein 90 (Hsp90) and Cdc37 and is destabilized by inhibitors of Hsp90 function. J Biol Chem 277:39858-39866

Beliakoff J, Bagatell R, Paine-Murrieta G, Taylor CW, Lykkesfeldt AE, Whitesell L (2003) Hormone-refractory breast cancer remains sensitive to the antitumor activity of heat shock protein 90 inhibitors. Clin Cancer Res 9:4961-4971

Bellacosa A, de Feo D, Godwin AK, Bell DW, Cheng JQ, Altomare DA, Wan M, Dubeau L, Scambia G, Masciullo V, et al. (1995) Molecular alterations of the AKT2 oncogene in ovarian and breast carcinomas. Int J Cancer 64:280-285

Bergo MO, Leung GK, Ambroziak P, Otto JC, Casey PJ, Young SG (2000) Targeted inactivation of the isoprenylcysteine carboxyl methyltransferase gene causes mislocalization of K-Ras in mammalian cells. J Biol Chem 275:17605-17610

Bergo MO, Leung GK, Ambroziak P, Otto JC, Casey PJ, Gomes AQ, Seabra MC, Young SG (2001) Isoprenylcysteine carboxyl methyltransferase deficiency in mice. J Biol Chem 276:5841-5845

Bergo MO, Ambroziak P, Gregory C, George A, Otto JC, Kim E, Nagase H, Casey PJ, Balmain A, Young SG (2002) Absence of the CAAX endoprotease Rce1: Effects on cell growth and transformation. Mol Cell Biol 22:171-181

Bergo MO, Gavino BJ, Hong C, Beigneux AP, McMahon M, Casey PJ, Young SG (2004a) Inactivation of ICMT inhibits transformation by oncogenic K-Ras and B-Raf. J Clin Invest 113:539-550

Bergo MO, Lieu HD, Gavino BJ, Ambroziak P, Otto JC, Casey PJ, Walker QM, Young SG (2004b) On the physiological importance of endoproteolysis of CAAX Proteins: Heart-specific Rce1 knockout mice develop a lethal cardiomyopathy. J Biol Chem 279:4729-4736

Bernhard EJ, Kao G, Cox AD, Sebti SM, Hamilton AD, Muschel RJ, McKenna WG (1996) The farnesyltransferase inhibitor FTI-277 radiosensitizes H-ras-transformed rat embryo fibroblasts. Cancer Res 56:1727-1730

Bernhard EJ, McKenna WG, Hamilton AD, Sebti SM, Qian Y, Wu JM, Muschel RJ (1998) Inhibiting Ras prenylation increases the radiosensitivity of human tumor cell lines with activating mutations of ras oncogenes. Cancer Res 58:1754-1761

Bernhard EJ, Stanbridge EJ, Gupta S, Gupta AK, Soto D, Bakanauskas VJ, Cerniglia GJ, Muschel RJ, McKenna

WG (2000) Direct evidence for the contribution of activated N-ras and K-ras oncogenes to increased intrinsic radiation resistance in human tumor cell lines. Cancer Res 60:6597–6600

Bisht KS, Bradbury CM, Mattson D, Kaushal A, Sowers A, Markovina S, Ortiz KL, Sieck LK, Isaacs JS, Brechbiel MW, Mitchell JB, Neckers LM, Gius D (2003) Geldanamycin and 17-allylamino-17-demethoxygeldanamycin potentiate the in vitro and in vivo radiation response of cervical tumor cells via the heat shock protein 90-mediated intracellular signaling and cytotoxicity. Cancer Res 63:8984–8995

Bos JL (1989) ras oncogenes in human cancer: a review. Cancer Res 49:4682–4689

Brodsky AL, Daley GQ, Hoover RR, Carr D, Kirschmeier P (2003) Apoptotic synergism between STI571 and the farnesyl transferase inhibitor SCH66336 on an imatinib-sensitive cell line. Blood 101:2070

Brognard J, Clark AS, Ni Y, Dennis PA (2001) Akt/protein kinase B is constitutively active in non-small cell lung cancer cells and promotes cellular survival and resistance to chemotherapy and radiation. Cancer Res 61:3986–3997

Busca R, Bertolotto C, Ortonne J-P, Ballotti R (1996) Inhibition of the phosphatidylinositol 3-kinase/p70S6-kinase pathway induces B16 melanoma cell differentiation. J Biol Chem 271:31824–31830

Chan S, Scheulen ME, Johnston S, Mross K, Cardoso F, Dittrich C, Eiermann W, Hess D, Morant R, Semiglazov V, Borner M, Salzberg M, Ostapenko V, Illiger H-J, Behringer D, Bardy-Bouxin N, Boni J, Kong S, Cincotta M, Moore L (2005) Phase II study of temsirolimus (CCI-779), a novel inhibitor of mTOR, in heavily pretreated patients with locally advanced or metastatic breast cancer. J Clin Oncol 23:5314–5322

Chardin P, Tavitian A (1986) The ral gene: a new ras related gene isolated by the use of a synthetic probe. EMBO J 5:2203–2208

Chen G, Oh S, Monia BP, Stacey DW (1996) Antisense oligonucleotides demonstrate a dominant role of c-Ki-RAS proteins in regulating the proliferation of diploid human fibroblasts. J Biol Chem 271:28259–28265

Cheng JQ, Altomare DA, Klein MA, Lee WC, Kruh GD, Lissy NA, Testa JR (1997) Transforming activity and mitosis-related expression of the AKT2 oncogene: evidence suggesting a link between cell cycle regulation and oncogenesis. Oncogene 14:2793–2801

Cho H, Mu J, Kim JK, Thorvaldsen JL, Chu Q, Crenshaw EB, 3rd, Kaestner KH, Bartolomei MS, Shulman GI, Birnbaum MJ (2001) Insulin resistance and a diabetes mellitus-like syndrome in mice lacking the protein kinase Akt2 (PKB beta). Science 292:1728–1731

Clark GJ, Kinch MS, Rogers-Graham K, Sebti SM, Hamilton AD, Der CJ (1997) The Ras-related protein Rheb is farnesylated and antagonizes ras signaling and transformation. J Biol Chem 272:10608–10615

Cloughesy TF, Kuhn J, Robins HI, Abrey L, Wen P, Fink K, Lieberman FS, Mehta M, Chang S, Yung A, DeAngelis L, Schiff D, Junck L, Groves M, Paquette S, Wright J, Lamborn K, Sebti SM, Prados M (2005) Phase I trial of tipifarnib in patients with recurrent malignant glioma taking enzyme-inducing antiepileptic drugs: A North American Brain Tumor Consortium Study. J Clin Oncol 23:6647–6656

Cohen-Jonathan E, Toulas C, Ader I, Monteil S, Allal C, Bonnet J, Hamilton AD, Sebti SM, Daly-Schveitzer N, Favre G (1999) The farnesyltransferase inhibitor FTI-277 suppresses the 24-kDa FGF2-induced radioresistance in HeLa cells expressing wild-type RAS. Radiat Res 152:404–411

Cohen-Jonathan E, Muschel RJ, Gillies McKenna W, Evans SM, Cerniglia G, Mick R, Kusewitt D, Sebti SM, Hamilton AD, Oliff A, Kohl N, Gibbs JB, Bernhard EJ (2000) Farnesyltransferase inhibitors potentiate the antitumor effect of radiation on a human tumor xenograft expressing activated HRAS. Radiat Res 154:125–132

Cortes J (2003) Farnesyltransferase inhibitors in acute myeloid leukemia and myelodysplastic syndromes. Clin Lymphoma 4 Suppl 1:S30–S35

Coudert B, Anthoney A, Fiedler W, Droz JP, Dieras V, Borner M, Smyth JF, Morant R, de Vries MJ, Roelvink M, Fumoleau P (2001) Phase II trial with ISIS 5132 in patients with small-cell (SCLC) and non-small cell (NSCLC) lung cancer. A European Organization for Research and Treatment of Cancer (EORTC) Early Clinical Studies Group report. Eur J Cancer 37:2194–2198

Cox AD, Der CJ (2002) Ras family signaling: therapeutic targeting. Cancer Biol Ther 1:599–606

Cripps MC, Figueredo AT, Oza AM, Taylor MJ, Fields AL, Holmlund JT, McIntosh LW, Geary RS, Eisenhauer EA (2002) Phase II Randomized study of ISIS 3521 and ISIS 5132 in patients with locally advanced or metastatic colorectal cancer: A National Cancer Institute of Canada Clinical Trials Group Study. Clin Cancer Res 8:2188–2192

Crul M, Rosing H, de Klerk GJ, Dubbelman R, Traiser M, Reichert S, Knebel NG, Schellens JHM, Beijnen JH, ten Bokkel Huinink WW (2002) Phase I and pharmacological study of daily oral administration of perifosine (D-21266) in patients with advanced solid tumours. Eur J Cancer 38:1615–1621

Cunningham CC, Holmlund JT, Geary RS, Kwoh TJ, Dorr A, Johnston JF, Monia B, Nemunaitis J (2001) A Phase I trial of H-ras antisense oligonucleotide ISIS 2503 administered as a continuous intravenous infusion in patients with advanced carcinoma. Cancer 92:1265–1271

da Rocha Dias S, Friedlos F, Light Y, Springer C, Workman P, Marais R (2005) Activated B-RAF Is an Hsp90 client protein that is targeted by the anticancer drug 17-allylamino-17-demethoxygeldanamycin. Cancer Res 65:10686–10691

Davies H, Bignell GR, Cox C, Stephens P, Edkins S, Clegg S, Teague J, Woffendin H, Garnett MJ, Bottomley W, Davis N, Dicks E, Ewing R, Floyd Y, Gray K, Hall S,

Hawes R, Hughes J, Kosmidou V, Menzies A, Mould C, Parker A, Stevens C, Watt S, Hooper S, Wilson R, Jayatilake H, Gusterson BA, Cooper C, Shipley J, Hargrave D, Pritchard-Jones K, Maitland N, Chenevix-Trench G, Riggins GJ, Bigner DD, Palmieri G, Cossu A, Flanagan A, Nicholson A, Ho JWC, Leung SY, Yuen ST, Weber BL, Seigler HF, Darrow TL, Paterson H, Marais R, Marshall CJ, Wooster R, Stratton MR, Futreal PA (2002) Mutations of the BRAF gene in human cancer. Nature 417:949–954

Delmas C, Heliez C, Cohen-Jonathan E, End D, Bonnet J, Favre G, Toulas C (2002) Farnesyltransferase inhibitor, R115777, reverses the resistance of human glioma cell lines to ionizing radiation. Int J Cancer 100:43–48

Demierre M-F, Higgins PDR, Gruber SB, Hawk E, Lippman SM (2005) Statins and cancer prevention. Nat Rev Cancer 5:930–942

Diel IJ, Solomayer EF, Bastert G (2000) Bisphosphonates and the prevention of metastasis: first evidences from preclinical and clinical studies. Cancer 88:3080–3088

Dolence EK, Dolence JM, Poulter CD (2000) Solid-phase synthesis of a farnesylated CaaX peptide library: inhibitors of the Ras CaaX endoprotease. J Comb Chem 2:522–536

Du W, Lebowitz PF, Prendergast GC (1999) Cell growth inhibition by farnesyltransferase inhibitors is mediated by gain of geranylgeranylated RhoB. Mol Cell Biol 19:1831–1840

Dudkin L, Dilling MB, Cheshire PJ, Harwood FC, Hollingshead M, Arbuck SG, Travis R, Sausville EA, Houghton PJ (2001) Biochemical correlates of mTOR inhibition by the rapamycin ester CCI-779 and tumor growth inhibition. Clin Cancer Res 7:1758–1764

Ellis CA, Vos MD, Wickline M, Riley C, Vallecorsa T, Telford WG, Zujewskil J, Clark GJ (2003) Tamoxifen and the farnesyl transferase inhibitor FTI-277 synergize to inhibit growth in estrogen receptor-positive breast tumor cell lines. Breast Cancer Res Treat 78:59–67

Emuss V, Garnett M, Mason C, The Cancer Genome Project, Marais R (2005) Mutations of C-RAF are rare in human cancer because C-RAF has a low basal kinase activity compared with B-RAF. Cancer Res 65:9719–9726

End DW, Smets G, Todd AV, Applegate TL, Fuery CJ, Angibaud P, Venet M, Sanz G, Poignet H, Skrzat S, Devine A, Wouters W, Bowden C (2001) Characterization of the antitumor effects of the selective protein farnesyl transferase inhibitor R115777 in vivo and in vitro. Cancer Res 61:131–137

Eng C (2003) PTEN: one gene, many syndromes. Hum Mutat 22:183–198

Enmon R, Yang WH, Ballangrud AM, Solit DB, Heller G, Rosen N, Scher HI, Sgouros G (2003) Combination treatment with 17-N-allylamino-17-demethoxy geldanamycin and acute irradiation produces supraadditive growth suppression in human prostate carcinoma spheroids. Cancer Res 63:8393–8399

Escudier B, Szczylik C, Eisen T, Oudard S, Stadler WM, Schwartz B, Shan M, Bukowski RM (2005a) Randomized Phase III trial of the multi-kinase inhibitor sorafenib (BAY 43-9006) in patients with advanced renal cell carcinoma (RCC). Eur J Cancer 3(S):226

Escudier B, Szczylik C, Eisen T, Stadler WM, Schwartz B, Shan M, Bukowski RM (2005b) Randomized phase III trial of the Raf kinase and VEGFR inhibitor sorafenib (BAY 43-9006) in patients with advanced renal cell carcinoma (RCC). J Clin Oncol (Meeting Abstracts) 23:LBA4510

Farnsworth C, Seabra M, Ericsson L, Gelb M, Glomset J (1994) Rab geranylgeranyl transferase catalyzes the geranylgeranylation of adjacent cysteines in the small GTPases Rab1A, Rab3A, and Rab5A. Proc Natl Acad Sci USA 91:11963–11967

Feig LA (2003) Ral-GTPases: approaching their 15 minutes of fame. Trends Cell Biol 13:419–425

Ferrarini M, Heltai S, Zocchi MR, Rugarli C (1992) Unusual expression and localization of heat-shock proteins in human tumor cells. Int J Cancer 51:613–619

Flaherty KT, Brose M, Schuchter L, Tuveson D, Lee R, Schwartz B, Lathia C, Weber B, O'Dwyer P (2004) Phase I/II trial of BAY 43-9006, carboplatin (C) and paclitaxel (P) demonstrates preliminary antitumor activity in the expansion cohort of patients with metastatic melanoma. J Clin Oncol (Meeting Abstracts) 22:7507

Frost P, Moatamed F, Hoang B, Shi Y, Gera J, Yan H, Frost P, Gibbons J, Lichtenstein A (2004) In vivo antitumor effects of the mTOR inhibitor CCI-779 against human multiple myeloma cells in a xenograft model. Blood 104:4181–4187

Gao Y, Dickerson JB, Guo F, Zheng J, Zheng Y (2004) Rational design and characterization of a Rac GTPase-specific small molecule inhibitor. Proc Natl Acad Sci USA 101:7618–7623

Geoerger B, Kerr K, Tang C-B, Fung K-M, Powell B, Sutton LN, Phillips PC, Janss AJ (2001) Antitumor activity of the rapamycin analog CCI-779 in human primitive neuroectodermal tumor/medulloblastoma models as single agent and in combination chemotherapy. Cancer Res 61:1527–1532

Gokhale PC, McRae D, Monia BP, Bagg A, Rahman A, Dritschilo A, Kasid U (1999) Antisense raf oligodeoxyribonucleotide is a radiosensitizer in vivo. Antisense Nucleic Acid Drug Dev 9:191–201

Gonzalez-Garcia A, Pritchard CA, Paterson HF, Mavria G, Stamp G, Marshall CJ (2005) RalGDS is required for tumor formation in a model of skin carcinogenesis. Cancer Cell 7:219–226

Graaf MR, Richel DJ, van Noorden CJ, Guchelaar HJ (2004) Effects of statins and farnesyltransferase inhibitors on the development and progression of cancer. Cancer Treat Rev 30:609–641

Grbovic OM, Basso AD, Sawai A, Ye Q, Friedlander P, Solit D, Rosen N (2006) V600E B-Raf requires the Hsp90 chaperone for stability and is degraded in response to Hsp90 inhibitors. Proc Natl Acad Sci USA 103:57–62

Hahn SM, Bernhard EJ, Regine W, Mohiuddin M, Haller DG, Stevenson JP, Smith D, Pramanik B, Tepper J, DeLaney TF, Kiel KD, Morrison B, Deutsch P, Muschel RJ, McKenna WG (2002) A Phase I trial of the farnesyltransferase inhibitor L-778,123 and radiotherapy for locally advanced lung and head and neck cancer. Clin Cancer Res 8:1065–1072

Hancock JF, Magee AI, Childs JE, Marshall CJ (1989) All ras proteins are polyisoprenylated but only some are palmitoylated. Cell 57:1167–1177

Hilgard P, Klenner T, Stekar J, Nossner G, Kutscher B, Engel J (1997) D-21266, a new heterocyclic alkylphospholipid with antitumour activity. Eur J Cancer 33:442–446

Hingorani SR, Jacobetz MA, Robertson GP, Herlyn M, Tuveson DA (2003) Suppression of BRAFV599E in human melanoma abrogates transformation. Cancer Res 63:5198–5202

Holmlund JT, Monia BP, Kwoh TJ, Dorr FA (1999) Toward antisense oligonucleotide therapy for cancer: ISIS compounds in clinical development. Curr Opin Mol Ther 1:372–385

Hotte SJ, Hirte HW (2002) BAY 43–9006: early clinical data in patients with advanced solid malignancies. Curr Pharm Des 8:2249–2253

Hu L, Zaloudek C, Mills GB, Gray J, Jaffe RB (2000) In vivo and in vitro ovarian carcinoma growth inhibition by a phosphatidylinositol 3-kinase inhibitor (LY294002). Clin Cancer Res 6:880–886

Hu L, Hofmann J, Lu Y, Mills GB, Jaffe RB (2002) Inhibition of phosphatidylinositol 3'-kinase increases efficacy of paclitaxel in in vitro and in vivo ovarian cancer models. Cancer Res 62:1087–1092

Humar R, Kiefer FN, Berns H, Resink TJ, Battegay EJ (2002) Hypoxia enhances vascular cell proliferation and angiogenesis in vitro via rapamycin (mTOR)-dependent signaling. FASEB J 16:771–780

Hussein D, Taylor SS (2002) Farnesylation of Cenp-F is required for G2/M progression and degradation after mitosis. J Cell Sci 115:3403–3414

Isakoff SJ, Engelman JA, Irie HY, Luo J, Brachmann SM, Pearline RV, Cantley LC, Brugge JS (2005) Breast cancer-associated PIK3CA mutations are oncogenic in mammary epithelial cells. Cancer Res 65:10992–11000

Jackson J, Cochrane C, Bourne J, Solski P, Buss J, Der C (1990) Farnesol modification of Kirsten-Ras exon 4B protein is essential for transformation. Proc Natl Acad Sci USA 87:3042–3046

Johnston SRD, Hickish T, Ellis P, Houston S, Kelland L, Dowsett M, Salter J, Michiels B, Perez-Ruixo JJ, Palmer P, Howes A (2003) Phase II study of the efficacy and tolerability of two dosing regimens of the farnesyl transferase inhibitor, R115777, in advanced breast cancer. J Clin Oncol 21:2492–2499

Karasarides M, Chiloeches A, Hayward R, Niculescu-Duvaz D, Scanlon I, Friedlos F, Ogilvie L, Hedley D, Martin J, Marshall CJ, Springer CJ, Marais R (2004) B-RAF is a therapeutic target in melanoma. Oncogene 23:6292–6298

Karp JE, Kaufmann SH, Adjei AA, Lancet JE, Wright JJ, End DW (2001) Current status of clinical trials of farnesyltransferase inhibitors. Curr Opin Oncol 13:470–476

Kato K, Cox A, Hisaka M, Graham S, Buss J, Der C (1992) Isoprenoid addition to Ras protein is the critical modification for its membrane association and transforming activity. Proc Natl Acad Sci USA 89:6403–6407

Kim E, Ambroziak P, Otto JC, Taylor B, Ashby M, Shannon K, Casey PJ, Young SG (1999) Disruption of the mouse Rce1 gene results in defective Ras processing and mislocalization of Ras within cells. J Biol Chem 274:8383–8390

Kohl NE, Mosser SD, deSolms SJ, Giuliani EA, Pompliano DL, Graham SL, Smith RL, Scolnick EM, Oliff A, Gibbs JB (1993) Selective inhibition of ras-dependent transformation by a farnesyltransferase inhibitor. Science 260:1934–1937

Kondapaka SB, Singh SS, Dasmahapatra GP, Sausville EA, Roy KK (2003) Perifosine, a novel alkylphospholipid, inhibits protein kinase B activation. Mol Cancer Ther 2:1093–1103

Kramer K, Harrington EO, Lu Q, Bellas R, Newton J, Sheahan KL, Rounds S (2003) Isoprenylcysteine carboxyl methyltransferase activity modulates endothelial cell apoptosis. Mol Biol Cell 14:848–857

Kurzrock R, Kantarjian HM, Cortes JE, Singhania N, Thomas DA, Wilson EF, Wright JJ, Freireich EJ, Talpaz M, Sebti SM (2003) Farnesyltransferase inhibitor R115777 in myelodysplastic syndrome: clinical and biologic activities in the phase 1 setting. Blood 102:4527–4534

Lebowitz PF, Casey PJ, Prendergast GC, Thissen JA (1997) Farnesyltransferase inhibitors alter the prenylation and growth-stimulating function of RhoB. J Biol Chem 272:15591–15594

Ling CC, Endlich B (1989) Radioresistance induced by oncogenic transformation. Radiat Res 120:267–279

Liu A-x, Du W, Liu J-P, Jessell TM, Prendergast GC (2000) RhoB alteration is necessary for apoptotic and anti-neoplastic responses to farnesyltransferase inhibitors. Mol Cell Biol 20:6105–6113

Lobell RB, Omer CA, Abrams MT, Bhimnathwala HG, Brucker MJ, Buser CA, Davide JP, deSolms SJ, Dinsmore CJ, Ellis-Hutchings MS, Kral AM, Liu D, Lumma WC, Machotka SV, Rands E, Williams TM, Graham SL, Hartman GD, Oliff AI, Heimbrook DC, Kohl NE (2001) Evaluation of farnesyl:protein transferase and geranylgeranyl:protein transferase inhibitor combinations in preclinical models. Cancer Res 61:8758–8768

Luo Y, Shoemaker AR, Liu X, Woods KW, Thomas SA, de Jong R, Han EK, Li T, Stoll VS, Powlas JA, Oleksijew A, Mitten MJ, Shi Y, Guan R, McGonigal TP, Klinghofer V, Johnson EF, Leverson JD, Bouska JJ, Mamo M, Smith RA, Gramling-Evans EE, Zinker BA, Mika AK, Nguyen PT, Oltersdorf T, Rosenberg SH, Li Q, Giranda VL (2005) Potent and selective inhibitors of

Akt kinases slow the progress of tumors in vivo. Mol Cancer Ther 4:977–986

Lyons J, Wilhelm S, Hibner B, Bollag G (2001) Discovery of a novel Raf kinase inhibitor. Endocr Relat Cancer 8:219–225

Mak BC, Yeung RS (2004) The tuberous sclerosis complex genes in tumor development. Cancer Invest 22:588–603

Malliri A, van der Kammen RA, Clark K, van der Valk M, Michiels F, Collard JG (2002) Mice deficient in the Rac activator Tiam1 are resistant to Ras-induced skin tumours. Nature 417:867–871

Mandler R, Kobayashi H, Hinson ER, Brechbiel MW, Waldmann TA (2004) Herceptin-geldanamycin immunoconjugates: pharmacokinetics, biodistribution, and enhanced antitumor activity. Cancer Res 64:1460–1467

Marcus AI, Zhou J, O'Brate A, Hamel E, Wong J, Nivens M, El-Naggar A, Yao T-P, Khuri FR, Giannakakou P (2005) The synergistic combination of the farnesyl transferase inhibitor lonafarnib and paclitaxel enhances tubulin acetylation and requires a functional tubulin deacetylase. Cancer Res 65:3883–3893

Martin GA, Viskochil D, Bollag G, McCabe PC, Crosier WJ, Haubruck H, Conroy L, Clark R, O'Connell P, Cawthon RM, et al. (1990) The GAP-related domain of the neurofibromatosis type 1 gene product interacts with ras p21. Cell 63:843–849

Martin NE, Brunner TB, Kiel KD, DeLaney TF, Regine WF, Mohiuddin M, Rosato EF, Haller DG, Stevenson JP, Smith D, Pramanik B, Tepper J, Tanaka WK, Morrison B, Deutsch P, Gupta AK, Muschel RJ, McKenna WG, Bernhard EJ, Hahn SM (2004) A Phase I trial of the dual farnesyltransferase and geranylgeranyltransferase inhibitor L-778,123 and radiotherapy for locally advanced pancreatic cancer. Clin Cancer Res 10:5447–5454

Mascaux C, Iannino N, Martin B, Paesmans M, Berghmans T, Dusart M, Haller A, Lothaire P, Meert AP, Noel S, Lafitte JJ, Sculier JP (2005) The role of RAS oncogene in survival of patients with lung cancer: a systematic review of the literature with meta-analysis. Br J Cancer 92:131–139

Mason CS, Springer CJ, Cooper RG, Superti-Furga G, Marshall CJ, Marais R (1999) Serine and tyrosine phosphorylations cooperate in Raf-1, but not B-Raf activation. EMBO J 18:2137–2148

Mavria G, Vercoulen Y, Yeo M, Paterson H, Karasarides M, Marais R, Bird D, Marshall CJ (2006) ERK-MAPK signaling opposes Rho-kinase to promote endothelial cell survival and sprouting during angiogenesis. Cancer Cell 9:33–44

McCoy MS, Bargmann CI, Weinberg RA (1984) Human colon carcinoma Ki-ras2 oncogene and its corresponding proto-oncogene. Mol Cell Biol 4:1577–1582

McKenna WG, Weiss MC, Bakanauskas VJ, Sandler H, Kelsten ML, Biaglow J, Tuttle SW, Endlich B, Ling CC, Muschel RJ (1990a) The role of the H-ras oncogene in radiation resistance and metastasis. Int J Radiat Oncol Biol Phys 18:849–859

McKenna WG, Weiss MC, Endlich B, Ling CC, Bakanauskas VJ, Kelsten ML, Muschel RJ (1990b) Synergistic effect of the v-myc oncogene with H-ras on radioresistance. Cancer Res 50:97–102

Micci F, Teixeira MR, Haugom L, Kristensen G, Abeler VM, Heim S (2004) Genomic aberrations in carcinomas of the uterine corpus. Genes Chromosomes Cancer 40:229–246

Michaloglou C, Vredeveld LCW, Soengas MS, Denoyelle C, Kuilman T, van der Horst CMAM, Majoor DM, Shay JW, Mooi WJ, Peeper DS (2005) BRAFE600-associated senescence-like cell cycle arrest of human naevi. Nature 436:720–724

Mijimolle N, Velasco J, Dubus P, Guerra C, Weinbaum CA, Casey PJ, Campuzano V, Barbacid M (2005) Protein farnesyltransferase in embryogenesis, adult homeostasis, and tumor development. Cancer Cell 7:313–324

Moasser MM, Sepp-Lorenzino L, Kohl NE, Oliff A, Balog A, Su D-S, Danishefsky SJ, Rosen N (1998) Farnesyl transferase inhibitors cause enhanced mitotic sensitivity to taxol and epothilones. Proc Natl Acad Sci USA 95:1369–1374

Monia BP, Johnston JF, Ecker DJ, Zounes MA, Lima WF, Freier SM (1992) Selective inhibition of mutant Ha-ras mRNA expression by antisense oligonucleotides. J Biol Chem 267:19954–19962

Monia BP, Johnston JF, Geiger T, Muller M, Fabbro D (1996a) Antitumor activity of a phosphorothioate antisense oligodeoxynucleotide targeted against C-raf kinase. Nat Med 2:668–675

Monia BP, Sasmor H, Johnston JF, Freier SM, Lesnik EA, Muller M, Geiger T, Altmann KH, Moser H, Fabbro D (1996b) Sequence-specific antitumor activity of a phosphorothioate oligodeoxyribonucleotide targeted to human C-raf kinase supports an antisense mechanism of action in vivo. Proc Natl Acad Sci USA 93:15481–15484

Morgan MA, Dolp O, Reuter CWM (2001) Cell-cycle-dependent activation of mitogen-activated protein kinase kinase (MEK-1/2) in myeloid leukemia cell lines and induction of growth inhibition and apoptosis by inhibitors of RAS signaling. Blood 97:1823–1834

Munster PN, Basso A, Solit D, Norton L, Rosen N (2001) Modulation of Hsp90 function by ansamycins sensitizes breast cancer cells to chemotherapy-induced apoptosis in an RB- and schedule-dependent manner. Clin Cancer Res 7:2228–2236

Nakajima A, Tauchi T, Sumi M, Bishop WR, Ohyashiki K (2003) Efficacy of SCH66336, a farnesyl transferase inhibitor, in conjunction with imatinib against BCR-ABL-positive cells. Mol Cancer Ther 2:219–224

Neckers L, Ivy SP (2003) Heat shock protein 90. Curr Opin Oncol 15:419–424

Nicol D, Hii SI, Walsh M, Teh B, Thompson L, Kennett C, Gotley D (1997) Vascular endothelial growth factor expression is increased in renal cell carcinoma. J Urol 157:1482–1486

Oza AM, Elit L, Swenerton K, Faught W, Ghatage P, Carey M, McIntosh L, Dorr A, Holmlund JT, Eisenhauer E (2003) Phase II study of CGP 69846A (ISIS 5132) in recurrent epithelial ovarian cancer: an NCIC clinical trials group study (NCIC IND.116)*. Gynecol Oncol 89:129–133

Podsypanina K, Ellenson LH, Nemes A, Gu J, Tamura M, Yamada KM, Cordon-Cardo C, Catoretti G, Fisher PE, Parsons R (1999) Mutation of Pten/Mmac1 in mice causes neoplasia in multiple organ systems. Proc Natl Acad Sci USA 96:1563–1568

Pollock PM, Harper UL, Hansen KS, Yudt LM, Stark M, Robbins CM, Moses TY, Hostetter G, Wagner U, Kakareka J, Salem G, Pohida T, Heenan P, Duray P, Kallioniemi O, Hayward NK, Trent JM, Meltzer PS (2003) High frequency of BRAF mutations in nevi. Nat Genet 33:19–20

Punt CJA, Boni J, Bruntsch U, Peters M, Thielert C (2003) Phase I and pharmacokinetic study of CCI-779, a novel cytostatic cell-cycle inhibitor, in combination with 5-fluorouracil and leucovorin in patients with advanced solid tumors. Ann Oncol 14:931–937

Rajagopalan H, Bardelli A, Lengauer C, Kinzler KW, Vogelstein B, Velculescu VE (2002) Tumorigenesis-RAF/RAS oncogenes and mismatch-repair status. Nature 418:934

Rao S, Cunningham D, de Gramont A, Scheithauer W, Smakal M, Humblet Y, Kourteva G, Iveson T, Andre T, Dostalova J, Illes A, Belly R, Perez-Ruixo JJ, Park YC, Palmer PA (2004) Phase III double-blind placebo-controlled study of farnesyl transferase inhibitor R115777 in patients with refractory advanced colorectal cancer. J Clin Oncol 22:3950–3957

Ratain MJ, Eisen T, Stadler WM, Flaherty KT, Gore M, Desai A, Patnaik A, Xiong HQ, Schwartz B, O'Dwyer P (2005) Final findings from a phase II, placebo-controlled, randomized discontinuation trial (RDT) of sorafenib (BAY 43–9006) in patients with advanced renal cell carcinoma (RCC). J Clin Oncol (Meeting Abstracts) 23:4544

Reuter CWM, Morgan MA, Bergmann L (2000) Targeting the Ras signaling pathway: a rational, mechanism-based treatment for hematologic malignancies? Blood 96:1655–1669

Rinehart J, Adjei AA, Lorusso PM, Waterhouse D, Hecht JR, Natale RB, Hamid O, Varterasian M, Asbury P, Kaldjian EP, Gulyas S, Mitchell DY, Herrera R, Sebolt-Leopold JS, Meyer MB (2004) Multicenter phase II study of the oral MEK inhibitor, CI-1040, in patients with advanced non-small-cell lung, breast, colon, and pancreatic cancer. J Clin Oncol 22:4456–4462

Risinger J, Hayes K, Maxwell G, Carney M, Dodge R, Barrett J, Berchuck A (1998) PTEN mutation in endometrial cancers is associated with favorable clinical and pathologic characteristics. Clin Cancer Res 4:3005–3010

Ross PJ, George M, Cunningham D, DiStefano F, Andreyev HJN, Workman P, Clarke PA (2001) Inhibition of Kirsten-ras expression in human colorectal cancer using rationally selected Kirsten-ras antisense oligonucleotides. Mol Cancer Ther 1:29–41

Rudin CM, Holmlund J, Fleming GF, Mani S, Stadler WM, Schumm P, Monia BP, Johnston JF, Geary R, Yu RZ, Kwoh TJ, Dorr FA, Ratain MJ (2001) Phase I Trial of ISIS 5132, an antisense oligonucleotide inhibitor of c-raf-1, administered by 24-hour weekly infusion to patients with advanced cancer. Clin Cancer Res 7:1214–1220

Samid D, Miller AC, Rimoldi D, Gafner J, Clark EP (1991) Increased radiation resistance in transformed and nontransformed cells with elevated ras proto-oncogene expression. Radiat Res 126:244–250

Samuels Y, Wang Z, Bardelli A, Silliman N, Ptak J, Szabo S, Yan H, Gazdar A, Powell SM, Riggins GJ, Willson JK, Markowitz S, Kinzler KW, Vogelstein B, Velculescu VE (2004) High frequency of mutations of the PIK3CA gene in human cancers. Science 304:554

Sansal I, Sellers WR (2004) The Biology and Clinical Relevance of the PTEN Tumor Suppressor Pathway. J Clin Oncol 22:2954–2963

Sarkaria JN, Tibbetts RS, Busby EC, Kennedy AP, Hill DE, Abraham RT (1998) Inhibition of phosphoinositide 3-kinase related kinases by the radiosensitizing agent wortmannin. Cancer Res 58:4375–4382

Schlitzer M, Winter-Vann A, Casey PJ (2001) Non-peptidic, non-prenylic inhibitors of the prenyl protein-specific protease Rce1. Bioorg Medicinal Chem Lett 11:425–427

Schulte TW, Blagosklonny MV, Romanova L, Mushinski JF, Monia BP, Johnston JF, Nguyen P, Trepel J, Neckers LM (1996) Destabilization of Raf-1 by geldanamycin leads to disruption of the Raf-1-MEK-mitogen-activated protein kinase signalling pathway. Mol Cell Biol 16:5839–5845

Schultz RM, Merriman RL, Andis SL, Bonjouklian R, Grindey GB, Rutherford PG, Gallegos A, Massey K, Powis G (1995) In vitro and in vivo antitumor activity of the phosphatidylinositol-3-kinase inhibitor, wortmannin. Anticancer Res 15:1135–1139

Sebolt-Leopold JS, Dudley DT, Herrera R, Van Becelaere K, Wiland A, Gowan RC, Tecle H, Barrett SD, Bridges A, Przybranowski S, Leopold WR, Saltiel AR (1999) Blockade of the MAP kinase pathway suppresses growth of colon tumors in vivo. Nat Med 5:810–816

Sebti SM, Adjei AA (2004) Farnesyltransferase inhibitors. Semin Oncol 31:28–39

Sebti SM, Hamilton AD (2000) Farnesyltransferase and geranylgeranyltransferase I inhibitors and cancer therapy: lessons from mechanism and bench-to-bedside translational studies. Oncogene 19:6584–6593

Senaratne SG, Pirianov G, Mansi JL, Arnett TR, Colston KW (2000) Bisphosphonates induce apoptosis in human breast cancer cell lines. Br J Cancer 82:1459–1468

Shayesteh L, Lu Y, Kuo WL, Baldocchi R, Godfrey T, Collins C, Pinkel D, Powell B, Mills GB, Gray JW (1999)

PIK3CA is implicated as an oncogene in ovarian cancer. Nat Genet 21:99–102

Shi Y, Gera J, Liping H, Jung-hsin H, Bookstein R, Weiqun L, Lichenstein A (2002) Enhanced sensitivity of multiple myeloma cells to CCI-779. Cancer Res 62:5027–5034

Singer G, Oldt R, III, Cohen Y, Wang BG, Sidransky D, Kurman RJ, Shih I-M (2003) Mutations in BRAF and KRAS characterize the development of low-grade ovarian serous carcinoma. J Natl Cancer Inst 95:484–486

Smith JS, Tachibana I, Passe SM, Huntley BK, Borell TJ, Iturria N, O'Fallon JR, Schaefer PL, Scheithauer BW, James CD, Buckner JC, Jenkins RB (2001) PTEN mutation, EGFR amplification, and outcome in patients with anaplastic astrocytoma and glioblastoma multiforme. J Natl Cancer Inst 93:1246–1256

Smith JW, Ko Y-J, Dutcher J, Hudes G, Escudier B, Motzer R, Negrier S, Duclos B, Galand L, Strauss L (2004) Update of a phase 1 study of intravenous CCI-779 given in combination with interferon-alpha to patients with advanced renal cell carcinoma. J Clin Oncol (Meeting Abstracts) 22:4513

Solit DB, Zheng FF, Drobnjak M, Munster PN, Higgins B, Verbel D, Heller G, Tong W, Cordon-Cardo C, Agus DB, Scher HI, Rosen N (2002) 17-Allylamino-17-demethoxygeldanamycin induces the degradation of androgen receptor and HER-2/neu and inhibits the growth of prostate cancer xenografts. Clin Cancer Res 8:986–993

Solit DB, Garraway LA, Pratilas CA, Sawai A, Getz G, Basso A, Ye Q, Lobo JM, She Y, Osman I, Golub TR, Sebolt-Leopold J, Sellers WR, Rosen N (2006) BRAF mutation predicts sensitivity to MEK inhibition. Nature 439:358–362

Sprang S (1997) G protein mechanisms: insights from structural analysis. Annu Rev Biochem 66:639–678

Stambolic V, Tsao M-S, Macpherson D, Suzuki A, Chapman WB, Mak TW (2000) High incidence of breast and endometrial neoplasia resembling human Cowden syndrome in pten+/- mice. Cancer Res 60:3605–3611

Sun J, Blaskovich MA, Knowles D, Qian Y, Ohkanda J, Bailey RD, Hamilton AD, Sebti SM (1999) Antitumor efficacy of a novel class of non-thiol-containing peptidomimetic inhibitors of farnesyltransferase and geranylgeranyltransferase I: combination therapy with the cytotoxic agents cisplatin, Taxol, and gemcitabine. Cancer Res 59:4919–4926

Sun M, Wang G, Paciga JE, Feldman RI, Yuan ZQ, Ma XL, Shelley SA, Jove R, Tsichlis PN, Nicosia SV, Cheng JQ (2001) AKT1/PKBalpha kinase is frequently elevated in human cancers and its constitutive activation is required for oncogenic transformation in NIH3T3 cells. Am J Pathol 159:431–437

Tassone P, Forciniti S, Galea E, Morrone G, Turco MC, Martinelli V, Tagliaferri P, Venuta S (2000) Growth inhibition and synergistic induction of apoptosis by zoledronate and dexamethasone in human myeloma cell lines. Leukemia 14:841–844

Tolcher AW, Reyno L, Venner PM, Ernst SD, Moore M, Geary RS, Chi K, Hall S, Walsh W, Dorr A, Eisenhauer E (2002) A randomized Phase II and pharmacokinetic study of the antisense oligonucleotides ISIS 3521 and ISIS 5132 in patients with hormone-refractory prostate cancer. Clin Cancer Res 8:2530–2535

Van Cutsem E, van de Velde H, Karasek P, Oettle H, Vervenne WL, Szawlowski A, Schoffski P, Post S, Verslype C, Neumann H, Safran H, Humblet Y, Perez Ruixo J, Ma Y, Von Hoff D (2004) Phase III trial of gemcitabine plus tipifarnib compared with gemcitabine plus placebo in advanced pancreatic cancer. J Clin Oncol 22:1430–1438

Van Ummersen L, Binger K, Volkman J, Marnocha R, Tutsch K, Kolesar J, Arzoomanian R, Alberti D, Wilding G (2004) A Phase I trial of perifosine (NSC 639966) on a loading dose/maintenance dose schedule in patients with advanced cancer. Clin Cancer Res 10:7450–7456

Vincenzi B, Santini D, Avvisati G, Baldi A, Cesa AL, Tonini G (2003) Statins may potentiate bisphosphonates anticancer properties: a new pharmacological approach? Med Hypotheses 61:98–101

Vivanco I, Sawyers CL (2002) The phosphatidylinositol 3-kinase AKT pathway in human cancer. Nat Rev Cancer 2:489–501

Wallace EM, Lyssikatos JP, Yeh T, Winkler JD, Koch K (2005) Progress towards therapeutic small molecule MEK inhibitors for use in cancer therapy. Curr Top Med Chem 5:215–229

Wan PT, Garnett MJ, Roe SM, Lee S, Niculescu-Duvaz D, Good VM, Jones CM, Marshall CJ, Springer CJ, Barford D, Marais R (2004) Mechanism of activation of the RAF-ERK signaling pathway by oncogenic mutations of B-RAF. Cell 116:855–867

West KA, Sianna Castillo S, Dennis PA (2002) Activation of the PI3K/Akt pathway and chemotherapeutic resistance. Drug Resistance Updates 5:234–248

Whitesell L, Lindquist SL (2005) Hsp90 and the chaperoning of cancer. Nat Rev Cancer 5:761–772

Whitesell L, Mimnaugh EG, De Costa B, Myers CE, Neckers LM (1994) Inhibition of heat shock protein HSP90-pp60v-src heteroprotein complex formation by benzoquinone ansamycins: essential role for stress proteins in oncogenic transformation. Proc Natl Acad Sci USA 91:8324–8328

Whyte DB, Kirschmeier P, Hockenberry TN, Nunez-Oliva I, James L, Catino JJ, Bishop WR, Pai J-K (1997) K- and N-Ras are geranylgeranylated in cells treated with farnesyl protein transferase inhibitors. J Biol Chem 272:14459–14464

Wilhelm SM, Carter C, Tang L, Wilkie D, McNabola A, Rong H, Chen C, Zhang X, Vincent P, McHugh M, Cao Y, Shujath J, Gawlak S, Eveleigh D, Rowley B, Liu L, Adnane L, Lynch M, Auclair D, Taylor I, Gedrich R, Voznesensky A, Riedl B, Post LE, Bollag G, Trail PA (2004) BAY 43-9006 exhibits broad spectrum oral antitumor activity and targets the RAF/MEK/ERK pathway and receptor tyrosine kinases involved in tumor progression and angiogenesis. Cancer Res 64:7099–7109

Xu GF, Lin B, Tanaka K, Dunn D, Wood D, Gesteland R, White R, Weiss R, Tamanoi F (1990a) The catalytic domain of the neurofibromatosis type 1 gene product stimulates ras GTPase and complements ira mutants of S. cerevisiae. Cell 63:835–841

Xu GF, O'Connell P, Viskochil D, Cawthon R, Robertson M, Culver M, Dunn D, Stevens J, Gesteland R, White R, et al. (1990b) The neurofibromatosis type 1 gene encodes a protein related to GAP. Cell 62:599–608

Yang JC, Haworth L, Sherry RM, Hwu P, Schwartzentruber DJ, Topalian SL, Steinberg SM, Chen HX, Rosenberg SA (2003) A randomized trial of bevacizumab, an anti-vascular endothelial growth factor antibody, for metastatic renal cancer. N Engl J Med 349:427–434

Yano M, Naito Z, Tanaka S, Asano G (1996) Expression and roles of heat shock proteins in human breast cancer. Jpn J Cancer Res 87:908–915

Zaal LH, Mooi WJ, Sillevis Smitt JH, van der Horst CMAM (2004) Classification of congenital melanocytic naevi and malignant transformation: a review of the literature. BrJ Plastic Surg 57:707–719

Zeng Q, Si X, Horstmann H, Xu Y, Hong W, Pallen CJ (2000) Prenylation-dependent association of protein-tyrosine phosphatases PRL-1, -2, and –3 with the plasma membrane and the early endosome. J Biol Chem 275:21444–21452

Zeng Q, Dong J-M, Guo K, Li J, Tan H-X, Koh V, Pallen CJ, Manser E, Hong W (2003) PRL-3 and PRL-1 promote cell migration, invasion, and metastasis. Cancer Res 63:2716–2722

The Mitogen-Activated Protein Kinase Pathway for Molecular-Targeted Cancer Treatment

Judith S. Sebolt-Leopold, Roman Herrera, and Jeffrey F. Ohren

Recent Results in Cancer Research, Vol. 172
© Springer-Verlag Berlin Heidelberg 2007

9.1 Introduction

The molecular characterization of key events associated with tumor initiation and progression has led to the identification of cellular signaling pathways that contribute not only to normal cell functioning but also to the overall phenotype associated with cancer. One such example is the Ras-regulated kinase pathway. This signaling module, comprising Raf, mitogen-activated protein kinase kinase (MEK), and extracellular signal-regulated kinase (ERK), plays a central role in regulating a broad range of cellular events. In response to a diverse group of extracellular stimuli including growth factors, cytokines, and proto-oncogenes, activation of this pathway results in alterations in cell proliferation, differentiation, and survival. It is therefore not surprising that this pathway has been found to be upregulated in a large percentage of human tumors. While contributing to the uncontrolled growth and enhanced survival of tumor cells, the Ras-MAP kinase pathway also plays a key role in their metastatic spread by regulating cell motility and invasion.

By virtue of its pivotal role in mediating these hallmarks of neoplasia, the Ras-MAP kinase signaling module provides molecular targets with the potential for broad therapeutic applications in oncology. As shown in Fig. 9.1 and reviewed elsewhere, activation of the small G protein Ras leads to a cascade of phosphorylation events, starting with activation of the serine/threonine kinase Raf (Downward 2003). Phosphorylated Raf, in turn, activates MEK, which then phosphorylates and activates ERK (also referred to as MAPK). Nuclear translocation of activated ERK is subsequently the trigger for the activation of a number of transcription factors, including ETS family members such as ELK1, resulting in a major impact on the phenotype of a given tumor. As a consequence of its role in transcriptional regulation, the expression of critical cell cycle regulatory proteins, for example, cyclin D, are under the control of the MAP kinase pathway. Activation of this pathway is therefore critical for enabling cells to progress through the G1 phase of the cell cycle (Pruitt and Der 2001). In addition, several other downstream kinases become activated in response to this signaling cascade, including 90-kDa ribosomal S6 protein kinase (RSK). Consequently, phosphorylation and inactivation of the proapoptotic protein BAD as well as phosphorylation of the transcription factor CREB serve to link MAP kinase pathway activation with survival response (Shimamura et al. 2000; Bonni et al. 1999).

Not unexpectedly, the MAPK pathway is subjected to tight control under physiological normal conditions. In addition to the major protein players, namely Ras, Raf, MEK, and ERK, a number of scaffolding proteins and endogenous inhibitors have been identified that play a role in determining the dynamics of this pathway (Kolch 2005). These proteins have been found to influence signal

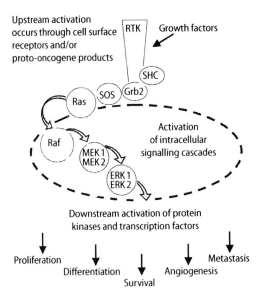

Fig. 9.1 Activation of the mitogen-activated protein kinase signaling pathway results in pleiotropic cellular responses

for members of the MAPK family of proteins (p38, Jun kinase, and ERK) and represent an unexplored field in the development of therapeutic strategies to control the Ras-Raf-ERK pathway (Farooq and Zhou 2004).

Over the last decade a number of drug discovery programs have been launched that target the downstream kinases in this signaling cascade. The reader is referred else for a comprehensive review on various therapeutic approaches that have been attempted for targeting the MAP kinase pathway (Sebolt-Leopold and Herrera 2004). These approaches encompass both nonkinase (e.g., farnesyltransferase) as well as kinase targets. We will review here the biology surrounding Raf and MEK, the rationale for targeting these proteins, and the progress to date in delivering clinical candidates that will hopefully provide answers on the validity of targeting the MAP kinase pathway for the therapeutic intervention of cancer.

flux, cross talk with other pathways, and subcellular localization of MEK/ERK complexes, thereby affording cells the flexibility to redirect signals away from the Ras-MAP kinase pathway. One such event that has implications for carcinogenesis is the cross talk interaction between the MAPK pathway and Smad-controlled signaling. Smad signaling is under control of the TGF-β family of growth factors. TGF-β plays a dual role in tumorigenesis. At an early stage of cancer development, TGF-β is known to induce cell cycle arrest and apoptosis. However, at later stages of tumorigenesis, TGF-β facilitates tumor metastasis by inducing expression of metalloproteinases and angiogenesis along with a downregulation of the immune system. The cooperation between the MAPK and Smad pathways can be illustrated, for example, in the induction of epithelial-mesenchymal transition (EMT), an event associated with aggressive invasion by certain tumors (Derynck et al. 2001).

Negative regulation of the MAPK pathway occurs in response to the dephosphorylation events that are controlled by the mitogen-induced MAPK phosphatases. These dual-specificity phosphatases have differential affinity

9.2 Structure and Biochemical Function of Raf and MEK

9.2.1 Raf

Members of the Raf serine/threonine kinase family, comprised of A-Raf, B-Raf, and C-Raf (Raf-1), share a common structure consisting of three conserved regions (Fig. 9.2). CR1 is the Ras binding region, CR2 is the regulatory domain negatively regulating Raf activity by virtue of phosphorylation by Akt or protein kinase A at a serine residue (S259), and CR3 is the kinase domain, with phosphorylation sites at S338 and tyrosine residues Y340 and Y341.

Raf isoforms, which vary in their cell-specific expression, have a number of overlapping as well as unique regulatory functions (Hagemann and Rapp 1999). Raf regulation is complex, with many questions still unanswered. The reader is referred elsewhere for a comprehensive review on this topic (Baccarini 2005). Clearly, the activation of B-raf appears to be much less complicated than that of Raf-1 and appears to only require Ras binding and

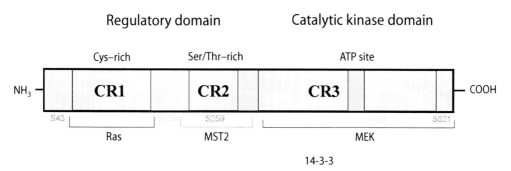

Fig. 9.2 Schematic diagram of the conserved structural elements of the Raf proteins. The three Raf isoforms, A-Raf, B-Raf and C-Raf (Raf-1) share multiple structural elements including the three conserved regions (CR), colored blue. CR1 contains the cysteine-rich (Cys-rich) domain that participates in both Ras binding and membrane recruitment. Phosphorylation of serine 43 (S43, C-Raf numbering) disrupts Ras binding to Raf. CR2 contains a serine and threonine-rich domain (Ser/Thr-rich) involved in negative regulatory interactions with the scaffolding/adapter proteins mammalian-sterile-like-2 (MST2) and 14-3-3. Phosphorylation of S338 activates Raf, while phosphorylation of S259 and S621 help to maintain Raf in an inactive conformation. CR3 consists of the kinase domain responsible for the phosphorylation and activation of MEK. The highly conserved ATP binding site (colored green) is where many of the activating, oncogenic mutants of Raf are found (see text for more details). Threonine 491 (T491) and S494 are the two conserved phosphorylation sites located in the activation segment of Raf. The pale purple areas depict regions of Raf that are variable among isoforms (Wellbrock et al. 2004; Kolch 2005; Beeram et al. 2005; Sridhar et al. 2005)

phosphorylation of the activation segment to disrupt intramolecular autoinhibition.

While most published work on the role of Raf in Ras-MAP kinase signaling has been carried out with Raf-1, emerging data have made a compelling case for B-raf serving as the primary MEK kinase in vivo. B-raf is the isoform that binds best to MEK and also exhibits the highest basal MEK kinase activity (Papin et al. 1996; Marais et al. 1997). Based on comparison of mammalian Raf kinases to those from lower organisms, it is now thought that A-Raf and Raf-1 have diverged to perform other functions (Baccarini 2005).

MEK is believed to be the sole physiological substrate for B-Raf. However, B-Raf mutant proteins that are unable to phosphorylate MEK in vitro have recently been shown to be capable of activating the MEK/ERK module in vivo by binding and activating Raf-1 (Wan et al. 2004). This finding provides yet more compelling evidence for the complexity that surrounds the central role of Raf regulatory events.

Determination of the crystal structure of B-Raf has led to significant advances in our understanding of the function of this protein (Wan et al. 2004). The overall structures of both wild-type and mutant (V599E) enzymes are comparable to other inactivated protein kinases like ABL and p38. The inhibitor BAY 43-9006, which will be discussed in a later section, binds to the ATP pocket and interacts with residues in both the P-loop and the kinase activation loop. Inhibition of Raf catalytic activity is most likely achieved by prevention of the activation loop and the catalytic residues from adopting a conformation that is competent to bind and phosphorylate substrate. As depicted in Fig. 9.3, binding of BAY43-9006 inhibits Raf activity by deforming the active site residues E593 and F594 that make up the conserved DFG motif (DFG). The proposed mechanism of action is that the inhibitor stabilizes an inactive conformation of Raf in which the side chain of F594 is rotated out into a DFG-out conformation. This mechanism is almost identical to that found for the inhibition of Abl kinase by Gleevec (Wan et al. 2004).

9.2.2 MEK

Conserved structural elements of the MEK proteins are depicted in Fig. 9.4. Both MEK ho-

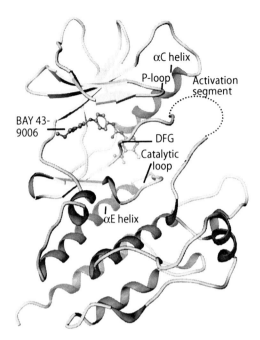

Fig. 9.3 Ribbon diagram of the B-Raf kinase domain bound to BAY43-9006. The wild-type B-Raf kinase domain structure (PDB code 1UWH) is shown here in the standard orientation with the typical bilobal architecture of a protein kinase. The amino terminus lobe is composed primarily of anti-parallel β-strands, including the glycine-rich or phosphate binding loop (P-loop) responsible for functional binding of ATP. A key structural component of the amino-terminus domain is α-helix C (αC helix). The kinase activation segment contains the Raf family conserved phosphorylation sites, T491 and S494. In this crystal structure, as in many other protein kinase structures, the Raf activation segment is disordered and indicated here with a dotted line. The carboxyl-terminal lobe is primarily composed of α-helices. The α-helix E (αE helix) functions to position the C-terminal catalytic residues (R574, E575, and N580) in the proper orientation for the binding of MEK substrate and the phosphotransfer reaction. The potent and selective Raf inhibitor BAY43-9006 is shown here binding in the kinase active site located between the two lobes

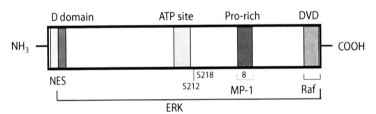

Fig. 9.4 Schematic diagram of the conserved structural elements of the MEK proteins. MEK1 and MEK2 are highly homologous and share most structural elements including the docking domain (D domain, colored light blue), a cluster of basic and hydrophobic residues that facilitates MEK binding to its ERK substrate. Removal of the D domain by the anthrax lethal factor completely disrupts ERK binding and subsequent activation by MEK. The nuclear export sequences (NES, colored purple) function to maintain MEK's cellular location in the cytoplasm. The conserved ATP binding site (colored green) is responsible for the phosphorylation and activation of ERK substrate. S212 is a negative regulatory element conserved among all MAPKKs that is located just amino-terminal to S218 and S222. Phosphorylation of S212 is performed by an unknown kinase and presumably inactivates MEK by folding the activation segment into an autoinhibited conformation. S218 and S222 (MEK1 numbering) are the two conserved sites of Raf phosphorylation located in the activation segment of MEK. The proline-rich domain (Pro-rich, colored blue) is unique to MEK1 and MEK2 and is not found in the other MAPKK family members. The Pro-rich domain contains several regulatory phosphorylation sites and mediates MEK binding to ERK as well as to the scaffolding/adaptor protein MP-1. The domain for versatile docking site (DVD, colored orange) has recently been identified as a highly conserved structural motif in all MAPKKs and functions to mediate binding of the MAPKKs with their upstream activators, in this case, MEK1 binding to Raf (Chen et al. 2001; Gopalbhai et al. 2003; Ohren et al. 2004; Takekawa et al. 2005)

mologs, MEK1 and MEK2, are phosphorylated and activated on two distinct serine residues, Ser218 and Ser222, by Raf kinases. These critical phosphorylation sites lie in a regulatory loop between conserved kinase subdomains (Alessi et al. 1994; Hanks and Quinn 1991). If these serine residues are substituted with negatively charged amino acids, for example, aspartate or glutamate, MEK becomes constitutively activated, presumably through stabilization of the regulatory loop, allowing MEK to retain an active conformation (Alessi et al. 1994). The location of a proline-rich region near the carboxyl terminus is critical for Raf association and contains a number of phosphorylation sites for various kinases, including MAP kinase, adding another dimension to the regulation of MEK activity (Catling et al. 1995; Frost et al. 1997). Finally, the amino-terminal end of MEK (amino acids 1–67) also plays a role in regulating kinase activity. The putative MAP kinase docking site is located within the first 32 amino acids of MEK and these residues alone are sufficient for in vitro binding of MAP kinase (Fukuda et al. 1997).

MEK proteins are dual-specificity kinases in nature, uniquely sharing the consensus kinase motifs of both serine/threonine as well as tyrosine kinases. The most notable feature distinguishing MEK1 and MEK2 from other dual-specificity kinases is the high level of stringency that they exhibit in phosphorylating their ERK substrates. Both MEK isoforms sequentially phosphorylate ERK1 and ERK2 at two sites, initially Tyr185 followed by Thr183 (Haystead et al. 1992). MEK2 is the most active ERK activator, being roughly seven times more catalytically active than MEK1 (Zheng and Guan 1993). Accessory factors, for example, MP1 (MEK Partner 1), have been shown to enhance the lowered activity of MEK1 by acting as adapters to increase its efficiency (Schaeffer et al. 1998).

MEK1 and MEK2 are ubiquitously expressed in mammals. Lower organisms, for example, C. elegans and Drosophila, have only one MEK gene to fulfill the function of both MEK1 and MEK2, suggesting both overlapping and distinct functions for the mammalian homologs, which are encoded by two distinct genes lo-

cated on different chromosomes (Brott et al. 1993). Multiple lines of evidence further point to distinctly different functions for MEK1 and MEK2. MEK1 appears to be more highly upregulated than MEK2 in ras-transformed cells and appears to be differentially regulated by Raf. MEK2 has never been detected in a Ras/Raf/MEK ternary complex, consistent with MEK1 showing a high degree of autophosphorylation in the proline-rich region, which has been shown to be absent in MEK2 (Catling et al. 1995).

No substrates for MEK have been identified other than ERK1 and ERK2 (Seger et al. 1992). This tight selectivity in addition to the ability to phosphorylate both tyrosine and threonine residues are consistent with this kinase playing a central role in the integration of signals into the MAPK pathway. Thus MEK regulates a crossover point in the MAP kinase pathway where the signaling cascade becomes less pleiotropic.

Structural analysis of human MEK1 and MEK2 has provided answers to how highly selective inhibitors of MEK, to be covered later in this review, can bind to MEK without perturbing the ATP site (Ohren et al. 2004; see Fig. 9.5). As in the case of Raf, the proposed mechanism of action for these highly selective inhibitors is that they stabilize an inactive conformation of the MEK activation loop. In contrast to the Raf-BAY43-9006 complex, the MEK ATP binding site is unaffected by the binding of one such highly selective MEK inhibitor, PD318088. This mechanism of inhibition is highly unusual and may be the result of PD318088 locking the kinase into an autoinhibitory conformation that mimics one caused by the phosphorylation of S212 (Gopalbhai et al. 2003; Ohren et al. 2004).

9.3 Role of the Ras-MAPK Pathway in Promoting Tumor Growth and Progression

Activating mutations of many of the components of this pathway have been found to be associated with a broad array of human can-

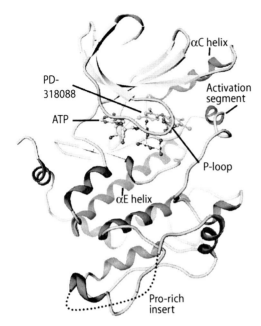

Fig. 9.5 Ribbon diagram of the MEK1 kinase domain bound to PD318088. The wild-type human MEK1 kinase domain structure (PDB code 1S9J) is shown here slightly rotated from the standard orientation in order to better show the concurrent binding of ATP and the small-molecule inhibitor PD318088. The role of the P-loop in ATP binding is evident from this view as the loop sits directly over the phosphates of ATP. As in the Raf structure the position of the αC helix is rotated slightly upward relative to the C-terminal lobe to accommodate the inhibitor-bound position of the activation segment. The kinase activation segment of MEK1 is unphosphorylated in this structure and contains the conserved phosphorylation sites, S218 and S222. The position of the αE helix is shown directly below the bound inhibitor, while the proline-rich insert, which is unique to MEK1 and MEK2, is shown as a dotted line. The potent and exquisitely selective MEK inhibitor PD318088 is shown here binding in the kinase active site directly behind ATP

cers. Mutations in any one of the three Ras proto-oncogenes, H-ras, K-ras, and N-ras, convert these genes into active oncogenes. The highest incidence of K-ras mutations is found in carcinomas of the pancreas (90%), colon (50%), and lung (30%). H-ras and N-ras mutations are found at a high frequency in thyroid tumors (50%) and myeloid leukemias (30%), respectively.

The oncogenic nature of B-raf has also recently been demonstrated, as evidenced by a 50%–70% incidence of B-raf mutations in melanomas and a 30% incidence in papillary thyroid carcinomas (Davies et al. 2002; Kimura et al. 2003; Pollock and Meltzer 2002). Particularly noteworthy is the fact that both melanocyte and thymocyte growth are positively regulated by cAMP. The vulnerability of both cell types to transformation by B-raf-activating mutations may be explained by B-raf's unique capability to transduce cAMP-dependent growth signals in these cells (Busca et al. 2000; Iacovelli et al. 2001). B-raf mutations, albeit at a lower frequency, also occur in a diverse array of other tumor types, including carcinomas of colorectal, lung, ovarian, and breast origin (Davies et al 2002; Singer et al. 2003; Brose et al. 2002). B-raf appears to fulfill the requirements of a classic oncogene, as mutations of this gene bestow significant elevation of kinase activity, constitutively activating MAP kinase in vivo in the absence of Ras activation. The association of activating mutations of components of the Ras-MAP kinase pathway with a wide array of human tumors clearly points to the important role of this signaling module in neoplastic transformation.

Irrespective of mutational status of upstream receptor tyrosine kinases, Ras, and Raf, upregulation of MAP kinase activity has been observed in a large percentage of human cancers. It has been reported that 50 of 138 tumor cell lines tested (36%) showed constitutive ERK activation, including lines of pancreatic, lung, and colon origin (Hoshino et al. 1999). Increased flux through the pathway may also lead to increased tumor cell expression of growth factors, further serving to stimulate activation of MAP kinase in an autocrine fashion (Steelman et al. 2004). The role of activated MAP kinase in cell cycle progression is well documented (Lavoie et al. 1996). Furthermore, MAP kinase signaling has been shown to be important in the regulation of cell motility and angiogenesis (Mercer and Pritchard 2003). Collectively, data point to a pivotal role for the Ras/Raf/MEK/ERK signaling module in driving tumorigenesis. Consequently, components of this pathway emerge as attractive therapeutic targets for the design of novel molecular-targeted cancer treatments.

9.4 Identification of Small-Molecule Inhibitors

Therapeutic strategies that target Raf seem ideally suited to address the high percentage of human cancers displaying constitutive activation of the MAP kinase pathway. An excellent review on this topic appears elsewhere and includes coverage of antisense oligonucleotide approaches (Beeram et al. 2005). Other therapeutic approaches include inhibitors of chaperone proteins, for example, Hsp90, which act to indirectly inhibit Raf by destabilization of the protein leading subsequently to its degradation. The impressive efficacy of geldanamycin analogs, which are naturally occurring antibiotics, is well documented but likely results from their broader pleiotropic effects (Maloney and Workman 2002).

Few small-molecule Raf kinase inhibitors have been reported. L-779450 and SB203580 have both been shown to be more effective at inhibiting c-Raf than B-Raf (Shelton et al. 2003; Lackey et al. 2000). Without question, the Raf kinase inhibitor that has received the most attention is BAY 43-9006 (Sorafenib, Fig. 9.6). High-throughput screening of small molecules against c-Raf kinase first uncovered this ATP-competitive bi-aryl urea class of Raf inhibitors (Thompson and Lyons 2005). Crystallographic analysis of wild-type and V599E B-raf kinase domains in complex with Sorafenib indicates that inhibition by this agent is most likely achieved by its ability to prevent the activation loop and the catalytic residues from adopting a conformation that is competent to bind and phosphorylate substrate (Wan et al. 2004). Interestingly, most oncogenic mutations of B-raf occur in either the activation loop or the P-loop. Therefore it is believed that B-raf mutations act to destabilize the inactive conformation of the protein kinase, thereby favoring an activated state of the enzyme. While Sofafenib, which targets c-Raf more potently than B-raf, was shown to inhibit the activation of MAP kinase in a wide array of tumor cell lines, it was later shown to inhibit a number of additional kinases important to tumor proliferation and angiogenesis. Other kinases potently inhibited by Sofafenib include VEGFR2, PDGFR, Flt-3, and c-Kit. As will be discussed in a later section, the multitargeted mechanistic nature of this agent clouds our ability to attribute its preclinical and clinical efficacy to B-raf inhibition.

The development of pharmacological inhibitors of MEK was launched with the identification of PD98059 as a highly selective small-molecule inhibitor of this kinase (Dudley et al. 1995). PD98059 proved to be the first of several non-ATP-competitive MEK inhibitors that have now been reported. However, owing to unfavorable pharmaceutical attributes including poor solubility, this compound was released to the academic community and has subsequently become a highly useful probe for exploring the role of the MAP kinase pathway in a broad array of physiological processes. U0126 subsequently emerged from cell-based screening efforts to identify inhibitors of phorbol ester-induced AP-1 activity (Favata et al. 1998). This inhibitor, which also exhibits non-ATP-competitive kinetics, results in significantly enhanced potency relative to PD98059 (Ahn et al. 2001). U0126 is believed to exert its cellular effects by suppressing MEK1 activation rather than by blocking its activity (Davies et al. 2000). Neither PD98059 nor U0126 has the requisite pharmaceutical profile to warrant clinical evaluation.

As reviewed elsewhere, a number of ATP-competitive MEK inhibitors have also been reported (Wallace et al. 2005). To the best of our knowledge, however, none of these compounds has proceeded into clinical development. We will now turn our attention to discussion of highly selective MEK inhibitors that have produced pharmaceutical profiles warranting advanced development. The remarkable selectivity of each of these agents, CI-1040, PD0325901, and ARRY-142886, is thought to be due to their unique noncompetitive mechanism of inhibition, which is now better understood based on crystallographic analysis of MEK bound to a small molecule inhibitor that is a close structural analog to CI-1040 (Fig. 9.5).

9.4.1 CI-1040 and PD0325901

PD184352 (CI-1040) was the first reported MEK inhibitor to inhibit tumor growth in animals.

Therefore this orally active compound, which is a substituted N-aryl anthranilic acid (Fig. 9.6) provided much-needed in vivo validation for targeting MEK in the cancer drug development arena. Owing to its non-ATP-competitive nature, CI-1040 was found to be highly selective against a broad panel of protein kinases (Sebolt-Leopold et al. 1999). Drug discovery efforts dedicated to optimizing the pharmaceutical profile of CI-1040 subsequently resulted in the clinical advancement of the structurally related PD0325901 (Fig. 9.6). The comparative preclinical profiles of these two agents will be described in the next section.

9.4.2 ARRY-142886 (AZD 6244)

Similarly reported to be a potent and highly selective MEK inhibitor, ARRY-142886 is also non-ATP-competitive (Wallace et al. 2005). Unfortunately, the exact chemical structure of this substituted benzimidazole has not been reported (Fig. 9.6). This agent, which shares a number of features exhibited by CI-1040 and PD0325901, is also currently undergoing clinical evaluation.

9.5 Preclinical Profile of MAP Kinase Pathway Inhibitors

9.5.1 Sorafenib

In cellular assays, Sorafenib has been shown to inhibit basal phosphorylation of MAP kinase in a panel of human melanoma, pancreatic, and colon cancer cell lines that were either wild type or expressed mutant K-ras or B-raf (Thompson and Lyons 2005). Generally, concentrations in the range of 1 μM were required to inhibit pERK signaling in these cell lines. Complete tumor stasis was observed in vivo for a number of tumor models, but in some cases activity appeared to be independent of K-ras status. Furthermore, Sorafenib did not always lower levels of MAP kinase phosphorylation in tumors despite tumor sensitivity, for example, the A549 lung model. It is likely that the contaminating receptor tyrosine kinase activities of Sorafenib account for this apparent disassociation of efficacy from effects on MAP kinase signaling. Furthermore, Sorafenib was found to decrease microvessel density in these same tumors, consistent with the notion that efficacy stems from the ability of this agent to

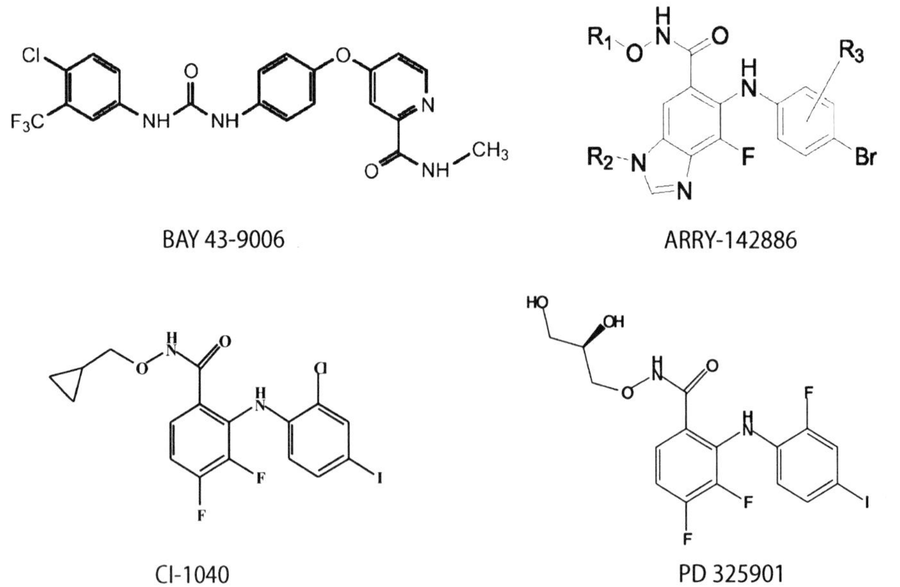

BAY 43-9006

ARRY-142886

CI-1040

PD 325901

Fig. 9.6 MAP kinase pathway inhibitors advanced into clinical testing

target VEGF-mediated angiogenesis (Wilhelm et al. 2004).

9.5.2 MEK Inhibitors

CI-1040, which was shown to inhibit purified MEK1 and MEK2 with an IC50 of 17 nM, was roughly one log less potent at inhibiting basal phosphorylation of MAP kinase in colon 26 carcinoma cells grown in culture (Sebolt-Leopold et al. 1999). Importantly, CI-1040 was shown to be orally active in tumor-bearing animals, possessing significant antitumor activity in a broad array of xenograft models, particularly carcinomas of the pancreas, colon, lung, and breast (Allen et al. 2003). Tumor regressions were commonly observed over a wide range of doses in this tumor panel, and evidence of apoptosis was obtained.

Consistent with ERK activation being required for growth factor-induced secretion of angiogenic factors from tumor cells, CI-1040 was also found to reduce VEGF secretion from A431 cells when tested at concentrations as low as 50 nM (Sebolt-Leopold 2004). CI-1040 has also been shown to effectively block HGF-induced activation of MAP kinase in colon carcinoma cells, profoundly affecting the ability of these cells to scatter. Corollary studies further showed that CI-1040 resulted in decreased invasiveness, consistent with the potential for this agent to inhibit tumor metastasis (Sebolt-Leopold et al. 1999).

Based on its promising preclinical profile, encompassing effects on proliferation, survival, invasion, and secretion of proangiogenic growth factors, CI-1040 was advanced into clinical trials. Meanwhile, as this agent was undergoing development, it possessed a number of properties for pharmaceutical improvement that served as the basis for a discovery program dedicated to identifying a back-up compound. Namely, issues surrounding its metabolic instability and poor bioavailability were key factors at the forefront of this research program. With the subsequent emergence of PD0325901, these limitations were successfully addressed. In addition, target potency relative to that of CI-1040 was greatly enhanced in PD0325901, as evidenced by its ability to effectively inhibit both purified MEK and basal MAP kinase phosphorylation at concentrations in the 1 nM range (Sebolt-Leopold and Herrera 2004).

ARRY-142886, with a cellular IC50 of 50 nM, was also shown to elicit antitumor activity when orally administered. Tumor growth was inhibited in a diverse panel of tumor xenografts of colon, breast, and skin origin (Wallace et al. 2005). As observed for CI-1040 and PD0325901, pancreatic adenocarcinoma xenografts proved to be especially sensitive to the effects of ARRY-142886. This agent also is currently undergoing clinical evaluation in cancer patients.

9.6 Role of Pharmacodynamic Assays in Target and Compound Validation

Pharmacodynamic markers are critical for providing proof of concept that a test agent is successfully modulating a given target and that modulation of that target translates into an efficacious outcome. The MAP kinase pathway is particularly amenable to pharmacodynamic evaluation, as commercially available antibodies exist that are specific for dually phosphorylated ERK1 and ERK2. Furthermore, in vivo evaluation of MEK inhibition can easily be measured in excised samples. Phosphorylated MAP kinase is the product of MEK activity and thus represents a direct measure of MEK inhibition. The utility of pharmacodynamic assays for measuring in vivo MEK inhibition was first demonstrated for CI-1040 administered to tumor-bearing animals (Sebolt-Leopold et al. 1999). These early studies were critical for demonstrating in preclinical samples a direct correlation between target suppression and antitumor response. At the preclinical stage, pharmacodynamic assays are also useful for optimizing dosing regimens so as to maximize therapeutic response. For example, early pharmacodynamic studies with CI-1040 in animals revealed that effective suppression of MAP kinase phosphorylation could only be achieved for a few hours after a single oral dose (Sebolt-Leopold et al. 1999). This finding led to the routine use of twice-a-day dosing regimens in order to keep the target suppressed for the duration of treatment.

Importantly, these assays were instrumental in showing that efficacy could be achieved at doses that were well tolerated and correlated with a reduction of the levels of activated MAP kinase in tumor samples. Pharmacodynamic assays also have the potential to be informative for preclinical toxicology assessment, as a wide range of tissues or cells can be tested for target modulation. Clearly the absence of target inhibition at exposure levels resulting in dose-limiting toxicity would evoke hesitation before proceeding into the clinic with a given drug candidate.

As will be described in the next section, the successful incorporation of robust pharmacodynamic assays in clinical trials is critical for addressing the extent of target modulation required for eliciting objective and meaningful patient responses. Therein lie the answers to the clinical validation of both the target and the clinical agent under study.

9.7 Clinical Trials

Sorafenib is currently the subject of an extensive number of clinical trials. The recent regulatory approval of this agent for advanced renal tumors signifies a major advance in the treatment of this refractory cancer. However, efficacy against renal cancer provides yet more compelling evidence for the activity of this agent being a consequence of its effective inhibition of VEGF receptors. This supposition is based on prior track records of other effective VEGF-directed therapies, for example, bevacizumab and Sutent, against human renal cancer. Thus it remains unclear whether the Raf kinase component of Sorafenib's profile contributes to the therapeutic outcome of these trials (Sebolt-Leopold and English 2006).

CI-1040 represents the first truly selective inhibitor of MAP kinase signaling to enter the clinic. Early evidence showing greater than 50% inhibition of tumor MAP kinase phosphorylation in evaluable phase I biopsies was encouraging. In addition, there were early hints of activity, as a pancreatic cancer patient exhibited a partial response and was on study for roughly 1 year (LoRusso et al. 2005). Because of its poor metabolic stability and bioavailability, large doses (800 mg administered twice a day) were required to see this degree of target modulation. Subsequent phase II trial results were discouraging, and development of this agent was terminated in favor of commencing clinical studies with PD0325901 (Rinehart et al. 2004).

PD0325901 and ARRY-142886 are currently undergoing clinical evaluation. A phase I study with PD0325901 demonstrated that this agent, as anticipated, is significantly more potent than CI-1040, as reflected by a starting dose of 1 mg in these trials (LoRusso et al. 2005). Two-thirds of the patients enrolled in this study had melanoma and therefore had highly accessible tumor tissue for monitoring target response to this agent. Consequently, it was determined that very low doses of PD0325901 in the 1–2 mg range were sufficient to inhibit phosphorylation of MAP kinase by greater than 90%. At this early stage of clinical testing, it is too soon to gauge the degree of clinical activity afforded by treatment with PD0325901. However, the high incidence of B-raf mutations in melanomas suggests that this patient population might prove highly susceptible to treatment with a MEK or B-raf inhibitor (Davies et al. 2002; Satyamoorthy et al. 2003). Preclinical data reported by Solit et al. for B-raf-mutated melanoma xenografts in mice treated with PD0325901 support this prediction (Solit et al. 2006). It is therefore encouraging that early signs of activity of PD0325901 have been noted in two melanoma patients, as reflected by their partial responses, as well as the notable incidence of stable disease in patients with melanoma, non-small-cell lung, or colorectal cancer (LoRusso et al. 2005).

9.8 Looking Forward

We now have available novel inhibitors selectively targeting the Raf/MEK/ERK pathway for providing ultimate clinical validation of this therapeutic approach.

The success of molecular targeted therapy will likely be facilitated as technological advances are made that aid us in steering patients toward a customized therapy that is predicated on the genetic and biochemical attributes of the given tumor. Tumors that exhibit mutations in either B-raf or one of the Ras proto-oncogenes may prove to be more susceptible to treatment with a MAP kinase pathway inhibitor than tumors without these defects. Gene expression signatures may also prove highly useful in determining the extent to which multiple signaling pathways are activated (Bild 2006; Downward 2006). As we increase our understanding of the cellular events regulated by the Ras/Raf/MEK/ERK signaling module, the design of rational combination therapy protocols using agents designed to impair multiple critical pathways will likely show greatest therapeutic gain. In the meantime, it is imperative that we persevere in developing a diverse array of highly potent, pharmaceutically attractive agents with demonstrated effectiveness against key targets. The pivotal role of the Ras-MAP kinase pathway in driving tumor proliferation and survival makes Raf and MEK inhibitors strong candidates for clinical development.

References

Ahn NG, Nahreini TS, Tolwinski NS, Resing KA (2001) Pharmacological inhibitors of MKK1 and MKK2. Methods Enzymol 332:417–431

Allen LF, Sebolt-Leopold J, Meyer MB (2003) CI-1040 (PD184352), a targeted signal transduction inhibitor of MEK (MAPKK). Semin Oncol 30:105–116

Alessi DR, Saito Y, Campbell DG, Cohen P, Sithanaandam G, Rapp U, Ashwort A, Marshall C, Cowley S (1994) Identification of the sites in MAP kinase kinase-1 phosphorylated by p74raf-1. EMBO J 13:1610–1619

Baccarini M (2005) Second nature: biological functions of the Raf-1 "kinase". FEBS Lett 579:3271–3277

Beeram M, Patnaik A, Rowinsky EK (2005) Raf:a strategic target for therapeutic development against cancer. J Clin Oncol 23:6771–6790

Bild AH, Yao G, Chang JT, Wang Q, Potti A, Chasse D, Joshi MB, Harpole D, Lancaster JM, Berchuck A, Olson JA Jr, Marks JR, Dressman HK, West M, Nevins JR (2006) Oncogenic pathway signatures in human cancers as a guide to targeted therapies. Nature 439:353–357

Bonni A, Brunet A, West AE, Datta SR, Takasu MA, Greenberg ME (1999) Cell survival promoted by the Ras-MAPK signaling pathway by transcription-dependent and -independent mechanisms. Science 286:1358–1362

Brose MS, Volpe P, Feldman M, Kumar M, Rishi I, Gerrero R, Einhorn E, Herlyn M, Minna J, Nicholson A, Roth JA, Albelda SM, Davies H, Cox C, Brignell G, Stephens P, Futreal PA, Wooster R, Stratton MR, Weber BL (2002) BRAF and RAS mutations in human lung cancer and melanoma. Cancer Res 62:6997–7000

Brott BK, Alessandrini A, Largaespada DA, Copeland NG, Jenkins NA, Crews CM, Erikson RL (1993) MEK2 is a kinase related MEK1 and is differentially expressed in murine tissues. Cell Growth Differ 4:921–929

Busca R, Abbe P, Mantoux F, Aberdam E, Peyssonnaux C, Eychene A, Ortonne JP, Ballotti R (2000) Ras mediates the cAMP-dependent activation of extracellular signal-regulated kinases (ERKs) in melanocytes. EMBO J 19:2900–2910

Catling AD, Schaeffer HJ, Reuter CW, Reddy GR, Weber MJ. (1995) A proline-rich sequence unique to MEK1 and MEK2 is required for Raf binding and regulates MEK function. Mol Cell Biol 15:5214–5225

Chen Z, Gibson TB, Robinson F, Silvestro L, Pearson G, Xu B, Wright A, Vanderbilt C, Cobb MH (2001) MAP kinases. Chem Rev 101:2449–2476

Davies H, Bignell GR, Cox C, Stephens P, Edkins S, Clegg S, Teague J, Woffendin H, Garnett MJ, Bottomley W, Davis N, Dicks E, Ewing R, Floyd Y, Gray K, Hall S, Hawes R, Hughes J, Kosmidou V, Menzies A, Mould C, Parker A, Stevens C, Watt S, Hooper S, Wilson R, Jayatilake H, Gusterson BA, Cooper C, Shipley J, Hargrave D, Pritchard-Jones K, Maitland N, Chenevix-Trench G, Riggins GJ, Bigner DD, Palmieri G, Cossu A, Flanagan A, Nicholson A, Ho JW, Leung SY, Yuen ST, Weber BL, Seigler HF, Darrow TL, Paterson H, Marais R, Marshall CJ, Wooster R, Stratton MR, Futreal PA (2002) Mutations of the BRAF gene in human cancer. Nature 417:949–954

Davies SP, Reddy H, Caivano M, Cohen P (2000) Specificity and mechanism of action of some commonly used protein kinase inhibitors. Biochem J 351:95–105

Derynck R, Akhurst RJ, Balmain A (2001) TGF-beta signaling in tumor suppression and cancer progression. Nat Genet 29:117–129

Downward J (2003) Targeting ras signalling pathways in cancer therapy. Nat Rev Cancer 3:11–22

Downward J (2006) Signatures guide drug choice. Nature 439:274–275

Dudley DT, Pang L, Decker SJ, Bridges AJ, Saltiel AR (1995) A synthetic inhibitor of the mitogen-activated protein kinase cascade. Proc Natl Acad Sci USA 92:7686–7689

Farooq A, Zhou MM (2004) Structure and regulation of MAPK phosphatases. Cell Signal 16:769–779.

Favata MF, Horiuchi KY, Manos EJ, Daulerio AJ, Stradley DA, Feeser WS, Van Dyk DE, Pitts WJ, Earl RA, Hobbs F, Copeland RA, Magolda RL, Scherle PA, Trzaskos JM (1998) Identification of a novel inhibitor of mitogen-activated protein kinase kinase. J Biol Chem 273:18623–18632

Frost JA, Steen H, Shapiro P, Lewis T, Ahn N, Shaw PE, Cobb MH (1997) Cross-cascade activation of ERKs and ternary complex factors by Rho family proteins. EMBO J 16:6426–6438

Fukuda M, Gotoh Y, Nishida E (1997) Interaction of MAP kinase with MAP kinase kinase:its possible role in the control of nucleocytoplasmic transport of MAP kinase. EMBO J 16:1901–1908

Gopalbhai K, Jansen G, Beauregard G, Whiteway M, Dumas F, Wu C, Meloche S (2003) Negative regulation of MAPKK by phosphorylation of a conserved serine residue equivalent to Ser212 of MEK1. J Biol Chem 278:8118–8125

Hagemann C and Rapp UR (1999) Isotype-specific functions of Raf kinases. Exp Cell Res 253:34–46

Hanks SK and Quinn AM (1991) Protein kinase catalytic domain sequence database: identification of conserved features of primary structure and classification of family members. Methods Enzymol 200:38–62

Haystead TA, Dent P, Wu J, Haystead CM, Sturgill TW (1992) Ordered phosphorylation of p42mapk by MAP kinase kinase. FEBS Lett 306:17–22

Hoshino R, Chatani Y, Yamori T, Tsuruo T, Oka H, Yoshida O, Shimada Y, Ari-I S, Wada H, Fujimoto J, Kohno M (1999) Constitutive activation of the 41-/43-Da mitogen-activated protein kinase signaling pathway in human tumors. Oncogene 18:813–822

Iacovelli L, Capobianco L, Salvatore L, Sallese M, D'Ancona GM, DeBlasi A (2001) Thyrotropin activates mitogen-activated protein kinase pathway in FRTL-5 by a cAMP-dependent protein kinase A-independent mechanism. Mol Pharmacol 60:924–933

Kimura ET, Nikiforova MN, Zhu Z, Knauf JA, Nikiforov YE, Fagin JA (2003) High prevalence of BRAF mutations in thyroid cancer: genetic evidence for constitutive activation of the RET/PTC-RAS-BRAF signaling pathway in papillary thyroid carcinoma. Cancer Res 63:1454–1457

Kolch W (2005) Coordinating ERK/MAPK signalling through scaffolds and inhibitors. Nat Rev Mol Cell Biol 6:827–837

Lackey K, Cory M, Davis R, Frye SV, Harris PA, Hunter RN, Jung DK, McDonald OB, McNutt RW, Peel MR, Rutkowske RD, Veal JM, Wood ER (2000) The discovery of potent cRaf1 kinase inhibitors. Bioorg Med Chem Lett 10:223–226

Lavoie JN, L'Allemain G, Brunet A, Muller R, Pouyssegur J (1996) Cyclin D1 expression is regulated positively by the p42/p44MAPK and negatively by the p38/HOGMAPK pathway. J Biol Chem 271:20608–20616

LoRusso PM, Adjei, AA, Varterasian M, Gadgeel S, Reid J, Mitchell DY, Hanson L, deLuca P, Bruzek L, Piens J, Asbury P, VanBecelaere K, Herrera R, Sebolt-Leopold JS, Meyer MB (2005) Phase 1 and pharmacodynamic study of the oral MEK inhibitor CI-1040 in patients with advanced malignancies. J Clin Oncol 23:5281–5293

LoRusso PM, Krishnamurthi S, Rinehart JR, Nabell L, Croghan G, Varterasian M, Sadis S, Menon SS, Leopold J, Spear MA, Meyer MB (2005) A phase 1–2 clinical study of a second generation oral MEK inhibitor, PD0325901 in patients with advanced cancer. Proc Am Soc Clin Oncol 24:Abst 3011

Maloney A and Workman P (2002) HSP90 as a new therapeutic target for cancer therapy:the story unfolds. Expert Opin Biol Ther 2:3–24

Marais R, Light Y, Paterson HF, Mason CS, Marshall CJ (1997) Differential regulation of Raf-1, A-Raf, and B-Raf by oncogenic ras and tyrosine kinases. J Biol Chem 272:4378–4383

Mercer KE and Pritchard CA (2003) Raf proteins and cancer:B-Raf is identified as a mutational target. Biochim Biophys Acta 1653:25–40

Ohren JF, Chen H, Pavlovsky A, Whitehead C, Zhang E, Kuffa P, Yan C, McConnell P, Spessard C, Banotai C, Mueller WT, Delaney A, Omer C, Sebolt-Leopold J, Dudley DT, Leung IK, Flamme C, Warmus J, Kaufman M, Barrett S, Tecle H, Hasemann CA (2004) Structures of human MAP kinase kinase 1 (MEK1) and MEK2 describe novel noncompetitive kinase inhibition. Nat Struct Mol Biol 11:1192–1197

Papin C, Denouel A, Calothy G, Eychene A (1996) Identification of signalling proteins interacting with B-Raf in the yeast two-hybrid system. Oncogene 12:2213–2221

Pollock PM and Meltzer PS (2002) A genome-based strategy uncovers frequent BRAF mutations in melanoma. Cancer Cell 2:5–7

Pruitt K, Der CJ (2001) Ras and Rho regulation of the cell cycle and oncogenesis. Cancer Lett. 171:1–10

Rinehart J, Adjei AA, LoRusso PM, Waterhouse D, Hecht JR, Natale RB, Hamid O, Varterasian M, Asbury P, Kaldjian EP, Gulyas S, Mitchell DY, Herrera R, Sebolt-Leopold JS, Meyer MB (2004) Multicenter phase II study of the oral MEK inhibitor, CI-1040, in patients with advanced non-small-cell lung, breast, colon, and pancreatic cancer. J Clin Oncol 22:4456–4462

Satyamoorthy K, Li G, Gerrero MR, Brose MS, Volpe P, Weber BL, VanBelle P, Elder DE, Herlyn M (2003) Constitutive mitogen-activated protein kinase activation in melanoma is mediated by both BRAF mutations and autocrine growth factor stimulation. Cancer Res 63:756–759

Schaeffer HJ, Catling AD, Eglen ST, Collier LS, Krauss A, Weber MJ (1998) MP1: a MEK binding partner that enhances enzymatic activation of the MAP kinase cascade. Science 281:1668–1671

Sebolt-Leopold JS (2004) MEK inhibitors:a therapeutic approach to targeting the Ras-MAP kinase pathway in tumors. Curr Pharm Design 10:1907–1914

Sebolt-Leopold JS and Herrera R (2004) Targeting the mitogen-activated protein kinase cascade to treat cancer. Nat Rev Cancer 4:937–947

Sebolt-Leopold JS and English JM (2006) Mechanisms of drug inhibition of signaling molecules. Nature, 441:457–462.

Sebolt-Leopold JS, Dudley DT, Herrera R, Van Becelaere K, Wiland A, Gowan RC, Tecle H, Barrett SD, Bridges A, Przybranowski S, Leopold WR, Saltiel AR (1999) Blockade of the MAP kinase pathway suppresses growth of colon tumors in vivo. Nature 5:810–816.

Seger R, Ahn NG, Posada J, Munar ES, Jensen AM, Cooper JA, Cobb MH, Krebs EG (1992) Purification and characterization of mitogen-activated protein kinase activator(s) from epidermal growth factor-stimulated A431 cells. J Biol Chem 267:14373–14381

Shelton JG, Moye PW, Steelman LS, Blalock WL, Lee JT, Franklin RA, McMahon M, McCubrey JA (2003) Differential effects of kinase cascade inhibitors on neoplastic and cytokine-mediated cell proliferation. Leukemia 17:1765–1782

Shimamura A, Ballif BA, Richards SA, Blenis J (2000) Rsk1 mediates a MEK-MAP kinase cell survival signal. Curr. Biol. 10:127–135

Singer G, Oldt RIII, Cohen Y, Wang BG, Sidransky D, Kurman RJ, Shih IeM (2003) Mutations in BRAF and KRAS characterize the development of low-grade ovarian serous carcinoma. J Natl Cancer Inst 95:484–486

Solit DB, Garraway LA, Pratilas CA, Sawai A, Getz G, Basso A, Ye Q, Lobo JM, She Y, Osman I, Golub TR, Sebolt-Leopold J, Sellers WR, Rosen N (2006) BRAF mutation predicts sensitivity to MEK inhibition. Nature 439:358–362

Sridhar SS, Hedley D, Siu LL (2005) Raf kinase as a target for anticancer therapeutics. Mol Cancer Ther 4:677–685

Steelman LS, Pohnert SC, Shelton JG, Franklin RA, Bertrand FE, McCubrey JA (2004) JAK/STAT, Raf/MEK/ERK, PI3K/Akt and BCR-ABL in cell cycle progression and leukemogenesis. Leukemia 18:189–218

Takekawa M, Tatebayashi K, Saito H (2005) Conserved docking site is essential for activation of mammalian MAP kinase kinases by specific MAP kinase kinases. Mol Cell 18:295–306

Thompson N and Lyons J (2005) Recent progress in targeting the Raf/MEK/ERK pathway with inhibitors in cancer drug discovery. Curr Opin Pharm 5:350–356

Wallace EM, Lyssikatos JP, Yeh T, Winkler JD, Koch K (2005) Progress towards therapeutic small molecule MEK inhibitors for use in cancer therapy. Curr Top Med Chem 5:215–229

Wan PT, Garnett MJ, Roe SM, Lee S, Niculescu-Duvaz D, Good VM, Jones CM, Marshall CJ, Springer CJ, Barford D, Marais R, Cancer Genome Project (2004) Mechanism of activation of the RAF-ERK signaling pathway by oncogenic mutations of B-RAF. Cell 116:855–867

Wellbrock C, Karasarides M, Marais R (2004) The Raf proteins take centre stage. Nat Rev Mol Cell Biol 5:875–885

Wilhelm SM, Carter C, Tang LY, Wilkie D, McNabola A, Rong H, Chen C, Zhang X, Vincent P, McHugh M, Cao Y, Shujath J, Gawlak S, Eveleigh D, Rowley B, Liu L, Adnane L, Lynch M, Auclair D, Taylor I, Gedrich R, Voznesensky A, Riedl B, Post LE, Bollag G, Trail PA (2004) BAY 43–9006 exhibits broad spectrum oral antitumor activity and targets the RAF/MEK/ERK pathway and receptor tyrosine kinases involved in tumor progression and angiogenesis. Cancer Res 64:7099–7109

Zheng CF and Guan KL (1993) Properties of MEKs, the kinases that phosphorylate and activate the extracellular signal-regulated kinases. J Biol Chem 268:23933–23939

Clinical Relevance of Targeted Interference with Src-Mediated Signal Transduction Events

Quan P. Ly and Timothy J. Yeatman

Recent Results in Cancer Research, Vol. 172
© Springer-Verlag Berlin Heidelberg 2007

10.1 Rationale for Targeting Src in Human Diseases

In the past decade, we have gained substantial insight into various signal transduction and molecular pathways regulating cancer cells. Moreover, we have recently been able to develop specific targeted therapies instead of classic chemotherapeutics that attempt to essentially provide more toxicity to the tumor than the normal cell. As a result, we have been able to decrease adverse side effects, thus improving the quality of life of cancer patients.

To better understand this concept of targeted therapy, we will focus on c-Src, a ubiquitous protein involved in multiple aspects of normal cell function as well as carcinogenesis, osteoporosis, and myocardial infarction. The clinical relevance of studying c-Src will be illustrated as we summarize its molecular structure, mechanisms of regulation, and new inhibitors targeting specific function.

In 1909, Peyton Rous first proposed that an infectious viral agent might transmit chicken sarcoma. It took almost 50 years for the scientific community to be convinced that the Rous sarcoma virus (RSV) produced infected tumor cells (Rubin 1955). Another 20 years passed before this viral genome (v-src) was sequenced. In 1976, researchers also sequenced cellular src (c-src) and found that it is a normal human proto-oncogene distinct from v-src. More importantly, there is evidence to show that transforming viruses capture cellular genes as well as inserting transforming genes into the host genomes (Martin 2004). Comparing the structures of these two nonreceptor kinases, v-src lacks the carboxy-terminal domain but contains numerous point mutations throughout the molecule, which explain the high level of activity of the protein. For the purpose of this chapter, we will only focus on c-src and its derivative protein, c-Src.

Although c-Src kinase has been linked to the development and progression of cancer for many years, only recently has there been renewed interest in this oncoprotein as a molecular target for cancer therapy, prevention of tissue injuries after myocardial infarction, as well as stopping the progression of osteoporosis. Before we can understand c-Src regulation, however, we need to understand its structure.

10.2 Structure and Function of Src

Both the avian and human forms of the c-Src protein are composed of a C-terminal tail containing a negative-regulatory tyrosine residue, four Src homology (SH) domains, and a unique amino-terminal domain (Fig. 10.1). The SH1 kinase domain contains the conserved tyrosine residue involved in autophosphorylation. The SH2 domain interacts with

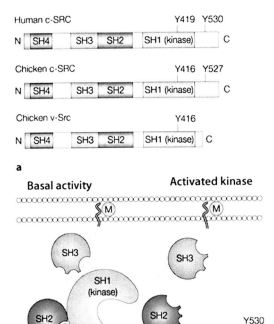

Fig. 10.1a, b. Structure and function of Src. (Reprinted from Yeatman 2004, Nature Reviews)

10.2.1 Src Activation

The activation of c-Src can be accomplished by protein phosphatases, receptor mediated kinases, nitric oxide, and a certain point mutation resulting in a truncated Src (Fig. 10.2).

There are several protein phosphatases that act as c-Src activators by removing the phosphate from the C-terminus. Protein tyrosine phosphatase-α (PTP-α) has been shown to activate c-Src by dephosphorylating the tyrosine residue in the Src C-terminus. By the same mechanism, it also activates other phosphatases involved in the regulation of c-Src like protein tyrosine phosphatase (PTP1), SH2-containing phosphatase 1 (SHP1), and SHP2. Alternatively, the phosphorylation of Tyr215 (homolog of Tyr213 in mouse and Tyr220 in rodents) in the SH2 domain in response to PDGF stimulation appears to prevent the binding of the Tyr530 of the C-terminus, thus increasing c-Src activity (Zhao et al. 2003).

Besides phosphorylation, extracellular signaling via receptor activation is another way to activate c-Src, probably by disrupting the intramolecular interaction and unfolding c-Src into an activated configuration (Yeatman 2004). Since several receptor tyrosine kinases have been linked with c-Src overexpression in many cancers, this implies that these kinases promote tumorigenesis by cooperative or synergistic interactions. Cotransfection of epithelial growth factor receptor (EGFR) and c-Src into murine fibroblasts results in increased proliferation, invasiveness, and tumorigenesis (Tice et al. 1999). Other ligand-activated receptor tyrosine kinases implicated in c-Src activation are PDGFR, ERBB2 (or HER2/NEU), fibroblast growth factor receptor (FGFR), colony-stimulating factor 1, and hepatocyte growth factor (Mao et al. 1997). With the current availability of a number of EGFR-targeted therapies, this raises the intriguing possibility that both the EGFR and Src may be simultaneously targeted for therapy, with a potential synergistic inhibition of tumor growth and progression.

Another proposed mechanism of c-Src regulation is nitric oxide. Nitric oxide activates v-Src by preferentially phosphorylating the tyrosine residue within the SH1 region but not that

the negative-regulatory tyrosine (Tyr530 in human and Tyr 527 in chicken) in the inactive or closed form, but in the active or open form this site may bind to platelet-derived growth factor receptor (PDGFR). The activation of Src by PDGFR stimulation is thought to induce cell proliferation in smooth muscle cells (Chen Z et al. 2006) as well as pancreatic stellate cells (Masamune et al. 2005). The SH3 domain promotes intramolecular contact with the kinase domain, resulting in a closed and inactive form of the protein. The SH4 domain has a myristoylation site, which is important in the localization of the protein in the cell membrane. Finally, the N-terminal domain is implicated in the transformating ability of the Src protein (Cross et al. 1985).

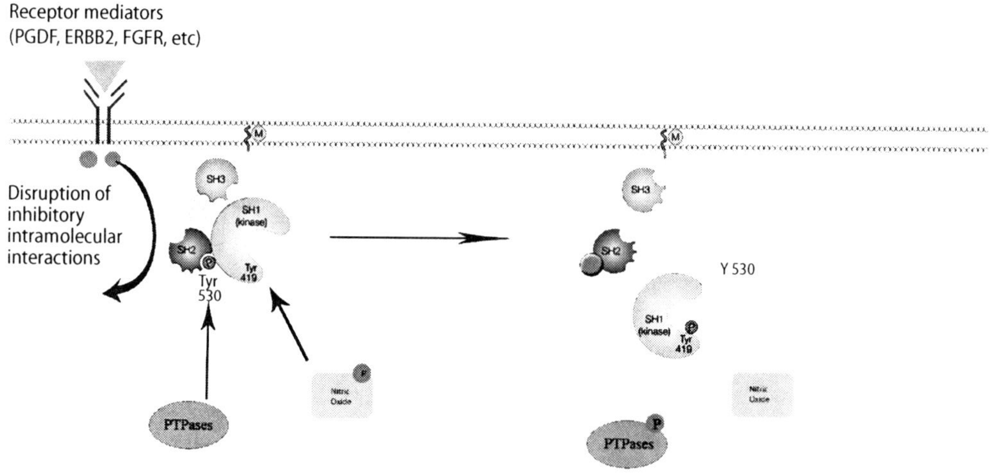

10 Clinical Relevance of Targeted Interference with Src-Mediated Signal Transduction Events

Fig. 10.2 Src activation

in the C-terminus, thus activating Src (Akhand et al. 1999).

And finally, a point mutation (Src531) that results in a truncated form of c-Src, one that has six amino acids deleted from the "negative-regulatory" C-terminus, was described in a subset of human colon cancers as constitutively activated (Yeatman 2004). While a rare occurrence, this finding provided the needed impetus to push Src forward in the drug development pipeline, resulting in the production of several new targeting agents now undergoing clinical trials.

10.2.2 Src Inactivation

As mentioned above, Src regulation is tightly controlled in normal cells. Understanding its precise mechanisms of inactivation would help us target these sites and reverse the effects of activated Src. Src inactivation is mostly accomplished by dephosphorylation and ubiquitylation (Fig. 10.3). C-terminal Src kinase (CSK) and its homolog (CHK) can inactivate c-Src protein by phosphorylating the tyrosine residue in the C-terminus. Structurally, CSK is similar to c-Src but lacks the negative-regulatory domain of the c-Src C-terminus. There is mounting evidence to suggest that reduced expression of CSK may be involved in human carcinogenesis (Masaki et al. 1999; Cam et al. 2001). Furthermore, the level of CSK expres-

sion has been shown to play a pivotal role in epithelial cell differentiation and metastatic potential (Boyer et al. 2002).

Another mechanism of c-SRC down-regulation is ubiquitylation (Kim et al. 2004). In normal cells, Src activation increases the extent of polyubiquitination and thus marks the proteins for proteasomic degradation. The presence of proteasome inhibitors increases the level of Src proteins (Hakak and Martin 1999). Furthermore, CBL ubiquitin ligase can suppress v-Src transformation in fibroblast through ubiquitin-dependent protein degradation (Kim et al. 2004).

10.2.3 Regulation of c-SRC Localization

Like Ras, the localization of c-Src within the cellular infrastructure is important to its function. The association of c-Src with the inner layer of the plasma membrane is considered essential for cellular transformation and the autophosphorylation of Tyr419 that occurs with membrane targeting. The phosphorylation of Tyr419, enabled by interactions with activated receptor tyrosine kinases, is associated with the highest level of c-Src transforming activity.

The inactive form of c-Src is localized at the perinuclear sites, but when activated its SH3 domain becomes indirectly associated with

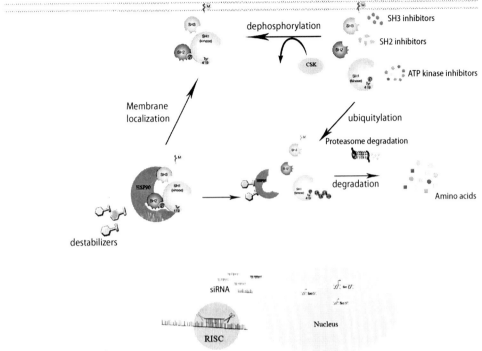

Fig. 10.3 Src inactivation

actin and is ultimately translocated to the cell periphery to sites of cell adhesion, where it attaches to the plasma membrane inner surface through its myristoylated SH4 domain. This tethered location allows for interactions with membrane-bound receptor tyrosine kinases and integrins associated with adhesion functions. The localization of c-Src at the membrane-cytoskeletal interface is an important interface in focal adhesions, formations of lamellipodia and filopodia. This localization process seems to be regulated by the G-proteins RhoA, RAC1, and CDC42 (Timpson et al. 2001).

10.2.4 Molecular Mechanism of Function

Src functions are multiple. Adhesion, invasion, and motility are related events that require several well-orchestrated molecular interactions. For example, motility, by definition, requires alterations in cell-cell and cell-matrix adhesion, and invasion requires alterations in both adhesion and motility. The assembly and dispersement of intercellular junctions that mediate adhesion is associated with both significant cytoskeletal alterations and integrin signaling, which allow morphological changes and alterations in motility and invasiveness.

10.2.5 Adhesion

Focal adhesions are dynamic structures that assemble to allow cells to adhere to the extracellular matrix, and dispersement would promote cell suspension. Besides providing the physical structures for cell-matrix attachment, focal adhesions also participate in cell-signaling processes that regulate proliferation and gene transcription. They are composed of over 50 different proteins – such as talin, vinulin, α-actinin, c-Src, FAK, CAS, and paxillin (Zamir and Geiger 2001). These cytoskeletal proteins are recruited to focal adhesions to mediate cellular migration. They are associated with cytoskeletal stress fibers, composed of actin and myosin, that control the shape and, ultimately, the motility of the cell.

The assembly of cell focal adhesions requires RhoA, a small GTP-binding protein that regulates actin cytoskeletal organization (Fujisawa et al. 1998). Specifically, for cells to adhere to each other, they must form stable junctions mediated by E-cadherin molecules on the cell surface (Chen et al. 1999). E-cadherin recruits first β-catenin then α-catenin, which binds to actin cytoskeleton (Aberle et al. 1994). This complex stabilizes the adherens junction. Thus, for a cell to move along or away from the ECM, c-Src is activated, which would disassemble the focal adhesions between the cell and its neighbor by suppressing E-cadherin localization and function at a crucial contact point. This process is seen in normal cellular migration and mitosis as well as during transformation (Hynes 1992).

10.2.6 Motility

Motility is a highly coordinated, multistep event that includes formation of cellular protrusions, their attachments to the ECM, traction and release of adhesions from other cells and from the basement membrane matrix. Cells are thought to move directionally by extending protrusions, forming stable attachments near the leading edge of these protrusions, propelling forward, releasing the adhesions, and retracting of the rear end (Lauffenburger and Horwitz 1996). The process whereby adhesions at the cell front disassemble as new adhesions form is called "adhesion turnover" (Laukaitis et al. 2001). Integrin-matrix contact is crucial in the stabilization of adhesions by recruiting cytoskeletal and signaling proteins. Cytoskeletal actin polymerization, sliding over myosin, propels the cell forward. c-Src not only disrupts the adherens junction but also enhances the adhesion turnover, thus increasing the cell motility. Many investigators are working on identifying the mechanisms for the formation and disassembly of these structures (Yeatman 2004).

10.2.7 Invasion

Cellular invasion occurs with the loss of E-cadherin expression. There are now data to show that E-cadherin reexpression suppresses invasion (Perl et al. 1998). As mentioned above, c-Src prevents E-cadherin localization to the cell membrane and thus inhibits focal adhesion and enhances motility. In addition, evidence indicates that FAK, a substrate of c-Src, signals to c-JUN N-terminal kinase, promoting the expression of matrix metalloproteases (MMP2 and MMP9) (Hsia et al. 2003). These matrix metalloproteases have been shown to degrade the matrix proteins, allowing cells to invade through the basement membrane (Crowe et al. 2001). These principles operate in both developmental and neoplastic processes.

10.3 SRC Expression Imparts a Metastatic Phenotype

10.3.1 Tumor Metastasis

In many cancers, c-Src kinase overexpression is associated with advancing stage, particularly in tumors that have metastasized. We now know that altered c-Src expression and activity may affect proliferation, cell adhesion, motility, and invasion, all of which directly influence the cell's metastatic potential. Interestingly, c-Src expression in cancer cells might have more significant effects on tumor growth rates in vivo (Irby et al. 1997) than on cell proliferation rates in vitro (Jones et al. 2002). Despite the effects on tumor growth rates, overexpression of wild-type c-Src does not seem to be sufficient to enhance metastatic potential (Irby et al. 1997). One of the more active forms, like c-Src531 (a truncated form that lacks six C-terminal inhibitory amino acids), appears to permit cells to achieve distant organ colonization (Boyer et al. 2002). Conversely, overexpression of Csk, a negative regulator of c-Src, suppresses metastasis in murine models (Nakagawa et al. 2000). Src expression and activity seem to be significantly increased in metastatic lesions compared to primary sites (Termuhlen et al. 1993).

10.3.2 Angiogenesis Promotion

Src proteins also seem to impart angiogenic activity. It has been shown that v-Src induces vascular endothelial growth factor (VEGF) expression through signal transducer and activator of transcription 3 (STAT3) activation (Yu et al. 1995; Niu et al. 2002). STAT3 activation by v-Src has also been shown to enhance cell proliferation and survival as well as immune evasion (Yu and Jove 2004). Furthermore, antisense c-src inhibits hypoxia-induced VEGF production and expression, thus indicating a direct relationship between Src and VEGF. Recent studies showed that endothelial cells with kinase-inactive c-SRC failed to spread and form cordlike structures (Kilarski et al. 2003). In addition, these cells have reduced phosphorylation of cortactin and paxillin, which would affect the stability of the actin cytoskeleton and thus motility. Inhibition of endothelial cell migration would prevent angiogenesis. To further demonstrate the relationship between VEGF and Src, many studies found that Src inhibitors, such as PP2, SU11333, and CGP77675 can inhibit invasive growth, sprouting of endothelial and vascular smooth muscle cells, as well as VEGF-induced vascular permeability (Laird et al. 2003).

10.3.3 Bone Resorption (Osteoporosis)

Despite the ubiquitous nature of Src in many cell types, Src-/- mice display osteopetrosis as the only observable phenotype(Soriano et al. 1991). Furthermore, osteoclasts isolated from Src-/- mice show abnormal cellular morphology and an unorganized actin cytoskeleton at the site of adhesion to the bone matrix (Boyce et al. 1992). These cells also lack the so-called ruffled border, which ultimately impairs their bone-resorbing activity resulting in osteopetrotic mice (Shakespeare et al. 2000). However, mice that lack only the Src-homology 2-containing inositol-5 phosphatase (SHIP), are severely osteoporetic. Interestingly, although these mice are viable and fertile, they all developed myeloproliferative disorder at 14 weeks (Helgason et al. 1998). Apparently the absence of SHIP enhances the sensitivity of marrow macrophages to M-CSF and RANKL, resulting in an increased number of large, hyperactive osteoclasts, which lead to severe osteoporosis (Takeshita et al. 2002). As mentioned above, the SH2 domain has a specific binding site for the Tyr530 of the C-terminus in the closed state, but in the opened form this is the site for receptor-mediated Src activation. Therefore, Src inhibitors, specifically SH2 inhibitors, would be predicted to reduce osteoclast activity and potentially reverse osteoporosis.

10.3.4 Postmyocardial Infarction Edema and Tissue Injury

Ischemia resulting from myocardial infarction (MI) has been associated with VEGF expression, leading to vascular permeability and edema, a process that contributes to tissue injury throughout the ventricle. At the cellular level, gaps are formed between adjacent endothelial cells. Within these gaps are activated platelets adhering to exposed basement membrane, thus reducing vessel patency. When VEGF is injected intravascularly into healthy animals, similar endothelial gaps, vascular permeability, platelet plugs, and myocyte damage are seen as the results. This effect was abrogated in Src-deficient mice. Mechanistically, the tight adherens junctions between the endothelial cells are transiently disrupted by VEGF; and blocking Src prevents the disassociation of this complex and thus the vascular permeability after VEGF exposure (Weis et al. 2004).

10.4 SRC Inhibitors and Clinical Application

Given the implication of c-Src in many pathways of carcinogenesis for numerous cancers, it seems prudent to employ various Src kinase inhibitors to block tumor progression and possibly promote tumor regression. There are currently three major classes of Src inhibitors being used in clinical trials: ATP-competitive kinase inhibitors, SH2/SH3 blockers, and c-Src destabilizing agents (Table 10.1).

10 Clinical Relevance of Targeted Interference with Src-Mediated Signal Transduction Events

Table 10.1 Src inhibitors and clinical application

Name	Company	Primary reference	Src kinase IC_{50} (nM)	Other kinase inhibited	Cell lines/ disease tested
ATP competitive Src kinase inhibitors					
PP1	Pfizer	Hanke et al. 1996	50–170	Hck, Fyn	T cells
PP2	Pfizer	Hanke et al. 1996	100	Lck, Fyn	T cells
AP23846	Ariad Pharmaceutical	Summy et al. 2005	0.5	Yes, Lyn, Lck and Hck	L3.6pl, HT29, PC3, endothelials
CGP76030	Novartis	Recchia et al. 2003	200	Lyn, Hck, Fgr	32D, COS7, K562, LAMA, U937, HL60 and OCI-AML5
CGP77675	Novartis	Missbach et al. 1999	5–20	Lck, Yes	MC3T3-E1, PC3
PD173955	Parke-Davis	Kraker et al. 2000	22	Yes	MDA-MBs
AZM475271	AstraZeneca	Yezhelyev et al. 2004	10	Lck, Yes	L3.6pl, 3T3
SU6656	Sugen	Blake et al. 2000	280	Fyn, Yes, Lyn, Lck, Abl	3T3, PMNs, B cells, glial cells
BMS354825	Bristol Myers	O'Hare et al. 2005	0.8	Lyn, Abl	BaF3
SKI-606	Wyeth	Boschelli et al. 2001	1.2	Lyn, Hck, Abl	K562, Ku812 (MOLT4, HL60, Ramos are not affected)
AZD0530	AstraZeneca	Hennequin et al. 2005	2.7	Abl	MCF7, MDA-MB231, NIH3T3,
SH2/SH3 inhibitors					
AP22408	Ariad Pharmaceutical	Shakespeare et al. 2000	300	Lck	Osteoclasts, Y527
UCS15A	Kyowa Hakko Kogyo Co	Oneyama et al. 2003	N/A–see text	Fyn	HCT116; 3T3
Src destabilizing agents					
Geldanamycin	Invitrogen	Uehara et al. 1988; An et al. 2000	<10 (bind HSP 90)	Lck, Hck	T cells, COS7, K562, PC12, N2A, HT29
Herbimycin	Calbiochem	Weinstein et al. 1991	12.000 (12 μM)	Bcr, Abl	3T3, HUVEC, CCL239,HT29

An WG, Schulte TW, Neckers LM (2000) The heat shock protein 90 antagonist geldanamycin alters chaperone association with p210bcr-abl and v-src proteins before their degradation by the proteasome. Cell Growth Differ 11:355–360

Blake RA, Broome MA, Liu X, Wu J, Gishizky M, Sun L, Courtneidge SA (2000) SU6656, a selective src family kinase inhibitor, used to probe growth factor signaling. Mol Cell Biol 20:9018–9027

Boschelli DH, Wang YD, Ye F, Wu B, Zhang N, Dutia M, Powell DW, Wissner A, Arndt K, Weber JM, Boschelli F (2001) Synthesis and Src kinase inhibitory activity of a series of 4-phenylamino-3-quinolinecarbonitriles. J Med Chem 44:822–833

Hanke JH, Gardner JP, Dow RL, Changelian PS, Brissette WH, Weringer EJ, Pollok BA, Connelly PA (1996) Discovery of a novel, potent, and Src family-selective tyrosine kinase inhibitor. Study of Lck- and FynT-dependent T cell activation. J Biol Chem 271:695–701

Hennequin LF, Allen J, Costello G, Fennell M, Green TP, Jacobs V, Morgentin R, Olivier A, Ple PA (2005) The discovery of AZD0530: a novel, oral, highly selective and dual-specific inhibitor of the Src and Abl family kinases. Proc Am Assoc Cancer Res 46:A2537

Kraker AJ, Hartl BG, Amar AM, Barvian MR, Showalter HD, Moore CW.(2000) Biochemical and cellular effects of c-Src kinase-selective pyrido[2, 3-d]pyrimidine

tyrosine kinase inhibitors. Biochem Pharmacol 60:885–898

Missbach M, Jeschke M, Feyen J, Muller K, Glatt M, Green J, Susa M (1999) A novel inhibitor of the tyrosine kinase Src suppresses phosphorylation of its major cellular substrates and reduces bone resorption in vitro and in rodent models in vivo. Bone 24:437–449

O'Hare T, Walters DK, Stoffregen EP, Jia T, Manley PW, Mestan J, Cowan-Jacob SW, Lee FY, Heinrich MC, Deininger MW, Druker BJ (2005) In vitro activity of Bcr-Abl inhibitors AMN107 and BMS-354825 against clinically relevant imatinib-resistant Abl kinase domain mutants. Cancer Res 65:4500–4505

Oneyama C, Agatsuma T, Kanda Y, Nakano H, Sharma S.V, Nakano S. Narazaki T, Tatsuta K (2003) Synthetic inhibitors of proline-rich ligand-mediated protein-protein interaction: potent analogs of UCS15A. Chem Biol 10:443–451

Oneyama C, Nakano H, Sharma SV (2002) UCS15A, a novel small molecule, SH3 domain-mediated protein-protein interaction blocking drug. Oncogene 21:2037–2050

Recchia I, Rucci N, Festuccia C, Bologna M, MacKay AR, Migliaccio S, Longo M, Susa M, Fabbro D, and Teti A (2003) Pyrrolopyrimidine c-Src inhibitors reduce growth, adhesion, motility and invasion of prostate cancer cells in vitro. Eur J Cancer 39:1927–1935

Shakespeare W, Yang M, Bohacek R, Cerasoli F, Stebbins K, Sundaramoorthi R, Azimioara M, Vu C, Pradeepan S, Metcalf C 3rd, Haraldson C, Merry T, Dalgarno D, Narula S, Hatada M, Lu X, van Schravendijk MR, Adams S, Violette S, Smith J, Guan W, Bartlett C, Herson J, Iuliucci J, Weigele M, Sawyer T (2000) Structure-based design of an osteoclast-selective, nonpeptide src homology 2 inhibitor with in vivo antiresorptive activity. Proc Natl Acad Sci USA 97:9373–9378

Summy JM, Trevino JG, Lesslie DP, Baker CH, Shakespeare WC, Wang Y, Sundaramoorthi R, Metcalf CA 3rd, Keats JA, Sawyer TK, Gallick GE (2005) AP23846, a novel and highly potent Src family kinase inhibitor, reduces vascular endothelial growth factor and interleukin-8 expression in human solid tumor cell lines

and abrogates downstream angiogenic processes. Mol Cancer Ther 4:1900–1911

Uehara Y, Murakami Y, Suzukake-Tsuchiya K, Moriya Y, Sano H, Shibata K, Omura S (1988) Effects of herbimycin derivatives on src oncogene function in relation to antitumor activity. J Antibiot (Tokyo) 41:831–834

Weinstein SL, Gold MR, DeFranco AL (1991) Bacterial lipopolysaccharide stimulates protein tyrosine phosphorylation in macrophages. Proc Natl Acad Sci USA 88:4148–4152

Yezhelyev MV, Koehl G, Guba M, Brabletz T, Jauch KW, Ryan A, Barge A, Green T, Fennell M, Bruns CJ (2004) Inhibition of SRC tyrosine kinase as treatment for human pancreatic cancer growing orthotopically in nude mice. Clin Cancer Res 10:8028–8036

Pyrimidines based

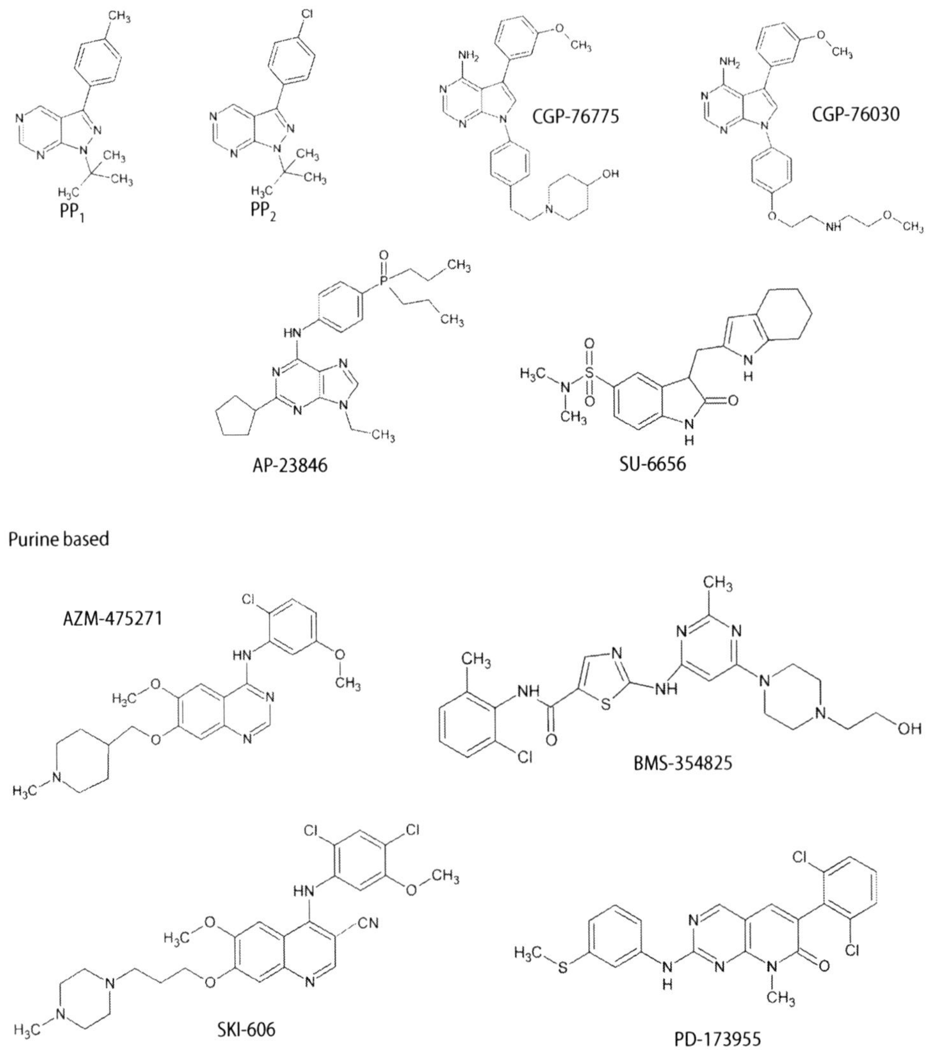

Purine based

Fig. 10.4 ATP-competitive Src kinase inhibitors

10.4.1 ATP-Competitive SRC Kinase Inhibitors

ATP-competitive SRC kinase inhibitors block the phosphotransferase activity of various phosphorylation sites of various kinase activities (Fig. 10.4). For an inhibitor to be effective, it must have high specificity due to significant homology in the primary as well as the tertiary structure of the ATP binding pockets of different kinases (Chen T et al. 2006).

PP1 (4-amino-5(4-methylphenyl)-7-(t-butyl) pyrazolo[3,4-d]pyrimidine) and PP2 (4-amino-5-(4-chlorophenyl)-7-(t-butyl)pyrazolo[3,4-d]pyrimidine) were first identified as ATP-competitive inhibitors of Src family kinases (Chen T et al. 2006). These two compounds have been used extensively to study the role of c-Src kinase in multiple cellular events. The specific site of PP1 activity corresponds to the Thr338 in c-Src. Mutation of this threonine in v-Src to methionine or phenylalanine would decrease PP1 affinity, while a substitution of alanine or glycine for the threonine would increase PP1 potency (Liu et al. 1999). Besides c-Src, PP1 was also found to strongly inhibit P21-activated kinase (PAK) at lower concentration than that required for c-Src inhibition, explaining PP1 inhibition of fibroblast anchorage-independent growth in soft agar (He et al. 2000). More recently, PP1 and PP2 were shown to inhibit c-Src not by competitively binding to ATP pocket, but by "mixed competition" for the space between the C-terminal and the N-terminal of the inactive Src form (Karni et al. 2003). Specifically, when PP1 or PP2 binds to c-Src, it causes a conformation change preventing ATP from binding. This mechanism of inhibition is different than that of other members in the Src kinase family like Hck and Lck (Karni et al. 2003). Despite their potency and wide use as Src inhibitors in in vitro studies, PP1 and/or PP2 have not been used in human clinical trials. They have, however, helped model the activity of other Src inhibitors.

CGP76030 and CGP77675 are both substituted 5,7-diphenyly-pyrrolo[2,3-d]pyrimidines (Chen T et al. 2006). CGP76030 is similar to PP1 in structure and function. Both are pyrimidine analogs and thus competitively inhibit the ATP site of Src kinase. Like PP1, CGP76030 also inhibits Bcr-Abl positive leukemia cells but at a much lower concentration (Warmuth et al. 2003). In addition, CGP76030 reduces osteoclast numbers by inhibiting osteoclastogenesis as well as induced apoptosis in mature osteoclasts (Recchia et al. 2004). In a recent study, CGP76030 was found to be more selective for Lyn, Hck, and Fgr of Src kinase family kinases than for Bcr-Abl (Hu et al. 2004), again supporting the idea of using a cocktail of inhibitors to treat patients with leukemia instead of a single agent. CGP77675 was found to be more potent than CGP76030, inhibiting Src kinase at nanomolar concentration. Interestingly, both of these compounds block the binding site of Src substrates, like Fak and paxillin, at a much lower concentration than that of the Src autophosphorylation site (Missbach et al. 1999). In MC3T3-E1 cells, CGP77675 prevents PDGFR activation of Src, but has minimal effect in blocking epithelial growth factor, basic fibroblast growth factor, and insulin-like growth factor, showing its high specificity. Similarly, CGP77675 inhibits parathyroid hormone-induced long bone resorption in culture and protects young oophorectomized rats against osteoporosis (Missbach et al. 1999). Besides cancer treatment, administering CGP77675 in conjunction with anti-CD154 allowed permanent cardiac graft acceptance in 60% of recipient mice showing acute rejection (Zhang et al. 2005). Despite promising preliminary animal studies, these drugs or their analogs have yet to be tested in human clinical trials.

SU6656 (2-oxo-3-(4,5,6,7-tetrahydro-1H-indol-2-ylmethylene)-2,3-dihydro-1H-indole-5-sulfonic acid dimethylamide) is a small-molecule inhibitor, designed to have selectivity for Src and other members of the Src family. According to Blake et al. (2000), SU6656 has a greater than 6.5-fold selectivity for Src relative to other kinases and did not inhibit PDGF receptor, and thus is a valuable tool to study Src activation pathways. Using SU6656 to treat NIH 3T3 fibroblasts, researchers found that Src family kinases are required for Myc induction as well as DNA synthesis in response to PDGF stimulation (Bowman et al. 2001). Another group studied the role of Src in polymorphonuclear leukocyte transmigration through human umbilical vein endothelium monolayers (Yang et al. 2006). Using two different Src inhibitors, PP2 and SU6656, to block the induced cortactin phosphorylation by Src, these investigators were able to show cortactin redistribution in endotheliocytes as well as a reduction in PMN transmigration. A third group of investigators examined B-cells from patients with chronic lymphocytic leukemia (B-CLL) and found that B-lymphocytes accumulate because they have uncontrolled growth and are resistant to apoptosis. These researchers analyzed proteins extracted from freshly isolated B-lymphocytes of 40 leukemic patients and found that the Src kinase Lyn is significantly overexpressed as compared to normal B-cells (Contri et al. 2005). Furthermore, when these malignant cells are treated with either PP2 or SU6656 in culture medium, Lyn activity and presence are significantly decreased and apoptosis is induced. Using SU6656 to define the role of Src in the dynamics of actin regulation and invasion of malignant glial cells in three dimensions was the interest of another group of scientists (Angers-Loustau et al. 2004). Again, despite its extensive use in laboratory research, SU6656 has yet to be tested in a clinical trial.

There are a host of other Src inhibitors being developed by various pharmaceutical companies but yet to be tested in humans. At the American Society of Clinical Oncology (ASCO) annual meeting in 2003, Sawyer et al. presented in vitro and in vivo data showing the potency of AP23451, a purine-based small molecule, in blocking Src kinase activity at nanomolar concentrations, as well as its specificity in preventing bone resorption and osteolytic lesions in murine models (Sawyer et al. 2003). AP23464, another purine-based small molecule, was designed to inhibit Src-dependent metastases (Dalgarno et al. 2006). Besides anti-Src activity, AP23464 also ablates Bcr-Abl tyrosine phosphorylation, thus halting cell cycle progression and promoting apoptosis in human CML cells (O'Hare et al. 2004). Similar to the previously mentioned inhibitors, AP23846 is a 2,6,9-trisubstituted purine (Wang et al. 2003). This novel compound is 10 times more potent than PP2 in blocking Src

activity, and it also inhibits VEGF and interleukin-8 expressions in pancreas, colon, and prostate cell lines (Summy et al. 2005). In laboratory studies, AP23846 decreases the proliferation and migration of pancreatic cancer cells (L3.6pl) without increasing apoptosis or other cytotoxicities. It also blocks endothelial cell migration in vitro and angiogenesis in vivo. Unfortunately, therapeutic levels have not been achieved in rodents (Summy et al. 2005). However, this novel small-molecule inhibitor presents promising possibilities for new therapeutic strategies. Perhaps a different substituted moiety will allow the compound to be more clinically useful.

PD173955 [6-(2,6-dichlorophenyl)-8-methyl-2-(3-methylsulfanylphenylamino)-8H-pyrido[2,3-d]pyrimidin-7-one] inhibits mitosis in early prophase in 13 cancer cell lines (Moasser et al. 1999) as well as nonmalignant cells, by blocking spindle formation and chromosome migration. In addition, this compound was also found to be more potent than imatinib in arresting Bcr-Abl-dependent growth in multiple leukemia cell lines (Wisniewski et al. 2002).

AZM475271 is a novel anilinoquinazoline inhibitor of Src (Ple et al. 2004) with an IC50 of 2.5 µM. This orally bioavailable compound could achieve a therapeutic level at a dosage of 50 mg/kg in mice laden with human pancreatic carcinoma xenografts, but the best result was seen when it was given in combination with gemcitabine. Moreover, these researchers found that AZM475271 inhibits cell proliferation, invasion, and migration of endothelial cells, but evidence showed that it achieved its therapeutic effect, especially in combination with gemcitabine, by blocking STAT3 signaling downstream of Src (Yezhelyev et al. 2004). Further preliminary studies are needed to verify safety and efficacy before human clinical studies.

SKI-606 (4-anilino-3-quinolinecarbonitrile) is an orally available compound with inhibitory activity against Src and Abl kinases. Preliminary studies showed SKI-606 to inhibit Src family kinase, Lyn, as well as Bcr-Abl tyrosine kinase activity [better known as Philadelphia chromosome t(9;22)– a cytogenetic marker for chronic myelogenous leukemia (CML)]. However, SKI-606 does not inhibit PDGF recep-

10 Clinical Relevance of Targeted Interference with Src-Mediated Signal Transduction Events

tor-mediated activation (Golas et al. 2003). In cell cultures, SKI-606 has potent antiproliferative activity against three leukemia cell lines, with an IC50 ranging from 5 nM to 20 nM. In animal studies, oral SKI-606 causes regression of HT29 (colon) xenografts (Boschelli et al. 2001) and K562 (CML) xenografts (Golas et al. 2003) in nude mice. There are two clinical studies currently recruiting patients to assess the safety and efficacy of SKI-606 in leukemias and advanced solid tumor malignancies. The phase I/II trials are treating patients in Houston, TX with Philadelphia chromosome (+) leukemia but are primarily refractory to imatinib or have failed with imatinib. Concurrently, a phase I trial is currently enrolling patients in Tampa, FL, Baltimore, MD, and Cleveland, OH to evaluate the safety and tolerability of oral SKI-606 in patients with advanced solid tumors, for which there is no effective alternative therapy available.

Dasatinib (formerly known as BMS-354825 or N-(2-chloro-6-methyl-phenyl)-2-(6-(4-(2-hydroxyethyl)- piperazin-1-yl)-2-methylpyrimidin-4-ylamino)thiazole-5-carboxamide) is an orally bioavailable small molecule, which competitively inhibits Src tyrosine ATP kinase as well as Abl tyrosine kinases. Dasatinib has been found to inhibit the PDGF-PDGFR activation cascade, reducing the activity of STAT3, Akt, and Erk2 in rat and human aortic smooth muscle cells at nanomolar concentrations (Chen Z et al. 2006). More importantly, dasatinib found to inhibit 14 of 15 Bcr-Abl mutants as well as wild-type Bcr-Abl (Doggrell 2005). In addition, dasatinib prolonged survival of mice with Bcr-Abl leukemia. In culture, dasatinib inhibited the proliferation of progenitor cells derived from bone marrow of imatinib-resistant CML patients (Shah et al. 2004). Furthermore, dasatinib appears to bind to a mutated KIT protein and selectively kills primary neoplastic bone marrow mast cells, sparing other hematopoietic cells (Shah et al. 2006).

At ASCO annual meeting in 2005, Talpaz et al. presented the results from a phase I study of BMS-354825 in 36 patients with imatinib-resistant and intolerant chronic phase CML. These investigators found that BMS-354825 achieved complete response in 86% of patients and major cytogenetic response in 31% of patients.

Moreover, the response was durable, with 33 of 36 patients remaining on the study. Adverse events noted were grade 4 thrombocytopenia, grade 4 neutropenia, one possibly related duodenal ulcer, and mild QTc prolongation (Talpaz et al. 2005). At the same meeting, Sawyer et al. presented slightly different aspects of the CA180002 phase I trial with BMS-354825. According to these researchers, BMS-354825 was also well tolerated in advanced stage CML, reporting grade 4 thrombocytopenia, grade 3–4 fluid retention, and tumor lysis syndrome as the only observed adverse events. Similarly, BMS-354825 appears to be an effective therapy, promoting durable hematologic and cytogenetic responses for more than half of patients with imatinib-resistant advanced disease CML and Ph+ ALL (Sawyers et al. 2005). During the same meeting, there was a third abstract reporting results from a phase I dose-escalating study of BMS-354825 in patients with gastrointestinal stromal tumor (GIST) and other solid tumor. As with the CA 180002, these researchers have yet defined a dose-limiting toxicity (DLT) for BMS-354825, but did list grade 3 lymphopenia, grade 3 anorexia, and a grade 3 elevation of alkaline phosphatase among the adverse symptoms. Although there were no objective responses on CT scan, there were some mixed responses found on FDG-PET and resolution of GIST-associated ascites in one patient (Evans et al. 2005). Because a DLT has not been reached, dose escalation is being continued. Thus far, two of nine resistant GIST patients are being continued on the study because of their response to BMS-354825. The scientific correlation of tumor biopsies and radiologic imaging are still being analyzed (Evans et al. 2005), but the clinical benefits noted so far are encouraging. Currently, there are 10 recruiting clinical trials around the country evaluating the use of dasatinib in leukemia (clinicaltrials. gov), most of which are relapsed or refractory cases. In addition, there is one dasatinib study evaluating the safety and efficacy of dasatinib in patients with advanced solid tumors.

AZD0530 is a novel aniline quinazoline that competitively inhibits ATP binding site of Src as well as Abl kinases and can inhibit invasion and migration in v-Src-transformed murine cell models (Hennequin et al. 2005). At the annual meeting of the American Association for Cancer Research held in Anaheim, CA, in April 2005, multiple preclinical studies were presented about this new compound. In estrogen receptor α-mutant and wild-type MCF7 breast cancer cell lines, AZD0530 dose-dependently inhibited Src tyrosine kinase phosphorylation and completely abolished Src activity at 5 μM (Herynk et al. 2005). Phenotypically, at 5 μM, AZD0530 effectively inhibited basal and estrogen-induced invasion and cell proliferation in MCF7 cells (Herynk et al. 2005). Furthermore, at 100 nM, AZD0530 reduced integrin expression, FAK Tyr861 phosphorylation, and fibronectin attachment in tamoxifen-resistant MCF7 cells, thus significantly reducing cell motility (Hiscox et al. 2005). Preclinical animal studies showed that AZD0530 reached a therapeutic level of tumor growth inhibition at 6 mg/kg/day in rats, and that the drug reached a maximal tumor tissue level of 44 μg per gram of tissue, which is 40 times higher than plasma (Logie et al. 2005). In a phase I trial, dose-limiting toxicities of diarrhea and vomiting were reached at 1,000 mg daily. Adverse side effects reported were usually mild and consisted of flu-ike symptoms, rash, myalgia, arthralgia, headache, loose stools, and nausea (Lockton et al. 2005). In addition to inhibition of tumor growth and invasion, AZD0530 also reduced osteoclast activities, reducing resorption area and decreasing the number of resorption pits and calcium released from mouse calvariae (Mullender et al. 2005). An early clinical study in healthy males showed that AZD0530 inhibits osteoclast-mediated bone resorption by suppressing Src kinase activity (Eastell et al. 2005). Currently, there is only one phase I/II study evaluating AZD0530. This Canadian study evaluating the safety and efficacy as well as the best dose of AZD0530 and gemcitabine is recruiting patients with locally advanced or metastatic pancreatic cancer that cannot be resected (clinicaltrials.gov).

10.5 SH2/SH3 Inhibitors

SH2 and SH3 are sites of receptor-mediated activation or protein recognition domains. While SH2 binds phosphotyrosine-specific sequences, SH3 prefers proline-rich sequences (Chen T et al. 2006). These domains enhance the interactions between Src and its substrate. In addition, the phosphorylation of the Tyr213 in the SH2 domain by PDGFR or other receptor kinases not only reactivates Src but also prevents Src from returning to its inactive state (Shakespeare et al. 2000). Thus inhibiting SH2 domains not only prevents receptor-mediated activation but also inactivates Src (Fig. 10.5). Intuitively, inhibitors of these specific domains would require a phosphotyrosine or a phosphotyrosine mimic. However, the difficulty in designing these inhibitors is that any phosphotyrosine-containing inhibitor is subjected to phosphatase activity, causing it to be inactivated. In addition, these inhibitors are poorly transported into the cells. As for the phosphotyrosine mimics, they have lower affinity and thus specificity to SH2 domains (Chen T et al. 2006).

AP22408 is an orally bioavailable phosphotyrosine mimic resulting from a structure-based design. In addition to its high affinity for SH2 domain, AP22408 has a 3',4'-diphosphono-phenylalanine (Dpp) moiety, making it highly selective for osteoclasts. Preliminary animal studies showed that AP22408 significantly reduced osteoclast resorptive activity in rats (Shakespeare et al. 2000). With its bone-targeting property, one would think AP22408 would be the drug of choice for treating bone tumors, multiple myeloma, or osteoporosis where osteoclasts are overactive. However, to date, AP22408 has not been tested in human clinical trials.

UCS15A is a proline-rich protein isolated from Streptomyces and found to inhibit the protein-protein interaction between SH3 domains and other proline-rich protein ligands (Oneyama et al. 2003). Unlike most Src inhibitors that alter the levels or the activity of Src

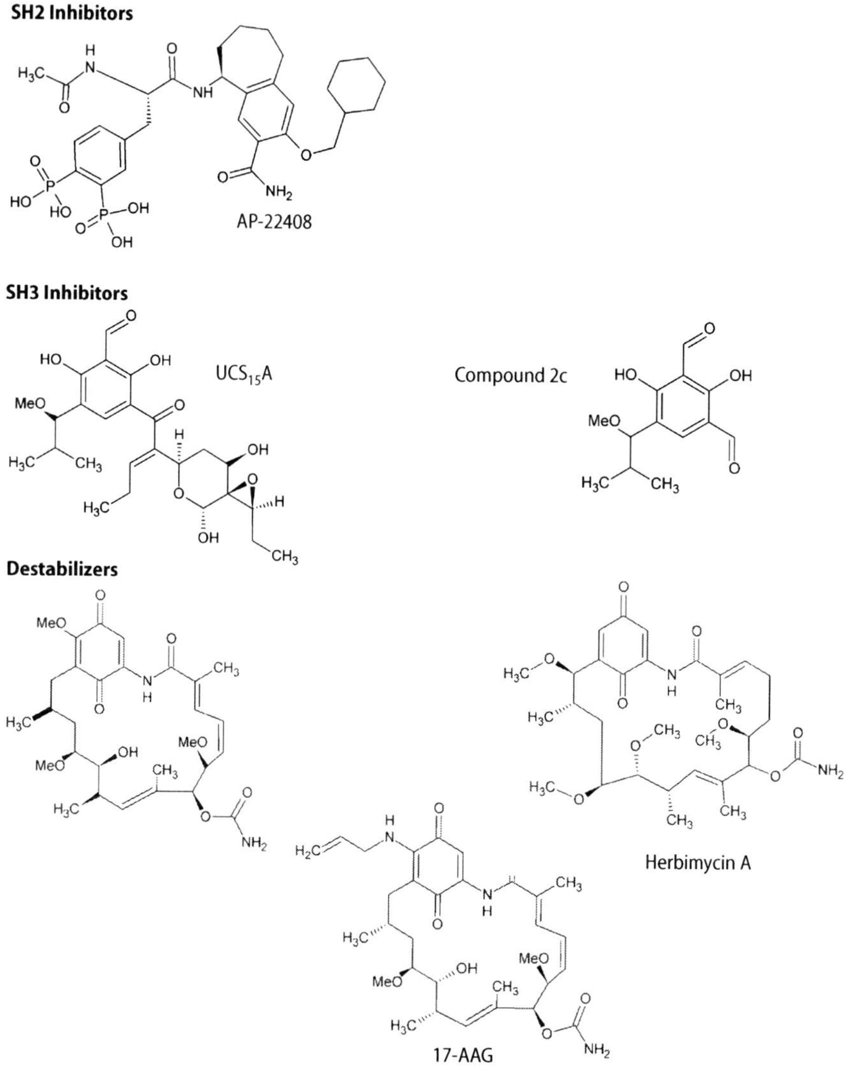

10 Clinical Relevance of Targeted Interference with Src-Mediated Signal Transduction Events

SH2 Inhibitors

SH3 Inhibitors

Destabilizers

Fig. 10.5 SH2/SH3 inhibitors, Destabilizers

tyrosine kinase, UCS15A disrupts the interaction between Src-SH3 and its substrates, like Sam68 and cortactin (Oneyama et al. 2002). Biologically, UCS15A decreased osteoclast bone resorption activity in vitro and effectively negated the stimulatory effects of parathyroid hormone on mouse calvaria at micromolar concentrations (Sharma et al. 2001). Besides its inhibition of the Src SH3 region, UCS15 also disrupts other similar SH3-mediated protein-protein interactions by competing with other proline-rich ligands (Oneyama et al. 2002).

Recently, a "simple analog" of UCS15A, compound 2c, was developed to be more potent and less cytotoxic. This compound appears to disrupt SH3-Sam68 association as well as inhibit the activation of MEK, but does not significantly change the cell morphology (Oneyama et al. 2003). Despite the potential promise, a more specific compound with nanomolar activity would further decrease cytotoxicity. In any case, preliminary animal studies need to be done to assess the safety and efficacy of these compounds before human trials.

10.6 SRC Destabilizers

After Src and its family members are synthesized in the cytoplasm, they require a chaperone until they are inserted or anchored into the cell membrane (Hartson and Matts 1994). Heat shock protein 90 (Hsp90), one of such chaperones, appears to keep Src in an inactive state but also to protect it from degradation. When Lck, a member of the Src family, was synthesized in the absence of Hsp90, it was degraded within 45 min (Bijlmakers and Marsh 2000). With this knowledge, researchers have looked for compounds that would destabilize the association between Src and Hsp90, and thus increase Src ubiquitylation and degradation (Fig. 10.6).

10.7 Geldanamycin

Geldanamycin is a benzoquinone antibiotic that has antineoplastic activity. It has been shown to bind to Hsp90, preventing its chaperone activity and allowing its client protein to be degraded (NCI drug definition). Because Hsp90 chaperone proteins are important in cell cycle, growth, survival, as well as apoptosis, inhibition with geldanamycin would have different effects on different cell types. For example, geldanamycin triggers apoptosis in rat pheochromocytoma cells (PC12) but causes differentiation with neurite outgrowth in murine neuroblastoma N2A (Lopez-Maderuelo et al. 2001). Because administering geldanamycin requires complex formulations, researchers have developed more

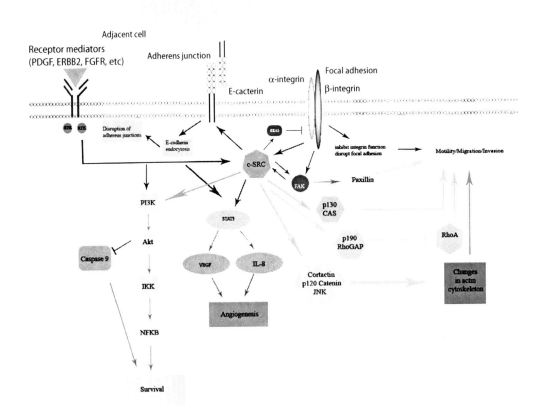

Fig. 10.6 Src destabilizers

hydrophilic analogs. In a preclinical study, the maximal therapeutic dose of 17-(allylamino)-17-demethoxygeldanamycin (17-DMAG) was found in rats and dogs, 12 mg/m2/day and 8/m2/day, respectively. In addition to gastrointestinal and bone marrow toxicities seen in rats, renal and gallbladder toxicities were also observed in dogs. Fortunately, all these toxicities are dose limiting and fully reversible after the completion of treatment (Glaze et al. 2005). At the ASCO annual meeting in 2004, the clinical results of a phase I trial using 17-AAG in 12 advanced cancer patients were presented. The maximal tolerated dose was 220 mg/m2 and the dose-limiting toxicities were hyperglycemia, dehydration, diarrhea, and elevation of hepatic enzymes (Erlichman et al. 2004). There is no currently open trial using geldanamycin analogs, but two phase I trials evaluating the safety and efficacy of 17-DMAG in treating patients with advanced cancer (UK) and solid tumors (USA) have recently been completed (clinicaltrials.gov).

10.8 Herbimycin

Herbimycin is also a benzoquinoid ansamycin antibiotic that shows antineoplastic properties. Presumably, like geldanamycin, herbimycin disrupts Src association with its chaperone, Hsp90, thus allowing Src to be ubiquitylated and degraded (Chen T et al. 2006). In culture, herbimycin inhibits growth of Philadelphia-positive leukemia cells. In animal studies, herbimycin A prolonged survival of mice inoculated with transformed FDC-P2 leukemia cells (Okabe et al. 1994). Besides cancer therapy, researchers have also found that herbimycin A reduces neoangiogenesis in rats with retinopathy of prematurity (McCollum et al. 2004). Similarly, when injected into the vitrea of rabbits, herbimycin decreases the inflammatory response and thus the development of traction retinal detachment (Imai et al. 2000). Like other Src inhibitors, herbimycin A also inhibits osteoclast activity in vitro and decreases recombinant human IL-1α stimulation of serum Ca2+ in vivo. In an interesting model in which mice

were implanted with human squamous cell tumor (MH-85), known to cause hypercalcemia, herbimycin significantly reduced the calcium level without showing any effect on tumor growth. Of note, subcutaneous injection of herbimycin at 100 µg/mouse/day is lethal within 3 days of treatment, but intraperitoneal injection of herbimycin at 200 µg/mouse/day was well tolerated. Unlike geldanamycin, herbimycin has not been tested in clinical trials.

Recent data found that Src is closely associated with histone deacetylases (HDAC) 3, one of four Class I HDACs. Like the others, HDAC3 are ubiquitously expressed in all cell types and bind with other corepressor proteins when active. These proteins downregulate gene expression by removing the acetyl groups from the lysine within the histones, thus preventing transcription (Longworth and Laimins 2006). But unlike other HDACs, HDAC3 can move in and out of the nucleus and binds with other cellular proteins like MAPK11 and Src (Yang et al. 2002). With immunostaining, these researchers showed that c-Src colocalized with HDAC3, whereas EGFR, E-cadherin, α-catenin, and β-catenin did not. With immunoprecipitation of different cell fractions, HDAC3 was demonstrated to complex with Src in the nuclear/cytoplasmic fraction as well as the membrane fraction. Furthermore, treatment of cells with PP1 decreased the phosphorylation of HDAC3 in the nuclear/cytoplasmic fraction, indicating that HDAC3 is a substrate of Src; however, the lack of phosphorylation by Src did not prevent HDAC3 from subsequently localizing to the cell membrane (Longworth and Laimins 2006). This new association between Src and HDAC3, a transcription modulator, may be a target for a novel therapeutic approach.

The last but definitely not least exciting class of Src inhibitors is small interfering RNA (siRNA). The concept of posttranscriptional gene silencing (PTGS) was first described by Vaucheret et al. in 1992 in plants. These researchers introduced antisense nitrite reductase cDNA into tobacco plants and found that the transgenic plants had underdeveloped and reduced chlorotic leaves when nitrate was given as the sole source of nitrogen. Furthermore, these plants accumulated nitrite five times more than wild type, and their nitrate reductase activity as well as mRNA levels were not detectable (Vaucheret et al. 1992). The idea of using siRNA to silence gene was demonstrated in C. elegans (Montgomery et al. 1998) and used to suppress hepatitis C viral RNA in Huh-7 hepatoma cell lines (Randall et al. 2003). Recently, the use of siRNA has been broadened to other virus-related diseases, like HIV (Cullen 2005) and large B cell lymphoma (Epstein-Barr virus) (Gururajan et al. 2005), neurodegenerative disease (Aronin 2006), and multiple myeloma (Hideshima et al. 2005).

More relevant to our purpose, siRNA to Src has also been studied. When Lyn siRNA was given to drug-resistant CML blast crisis cells, Lyn protein level was reduced 80%–95% and within 48 h the Brc-Abl(+) blasts underwent apoptosis (Ptasznik et al. 2004). When c-Src-specific siRNA was introduced to pancreatic adenocarcinoma cell lines (MiaPaCa2, PANC1, BxPC3, and Capan2), cellular Akt activity was correspondingly reduced with Src activity and the cells became more sensitive to gemcitabine-induced caspase-mediated apoptosis (Duxbury et al. 2004). According to the NCI, there are currently three trials around the world evaluating the effect of siRNA. In Israel, the efficacy of using a simian virus vector to deliver siRNA of a drug-resistant gene in CML patients is being evaluated. In the United States, a phase II trial is being conducted to test the efficacy of cand5, a synthetic double-stranded RNA of VEGF encoded gene, in treating diabetic macular edema. And in Taiwan, interleukin 10 siRNA is being tested to reverse the adverse effects of preeclamsia. Despite all the positive results with Src-specific siRNA in the laboratory, there is no clinical trial yet using Src-specific siRNA (clinicaltrials.gov).

10.9 Conclusion

Because c-Src overexpression is only weakly transforming and does not appear to be the primary cause in any specific tumor type, targeting c-Src alone would not seem to be an effective therapeutic option. However, because c-Src appears to be associated more with invasion and metastases, adding small-molecule c-Src inhibitors to other targeted therapy like EGFR inhibitors and/or VEGF inhibitors would be an effective means to block multiple, but specific, kinases in these cancer cells. The concept of utilizing targeted therapies, as opposed to therapies that treat cancer by means of exploiting the relative toxicity of drug in tumor vs. normal tissue, has come of age and holds promise to substantially reduce cancer therapy side effects. Because these targeted therapies are substantially more selective than standard chemotherapeutic agents, there is a burgeoning need to develop pretreatment diagnostic and prognostic tests predicting the presence of the target or surrogates for it. The application of whole genome analysis via expression microarrays is now being explored as a means to match the right patients to the right therapy through molecular fingerprint assessment before treatment.

References

Aberle H, Butz S, Stappert J, Weissig H, Kemler R, Hoschuetzky H (1994) Assembly of the cadherin-catenin complex in vitro with recombinant proteins. J Cell Sci 107:3655–3663

Akhand A A, Pu M, Senga T, Kato M, Suzuki H, Miyata T, Hamaguchi M, Nakashima I (1999) Nitric oxide controls src kinase activity through a sulfhydryl group modification-mediated Tyr-527-independent and Tyr-416-linked mechanism. J Biol Chem 274:25821–25826

Angers-Loustau A, Hering R, Werbowetski TE, Kaplan DR, Del Maestro RF (2004) SRC regulates actin dynamics and invasion of malignant glial cells in three dimensions. Mol Cancer Res 2:595–605

Aronin N (2006) Target selectivity in mRNA silencing. Gene Ther 13:509–516

Bijlmakers MJ, and Marsh M (2000) Hsp90 is essential for the synthesis and subsequent membrane association, but not the maintenance, of the Src-kinase p56(lck). Mol Biol Cell 11:1585–1595

Blake RA, Broome MA, Liu X, Wu J, Gishizky M, Sun L, Courtneidge SA (2000) SU6656, a selective src family kinase inhibitor, used to probe growth factor signaling. Mol Cell Biol 20:9018–9027

Boschelli DH, Ye F, Wang YD, Dutia M, Johnson SL, Wu B, Miller K, Powell DW, Yaczko D, Young M, Tischler M, Arndt K, Discafani C, Etienne C, Gibbons J, Grod J, Lucas J, Weber JM, Boschelli F (2001) Optimization of 4-phenylamino-3-quinolinecarbonitriles as potent inhibitors of Src kinase activity. J Med Chem 44:3965–3977

Bowman T, Broome MA, Sinibaldi D, Wharton W, Pledger WJ, Sedivy JM, Irby R, Yeatman T, Courtneidge SA, Jove R (2001) Stat3-mediated Myc expression is required for Src transformation and PDGF-induced mitogenesis. Proc Natl Acad Sci USA 98:7319–7324

Boyce BF, Yoneda T, Lowe C, Soriano P, Mundy GR (1992) Requirement of pp60c-src expression for osteoclasts to form ruffled borders and resorb bone in mice. J Clin Invest 90:1622–1627

Boyer B, Bourgeois Y, Poupon MF (2002) Src kinase contributes to the metastatic spread of carcinoma cells. Oncogene 21:2347–2356

Cam WR, Masaki T, Shiratori Y, Kato N, Ikenoue T, Okamoto M, Igarashi K, Sano T, Omata M (2001) Reduced C-terminal Src kinase activity is correlated inversely with pp60(c-src) activity in colorectal carcinoma. Cancer 92:61–70

Chen T, George JA, Taylor CC (2006) Src tyrosine kinase as a chemotherapeutic target: is there a clinical case? Anticancer Drugs 17:123–131

Chen YT, Stewart DB, Nelson WJ (1999) Coupling assembly of the E-cadherin/beta-catenin complex to efficient endoplasmic reticulum exit and basal-lateral membrane targeting of E-cadherin in polarized MDCK cells. J Cell Biol 144:687–699

Chen Z, Lee FY, Bhalla KN, Wu J (2006) Potent inhibition of platelet-derived growth factor-induced responses in vascular smooth muscle cells by BMS-354825. Mol Pharmacol

Contri A, Brunati AM, Trentin L, Cabrelle A, Miorin M, Cesaro L, Pinna LA, Zambello R, Semenzato G, Donella-Deana A (2005) Chronic lymphocytic leukemia B cells contain anomalous Lyn tyrosine kinase, a putative contribution to defective apoptosis. J Clin Invest 115:369–378

Cross FR, Garber EA, Hanafusa H (1985) N-terminal deletions in Rous sarcoma virus p60src:effects on tyrosine kinase and biological activities and on recombination in tissue culture with the cellular src gene. Mol Cell Biol 5:2789–2795

Crowe DL, Tsang KJ, Shemirani B (2001) Jun N-terminal kinase 1 mediates transcriptional induction of matrix metalloproteinase 9 expression. Neoplasia 3:27–32

Cullen B R (2005) Does RNA interference have a future as a treatment for HIV-1 induced disease? AIDS Rev 7:22–25

Dalgarno D, Stehle T, Narula S, Schelling P, van Schravendijk MR, Adams S, Andrade L, Keats J, Ram M, Jin L, Grossman T, MacNeil I, Metcalf C 3rd, Shakespeare W, Wang Y, Keenan T, Sundaramoorthi R, Bohacek R, Weigele M, Sawyer T (2006) Structural basis of Src tyrosine kinase inhibition with a new class of potent and selective trisubstituted purine-based compounds. Chem Biol Drug Des 67:46–57

Doggrell SA (2005) BMS-354825:a novel drug with potential for the treatment of imatinib-resistant chronic myeloid leukaemia. Expert Opin Investig Drugs 14:89–91

Duxbury MS, Ito H, Zinner MJ, Ashley SW, and Whang EE (2004) siRNA directed against c-Src enhances pancreatic adenocarcinoma cell gemcitabine chemosensitivity. J Am Coll Surg 198:953–959

Eastell R, Hannon RA, Gallagher NJ, Clack G, Macpherson M, Marshall AL (2005) The effect of AZD0530, a highly selective, orally available Src/Abl kinase inhibitor, on biomarkers of bone resorption in healthy males. American Society of Clinical Oncology, Orlando, FL

Erlichman C, Toft D, Reid J, Goetz M, Ames M, Mandrekar S, Ajei A, McCollum A, Ivy P (2004) A phase I trial of 17-allylamino-geldanamycin (17AAG) in patients with advanced cancer. American Society of Clinical Oncology, New Orleans, LA

Evans TR, Morgan JA, van den Abbeele AD, McPherson IR, George S, Crawford D, Mastrullo M, Cheng S, Fletcher JA, and Demetri GD (2005) Phase I doseescalation study of the Src and multi-kinase inhibitor BMS-354825 in patients (pts) with GIST and other solid tumors. American Society of Clinical Oncology, Orlando, FL

Fujisawa K, Madaule P, Ishizaki T, Watanabe G, Bito H, Saito Y, Hall A, Narumiya S (1998) Different regions of Rho determine Rho-selective binding of different classes of Rho target molecules. J Biol Chem 273:18943–18949

Glaze ER, Lambert AL, Smith AC, Page JG, Johnson WD, McCormick DL, Brown AP, Levine BS, Covey JM, Egorin MJ, Eiseman JL, Holleran JL, Sausville EA, and Tomaszewski JE (2005) Preclinical toxicity of a geldanamycin analog, 17-(dimethylaminoethylamino)-17-demethoxygeldanamycin (17-DMAG), in rats and dogs:potential clinical relevance. Cancer Chemother Pharmacol 56:637–647

Golas JM, Arndt K, Etienne C, Lucas J, Nardin D, Gibbons J, Frost P, Ye F, Boschelli DH, Boschelli F (2003) SKI-606, a 4-anilino-3-quinolinecarbonitrile dual inhibitor of Src and Abl kinases, is a potent antiproliferative agent against chronic myelogenous leukemia cells in culture and causes regression of K562 xenografts in nude mice. Cancer Res 63:375–381

Gururajan M, Chui R, Karuppannan AK, Ke J, Jennings CD, Bondada S (2005) c-Jun N-terminal kinase (JNK) is required for survival and proliferation of B-lymphoma cells. Blood 106:1382–1391

Hakak Y, Martin GS (1999) Ubiquitin-dependent degradation of active Src. Curr Biol 9:1039–1042

Hartson SD, Matts RL (1994) Association of Hsp90 with cellular Src-family kinases in a cell-free system correlates with altered kinase structure and function. Biochemistry 33:8912–8920

He H, Hirokawa Y, Levitzki A, and Maruta H (2000) An anti-Ras cancer potential of PP1, an inhibitor specific for Src family kinases: in vitro and in vivo studies. Cancer J 6:243–248

Helgason CD, Damen JE, Rosten P, Grewal R, Sorensen P, Chappel SM, Borowski A, Jirik F, Krystal G,

Humphries RK (1998) Targeted disruption of SHIP leads to hemopoietic perturbations, lung pathology, and a shortened life span. Genes Dev 12:1610–1620

Hennequin LF, Allen J, Costello G, Fennell M, Green TP, Jacobs V, Morgentin R, Olivier A, Ple PA (2005) The discovery of AZD0530:a novel, oral, highly selective and dual-specific inhibitor of the Src and Abl family kinases. Proc Am Assoc Cancer Res 46:A2537

Herynk MH, Beyer A, Cui Y, Green TP, Fuqua SAW (2005) c-Src inhibition with AZD0530 reduces estrogen mediated growth and invasion in breast cancer cells expressing the K303R ERα mutant. Proc Am Assoc Cancer Res 46:A264

Hideshima T, Bradner JE, Wong J, Chauhan D, Richardson P, Schreiber SL, and Anderson KC (2005) Small-molecule inhibition of proteasome and aggresome function induces synergistic antitumor activity in multiple myeloma. Proc Natl Acad Sci USA 102:8567–8572

Hiscox S, Barrow D, Green T, Nicholson RI (2005) Adhesion-independent focal adhesion kinase activation involves Src and promotes cell adhesion and motility in tamoxifen-resistant MCF-7 cells and is inhibited by the Src/Abl kinase inhibitor AZD0530. Proc Am Assoc Cancer Res 46:A266

Hsia DA, Mitra SK, Hauck CR, Streblow DN, Nelson JA, Ilic D, Huang S, Li E, Nemerow GR, Leng J, Spencer KS, Cheresh DA, Schlaepfer DD (2003) Differential regulation of cell motility and invasion by FAK. J Cell Biol 160:753–767

Hu Y, Liu Y, Pelletier S, Buchdunger E, Warmuth M, Fabbro D, Hallek M, Van Etten RA, Li S (2004) Requirement of Src kinases Lyn, Hck and Fgr for BCR-ABL1-induced B-lymphoblastic leukemia but not chronic myeloid leukemia. Nat Genet 36:453–461

Hynes RO (1992) Integrins: versatility, modulation, and signaling in cell adhesion. Cell 69:11–25

Imai K, Loewenstein A, Koroma B, Grebe R, de Juan E Jr (2000) Herbimycin A in the treatment of experimental proliferative vitreoretinopathy: toxicity and efficacy study. Graefes Arch Clin Exp Ophthalmol 238:440–447

Irby R, Mao W, Coppola D, Jove R, Gamero A, Cuthbertson D, Fujita D, Yeatman TJ (1997) Overexpression of normal c-Src in poorly metastatic human colon cancer cells enhances primary tumor growth but not metastatic potential. Cell Growth Differ 8:1287–1295

Jones RJ, Avizienyte E, Wyke AW, Owens DW, Brunton VG, Frame MC (2002) Elevated c-Src is linked to altered cell-matrix adhesion rather than proliferation in KM12C human colorectal cancer cells. Br J Cancer 87:1128–1135

Karni R, Mizrachi S, Reiss-Sklan E, Gazit A, Livnah O, Levitzki A (2003) The pp60c-Src inhibitor PP1 is noncompetitive against ATP. FEBS Lett 537:47–52

Kilarski WW, Jura N, Gerwins P (2003) Inactivation of Src family kinases inhibits angiogenesis in vivo: implications for a mechanism involving organization of the actin cytoskeleton. Exp Cell Res 291:70–82

Kim M, Tezuka T, Tanaka K, Yamamoto T (2004) Cbl-c suppresses v-Src-induced transformation through ubiquitin-dependent protein degradation. Oncogene 23:1645–1655

Laird AD, Li G, Moss KG, Blake RA, Broome MA, Cherrington JM, Mendel DB (2003) Src family kinase activity is required for signal tranducer and activator of transcription 3 and focal adhesion kinase phosphorylation and vascular endothelial growth factor signaling in vivo and for anchorage-dependent and -independent growth of human tumor cells. Mol Cancer Ther 2:461–469

Lauffenburger DA Horwitz AF (1996) Cell migration: a physically integrated molecular process. Cell 84:359–369

Laukaitis CM, Webb DJ, Donais K, Horwitz AF (2001) Differential dynamics of alpha 5 integrin, paxillin, and alpha-actinin during formation and disassembly of adhesions in migrating cells. J Cell Biol 153:1427–1440

Liu Y, Bishop A, Witucki L, Kraybill B, Shimizu E, Tsien J, Ubersax J, Blethrow J, Morgan DO, Shokat KM (1999) Structural basis for selective inhibition of Src family kinases by PP1. Chem Biol 6:671–678

Lockton JA, Smethurst D, Macpherson M, Tootell R, Marshall AL, Clack G, Gallagher NJ (2005) Phase I ascending single and multiple dose studies to assess the safety, tolerability and pharmacokinetics of AZD0530, a highly selective, dual-specific Src-Abl inhibitor. American Society of Clinical Oncology, Orlando, FL

Logie A, Martin PD, Partridge EA, Byatt SL, Whittaker RD, Green TP (2005) Pharmacokinetics, tissue distribution and anti-tumor activity of the Src/Abl kinase inhibitor AZD0530 in rat xenograft model. Proc Am Assoc Cancer Res 43:A5989

Longworth MS, Laimins LA (2006) Histone deacetylase 3 localizes to the plasma membrane and is a substrate of Src. Oncogene

Lopez-Madderuelo MD, Fernandez-Renart M, Moratilla C, Renart J (2001) Opposite effects of the Hsp90 inhibitor Geldanamycin: induction of apoptosis in PC12, and differentiation in N2A cells. FEBS Lett 490:23–27

Mao W, Irby R, Coppola D, Fu L, Wloch M, Turner J, Yu H, Garcia R, Jove R, Yeatman TJ (1997) Activation of c-Src by receptor tyrosine kinases in human colon cancer cells with high metastatic potential. Oncogene 15:3083–3090

Martin GS (2004) The road to Src. Oncogene 23:7910–7917

Masaki T, Okada M, Tokuda M, Shiratori Y, Hatase O, Shirai M, Nishioka M, Omata M (1999) Reduced C-terminal Src kinase (Csk) activities in hepatocellular carcinoma. Hepatology 29:379–384

Masamune A, Satoh M, Kikuta K, Suzuki N, Shimosegawa T (2005) Activation of JAK-STAT pathway is required for platelet-derived growth factor-induced proliferation of pancreatic stellate cells. World J Gastroenterol 11:3385–3391

McCollum GW, Rajaratnam VS, Bullard LE, Yang R, Penn JS (2004) Herbimycin A inhibits angiogenic activity in endothelial cells and reduces neovascularization in a rat model of retinopathy of prematurity. Exp Eye Res 78:987–995

Missbach M, Jeschke M, Feyen J, Muller K, Glatt M, Green J, Susa M (1999) A novel inhibitor of the tyrosine kinase Src suppresses phosphorylation of its major cellular substrates and reduces bone resorption in vitro and in rodent models in vivo. Bone 24:437–449

Moasser MM, Srethapakdi M, Sachar KS, Kraker AJ, Rosen N (1999) Inhibition of Src kinases by a selective tyrosine kinase inhibitor causes mitotic arrest. Cancer Res 59:6145–6152

Montgomery MK, Xu S, Fire A (1998) RNA as a target of double-stranded RNA-mediated genetic interference in Caenorhabditis elegans. Proc Natl Acad Sci USA 95:15502–15507

Mullender MG, Everts V, Green TP, Klein-Nulend J (2005) Inhibition of osteoclastic bone resorption by the novel, potent, and selective c-Src/Abl kinase inhibitor, AZD0530. Proc Am Assoc Cancer Res 46:A2923

Nakagawa T, Tanaka S, Suzuki H, Takayanagi H, Miyazaki T, Nakamura K, Tsuruo T (2000) Overexpression of the csk gene suppresses tumor metastasis in vivo. Int J Cancer 88:384–391

Niu G, Wright KL, Huang M, Song L, Haura E, Turkson J, Zhang S, Wang T, Sinibaldi D, Coppola D, Heller R, Ellis LM, Karras J, Bromberg J, Pardoll D, Jove R, Yu H (2002) Constitutive Stat3 activity up-regulates VEGF expression and tumor angiogenesis. Oncogene 21:2000–2008

O'Hare T, Pollock R, Stoffregen EP, Keats JA, Abdullah OM, Moseson EM, Rivera VM, Tang H, Metcalf CA 3rd, Bohacek RS, Wang Y, Sundaramoorthi R, Shakespeare WC, Dalgarno D, Clackson T, Sawyer TK, Deininger MW, Druker BJ (2004) Inhibition of wild-type and mutant Bcr-Abl by AP23464, a potent ATP-based oncogenic protein kinase inhibitor:implications for CML. Blood 104:2532–2539

Okabe M, Uehara Y, Noshima T, Itaya T, Kunieda Y, Kurosawa M (1994) In vivo antitumor activity of herbimycin A, a tyrosine kinase inhibitor, targeted against BCR/ABL oncoprotein in mice bearing BCR/ABL-transfected cells. Leuk Res 18:867–873

Oneyama C, Agatsuma T, Kanda Y, Nakano H, Sharma SV, Nakano S, Narazaki F, Tatsuta K (2003) Synthetic inhibitors of proline-rich ligand-mediated protein-protein interaction:potent analogs of UCS15A. Chem Biol 10:443–451

Oneyama C, Nakano H, Sharma SV (2002) UCS15A, a novel small molecule, SH3 domain-mediated protein-protein interaction blocking drug. Oncogene 21:2037–2050

Perl AK, Wilgenbus P, Dahl U, Semb H, Christofori G (1998) A causal role for E-cadherin in the transition from adenoma to carcinoma. Nature 392:190–193

Ple PA, Green TP, Hennequin LF, Curwen J, Fennell M, Allen J, Lambert-Van Der Brempt C, Costello G (2004) Discovery of a new class of anilinoquinazoline inhibitors with high affinity and specificity for the tyrosine kinase domain of c-Src. J Med Chem 47:871–887

Ptasznik A, Nakata Y, Kalota A, Emerson SG, and Gewirtz AM (2004) Short interfering RNA (siRNA) targeting the Lyn kinase induces apoptosis in primary, and drug-resistant, BCR-ABL1(+) leukemia cells. Nat Med 10:1187–1189

Randall G, Grakoui A, Rice CM (2003) Clearance of replicating hepatitis C virus replicon RNAs in cell culture by small interfering RNAs. Proc Natl Acad Sci USA 100:235–240

Recchia I, Rucci N, Funari A, Migliaccio S, Taranta A, Longo M, Kneissel M, Susa M, Fabbro D, Teti A (2004) Reduction of c-Src activity by substituted 5,7-diphenyl-pyrrolo[2,3-d]-pyrimidines induces osteoclast apoptosis in vivo and in vitro. Involvement of ERK1/2 pathway. Bone 34:65–79

Rubin H (1955) Quantitative relations between causative virus and cell in the Rous no. 1 chicken sarcoma. Virology 1:445–73

Sawyer T, Shakespeare W, Wang Y, Metcalf CA 3rd, Sundaramoorthi R, Keenan T, Bohacek R, Dalgarno D, Xing L, and Boyce B (2003) A new class of small-molecule therapeutics for osteolytic bone metastasis:discovery of novel bone-targeted Src tyrosine kinase inhibitors having potent in vitro and in vivo activities. American Society of Clinical Oncology, Chicago, IL

Sawyers CL, Shah NP, Kantarjian HM, Cortes J, Paquette R, Nicoll J, Bai SA, Clark E, Decillis AP, Talpaz M (2005) A phase I study of BMS-354825 in patients with imatinib-resistant and intolerant accelerated and blast phase chronic myeloid leukemia (CML): results from CA 180002. American Society of Clinical Oncology, Orlando, FL

Shah NP, Lee FY, Luo R, Jiang Y, Donker M, Akin C (2006) Dasatinib (BMS-354825) inhibits KITD816V, an imatinib-resistant activating mutation that triggers neoplastic growth in the majority of patients with systemic mastocytosis. Blood

Shah NP, Tran C, Lee FY, Chen P, Norris D, Sawyers CL (2004) Overriding imatinib resistance with a novel ABL kinase inhibitor. Science 305:399–401

Shakespeare W, Yang M, Bohacek R, Cerasoli F, Stebbins K, Sundaramoorthi R, Azimioara M, Vu C, Pradeepan S, Metcalf C 3rd, Haraldson C, Merry T, Dalgarno D, Narula S, Hatada M, Lu X, van Schravendijk MR, Adams S, Violette S, Smith J, Guan W, Bartlett C, Herson J, Iuliucci J, Weigele M, T Sawyer (2000) Structure-based design of an osteoclast-selective, nonpeptide src homology 2 inhibitor with in vivo antiresorptive activity. Proc Natl Acad Sci USA 97:9373–9378

Sharma SV, Oneyama C, Yamashita Y, Nakano H, Sugawara K, Hamada M, Kosaka N, Tamaoki T (2001) UCS15A, a non-kinase inhibitor of Src signal transduction. Oncogene 20:2068–2079

Soriano P, Montgomery C, Geske R, Bradley A (1991) Targeted disruption of the c-src proto-oncogene leads to osteopetrosis in mice. Cell 64:693–702

Summy JM, Trevino JG, Lesslie DP, Baker CH, Shakespeare WC, Wang Y, Sundaramoorthi R, Metcalf CA 3rd, Keats JA, Sawyer TK, Gallick GE (2005) AP23846, a novel and highly potent Src family kinase inhibitor, reduces vascular endothelial growth factor and interleukin-8 expression in human solid tumor cell lines and abrogates downstream angiogenic processes. Mol Cancer Ther 4:1900–1911

Takeshita S, Namba N, Zhao JJ, Jiang Y, Genant HK, Silva MJ, Brodt MD, Helgason CD, Kalesnikoff J, Rauh MJ, Humphries RK, Krystal G, Teitelbaum SL, Ross FP (2002) SHIP-deficient mice are severely osteoporotic due to increased numbers of hyper-resorptive osteoclasts. Nat Med 8:943–949

Talpaz M, Kantarjian HM, Paquette R, Shah NP, Cortes J, Nicoll J, Bai SA, Huang F, Decillis AP, Sawyers CL (2005) A phase I study of BMS-354825 in patients with imatinib-resistant and intolerant chronic phase chronic myeloid leukemia (CML): results from CA180002. American Society of Clinical Oncology, Orlando, FL

Termuhlen PM, Curley SA, Talamonti MS, Saboorian MH, Gallick GE (1993) Site-specific differences in pp60c-src activity in human colorectal metastases. J Surg Res 54:293–298

Tice DA, Biscardi JS, Nickles AL, Parsons SJ (1999) Mechanism of biological synergy between cellular Src and epidermal growth factor receptor. Proc Natl Acad Sci U S A 96:1415–1420

Timpson P, Jones GE, Frame MC, Brunton VG (2001) Coordination of cell polarization and migration by the Rho family GTPases requires Src tyrosine kinase activity. Curr Biol 11:1836–1846

Vaucheret H, Kronenberger J, Lepingle A, Vilaine F, Boutin JP, Caboche M (1992) Inhibition of tobacco nitrite reductase activity by expression of antisense RNA. Plant J 2:559–569

Wang Y, Metcalf CA 3rd, Shakespeare WC, Sundaramoorthi R, Keenan TP, Bohacek RS, van Schravendijk MR, Violette SM, Narula SS, Dalgarno DC, Haraldson C, Keats J, Liou S, Mani U, Pradeepan S, Ram M, Adams S, Weigele M, Sawyer TK (2003) Bone-targeted 2,6,9-trisubstituted purines:novel inhibitors of Src tyrosine kinase for the treatment of bone diseases. Bioorg Med Chem Lett 13:3067–3070

Warmuth M, Simon N, Mitina O, Mathes R, Fabbro D, Manley PW, Buchdunger E, Forster K, Moarefi I, Hallek M (2003) Dual-specific Src and Abl kinase

inhibitors, PP1 and CGP76030, inhibit growth and survival of cells expressing imatinib mesylate-resistant Bcr-Abl kinases. Blood 101:664–672

Weis S, Shintani S, Weber A, Kirchmair R, Wood M, Cravens A, McSharry H, Iwakura A, Yoon YS, Himes N, Burstein D, Doukas J, Soll R, Losordo D, Cheresh D (2004) Src blockade stabilizes a Flk/cadherin complex, reducing edema and tissue injury following myocardial infarction. J Clin Invest 113:885–894

Wisniewski D, Lambek CL, Liu C, Strife A, Veach DR, Nagar B, Young MA, Schindler T, Bornmann WG, Bertino JR, Kuriyan J, Clarkson B (2002) Characterization of potent inhibitors of the Bcr-Abl and the c-kit receptor tyrosine kinases. Cancer Res 62:4244–4255

Yang L, Kowalski JR, Zhan X, Thomas SM, Luscinskas FW (2006) Endothelial cell cortactin phosphorylation by Src contributes to polymorphonuclear leukocyte transmigration in vitro. Circ Res 98:394–402

Yang WM, Tsai SC, Wen YD, Fejer G, Seto E (2002) Functional domains of histone deacetylase-3. J Biol Chem 277:9447–9454

Yeatman TJ (2004) A renaissance for SRC. Nat Rev Cancer 4:470–480

Yezhelyev MV, Koehl G, Guba M, Brabletz T, Jauch KW, Ryan A, Barge A, Green T, Fennell M, Bruns CJ (2004) Inhibition of SRC tyrosine kinase as treatment for human pancreatic cancer growing orthotopically in nude mice. Clin Cancer Res 10:8028–8036

Yu CL, Meyer DJ, Campbell GS, Larner AC, Carter-Su C, Schwartz J, Jove R (1995) Enhanced DNA-binding activity of a Stat3-related protein in cells transformed by the Src oncoprotein. Science 269:81–83

Yu H, Jove R (2004) The STATs of cancer–new molecular targets come of age. Nat Rev Cancer 4:97–105

Zamir E, Geiger B (2001) Molecular complexity and dynamics of cell-matrix adhesions. J Cell Sci 114:3583–3590

Zhang Q, Fairchild RL, Reich MB, Miller GG (2005) Inhibition of Src kinases combined with CD40 ligand blockade prolongs murine cardiac allograft survival. Transplantation 80:1112–1120

Zhao WQ, Alkon DL, Ma W (2003) c-Src protein tyrosine kinase activity is required for muscarinic receptor-mediated DNA synthesis and neurogenesis via ERK1/2 and c-AMP-responsive element-binding protein signaling in neural precursor cells. J Neurosci Res 72:334–342

CPSIA information can be obtained at www.ICGtesting.com
Printed in the USA
LVOW120500160911

246538LV00004B/1/P